Deutsche Gesellschaft für Pharmakologie und Toxikologie

Abstracts

of the Autumn Meeting

10–14 September 1991, Berlin

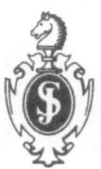

Springer-Verlag Berlin Heidelberg GmbH

ISBN 978-3-662-38798-6   ISBN 978-3-662-39701-5 (eBook)
DOI 10.1007/978-3-662-39701-5

Deutsche Gesellschaft für Pharmakologie und Toxikologie
Autumn Meeting
Berlin, September 10 - 14, 1991

Contents   Abstract Numbers

RUDOLF-BUCHHEIM-LECTURE   S1

SYMPOSIA

COMMUNICATIONS

S1

DRUGS AND GENETIC FACTORS
Michel Eichelbaum

Already in 1902 Garrod the founder of modern biochemical genetics, postulated that abnormal reactions to drugs and food are caused by genetic variations of certain biochemical processe. It was not until the late 1950's when it was proven that his hypothesis was correct. At that time it was demonstrated that hemolytic aenemias observed after the consumption of fava beans and certain drugs such as primaquine were due to agenetic determined glucose 6-phosphate dehydrogenase deficiency.

Since that time it has been realised that genetic variability of enzymes involved in the action and metabolism of drugs critically influences the metabolism, disposition, and response to numerous drugs and significantly contributes to variability in drug response. The discovery of several genetic polymorphisms of glucose-6-phosphate-dehydrogenase, hemoglobins, N-acetyltransferase and P-450 isozymes has provided an explanation why some patients do not obtain the expected drug effects or why some patients show serious toxicity and unusual drug effects after taking the "standard and safe" dose of a drug.

The first evidence for a genetic polymorphism of cytochrome P-450 isozymes was presented in the mid-1970's for the oxytocic and antiarrhythmic alkaloid sparteine and for the antihypertensive drug debrisoquine (Eichelbaum 1975, 1979, Mahghoub 1977). Cytochrome P-450 isozymes of the liver play an important role in the biotransformation of many drugs. The activity of these drug-metabolizing enzymes is a major determinant of the intensity and duration of drug effects. In addition these enzymes are of paramount importance in chemical mutagenesis, carcinogenesis and toxicity mediated via metabolic activation of xenobiotics. Thus genetically determined differences in the activity of these enzymes can influence individual susceptibility to the action of drugs adverse drug reactions and drug induced diseases. The genetic polymorphisms of three human drug metabolizing enzymes, namely N-acetyltransferase and two cytochrome P-450 isozymes (P-450 II D6: sparteine/debrisoquine polymorphism, P-450 IIC8/10; mephenytoin polymorphism) have been firmly established. Based on the metabolic handling of certain probe drugs the population can be divided into two phenotypes: the extensive (EM) and poor metabolizer (PM). The PM phenotype of the sparteine/debrisoquine polymorphism which occurs with a frequency of 5 to 10% in the European population has a severely impaired capacity to metabolize about 30 clinically widely used drugs such as antiarrhythmics, some ß-adrenoceptor antagonists, tricyclic antidepressants, neuroleptics and opioid alkaloids. Defective drug metabolism is inherited as an autosomal recessive trait. The gene encoding for the synthesis of cytochrome P-450IID6 is located on the long arm of chromosome 22 (Eichelbaum et al. 1987). The gene locus (CYP2D) consists of two pseudogenes (D8 and D7) and one functional gene (D6) (Kimura et al. 1989). The CYP2D6 gene locus is highly polymorphic and several mutations causing the PM phenotype have been discovered (Skoda et al. 1988; Gonzalez et al. 1988a; Kagimoto et al. 1990; Heim and Meyer, 1990).

The most common mutant allele 29B has multiple mutations with base changes in exons 1, 2 and 9 and a point mutation at the consensus sequence of the splice site of the 3rd intron. The 29A mutant allele is characterized by a simple nucleotide deletion in the 5th exon with consequent frameshift (Kagimoto et al. 1990; Heim and Meyer, 1990). Another mutant allele of 44 kb size after XbaI digestion has the same mutation as mutant allele 29B. The mutant allele of 11.5 kb after XbaI digestion is due to the deletion of the entire functional IID6 gene (Gaedigk et al. 1991). In addition another rare mutation which results in a 16 + 9 kb XbaI fragment is associated with the PM phenotype (Evans and Relling, 1990).

Thus there are at least 12 genotypes responsible for the PM phenotype. Despite the diversity of genotypes causing the PM phenotype all these mutations result in the absence of P450IID6 in the liver of PMs (Gonzalez et al. 1988b; Zanger et al. 1988). The clinical implications of polymorphism drug metabolism are as such that in the PM phenotype administration of standard doses of drugs affected will result in elevated concentrations which in turn produce exaggerated pharmacological effects and side effects. This has been clearly demonstrated for some antiarrhythmic drugs, tricyclic antidepressants and neuroleptics. If formation of an active metabolite is affected then poor metabolisers will have diminished pharmacological response as for example with metabolism of codeine to morphine (Eichelbaum & Gross 1990, Brosen & Gram 1989). There can be no doubt that the discovery of genetic polymorphisms in drug metabolism has contributed a great deal to our understanding of the influence of genetic factors on the disposition and effects of drugs and has enabled us to elucidate the mechanisms responsible for certain adverse drug reactions. It is hoped that this knowledge will find its way into clinical practice in order to achieve our ultimate goal of making drug therapy more effective and safer for the benefit of the patient.

References

1. Eichelbaum M (1975). Ein neuentdeckter Defet im Arzneimittelstoffwechsel des Menschen: Die fehlende N-Oxidation des Spartein. Habilitationsschrift, Medizinische Fakultät Rheinischen Friedrich-Wilhelms-Universität, Bonn.

2. Eichelbaum M, Spannbrucker N, Steincke B and Dengler HJ (1979). Defective N-oxidation of sparteine in man: A new pharmacogenetic defect. Eur J Clin Pharmacol. 16, 183-187.

3. Maghoub A, Idle JR, Dring LG, Lancester R and Smith RL (1977). Polymorphic hydroxylation of debrisoquine in man. Lancet II, 584-586.

4. Eichelbaum M, Baur MP, Osikowska-Evers, BO, Tieves G, Zekorn C and Rittner C (1987). Chromosomal assignement of human cytochrome P450 (debrisoquine/sparteine type) to chromosome 22. Br J Clin Pharmac 23, 455-458

5. Skoda RC, Gonzalez FJ, Demierre A and Meyer UA (1988). Two mutant alleles of the human cytochrome P 450 db1-gene (P450 C2D1) associated with genetically deficient metabolism of debrisoquine and other drugs. Proc Natl Acad Sci. USA 85, 5240-5243

6. Gonzalez FJ, Skoda RC, Kimura S, Umeno M, Zanger UM, Nebert DW, Gelboin HV, Handwick JP and Meyer UA (1988a). Characterization of the common genetic defect in humans deficient in debrisoquin metabolism. Nature 331, 442-446.

7. Kagimoto M, Heim M, Kagimoto K, Zeugin T and Meyer UA (1990). Multiple mutations of the human cytochrome P450IID6 gene (CYP2D6) in poor metabolizers of debrisoquine. Study of the functional significance of individual mutations by expression of chimeric genes. J Biol Chem 265, 17209-17214.

8. Heim M and Meyer UA (1990). Genotyping of poor metabolisers of debrisoquine by allele-specific PCR amplification. Lancet 336, 529-532.

9. Gaedigk A, Blum M, Gaedigk R, Eichelbaum M, and Meyer UA (1991). Deletion of the entire cytochrome P450 CYP2D6 gene as a cause of impaired drug metabolism in poor metabolizers of the debrisoquine/sparteine polymorphism. Am J Human Genet. 48, 943-950.

10. Evans,WE and Relling MV (1990). Xba1 16-plus 9-kilobase DNA restriction fragments identify a mutant allele for debrisoquin hydroxylase: report of a family study. Mol. Pharmac 37, 639-642.

11. Gonzalez FJ, Vilbois F, Hardwick JP, McBride OW, Gelboin HV and Meyer UA (1988b). Human debrisoquine 4-hydroxylase (P450IID1): cDNA and deduced amino acid sequence and assignement of the CYP2D locus to chromosome 22. Genomics 2, 174-179.

12. Zanger UM, Vilbois F, Hardwick JP and Meyer UA (1988). Absence of hepatic cytochrome P450-bufl causes genetically deficient debrisoquine hydroxylation in man. Biochemistry 27, 5447-5454.

13. Eichelbaum M and Gross AS (1990). The genetic polymorphism of debrisoquine/sparteine metabolism clinical aspects. Pharmac Ther 46, 377-394.

14. Brosen K and Gram LF (1989). Clinical significance of the sparteine/debrisoquine oxidation polymorphism. Eur. J. Clin. Pharmacol. 36, 537-547.

Dr. Margarete Fischer-Bosch-Institut, für Klinische Pharmakologie, Auerbachstr. 112, D-7000 Stuttgart - 50, Germany.

S2

THE NICOTINIC ACETYLCHOLINE RECEPTOR : STRUCTURE, FUNCTION AND REGULATION OF GENE EXPRESSION DURING ENDPLATE DEVELOPMENT. J.P. Changeux

The acetylcholine (ACh) receptor 300 KD light form from fish electric organ and vertebrate neuromuscular junction is an heterologous pentamer $\alpha_2\beta\gamma\delta$ which contains the ion channel and all the structural elements engaged in the fast (activation) and slow (desensitization) regulation of its opening by ACh. The amino acids which compose the ACh binding sites have been identified, on the native α-subunit from Torpedo marmorata, with a photolabile competitive antagonist p-[^{3}H] (dimethylamino)-benzenediazonium fluoroborate (DDF) as [Tyr 190, Cys 192-193], [Trp 149], [Tyr 93]. They belong to three distinct loops within the large NH2-terminal hydrophilic domain of the α-subunit. Their relative contribution, as that of the non-α subunits, change upon stabilization of the high affinity desensitized state by the allosteric effector meproadifen. The channel blocker ^{3}H-chlorpromazine covalently labels, upon UV irradiation, all the subunits when bound to its unique high affinity site, suggesting that this site is located in the axis of symmetry of the AChR. The labeled amino acids (α-Ser 248, β-Ser 254, β-Leu 257, γ-Thr 253, γ-Ser 257, γ-Leu 260 and δ-Ser 262) all belong to the hydrophobic segment MII and their distribution is consistent with its α-helical organization. These results, together with site-directed mutagenesis experiments, support the notion that the MII segments are involved in ion permeation. At the adult motor endplate, the AChR protein and the α-subunit mRNA localized under the nerve ending, while in the non innervated myotube, they are distributed all over the cell. Denervation causes a reappearance of unspliced and mature mRNA in extrajunctional areas. A compartmentalisation of gene expression at the level of subneural "fundamental" nuclei takes place and is analyzed by the methods of recombinant DNA technology and cell biology with both cultured and developing muscles in situ. The data are interpreted in terms of a model which assumes that : 1) in the adult muscle fiber, nuclei may exist in different stages of gene expression in subneural and extrajunctional areas, different second messengers elicited by neural factors such as 2) CGRP (cAMP) (under the nerve endings) or electrical activity (Ca^{++}, protein kinase C) (outside the endplate) regulate the state of transcription of these nuclei via trans-acting allosteric proteins (e.g. from MyoD1 family) binding to cis-acting DNA regulatory elements to the α-subunit 5'-upstream sequences.

UA CNRS D1284 "Neurobiologie Moléculaire", Département des Biotechnologies, Institut Pasteur, 25 rue du Dr. Roux, 75724 Paris Cedex 15, France

S3

THE GLUTAMATE RECEPTOR GENES: SUBUNIT COMPOSITION DETERMINES RECEPTOR PROPERTIES

Heinemann, S.*, Bettler, B., Boulter, J.*, Duvoisin, R., Edgebjerg, J., Gasic, G.**, Hartley, M., Hermans-Borgmeyer, I., Hollmann, M.*, Hughes, T.E.***, Moll, C., and Rogers, S.*

The mammalian glutamate receptor system is thought to be involved in the first steps of learning and memory acquisition and is perhaps the most important excitatory receptor system in the mammalian brain. The glutamate receptor system has also been implicated in a number of degenerative diseases as well as the neuronal cell death that takes place after insults to the brain such as head trauma, epileptic seizures and stroke.

In order to study the glutamate receptor system at the molecular and physiological level we have an expression cloning approach to identify and clone a family of glutamate receptor genes. One gene that we have called GluR1, codes for a functional glutamate receptor which is also activated by AMPA and kainate. The primary structure and the physiology of the GluR1 glutamate receptor indicates that it is a member of the ligand-gated channel family (1). Five additional genes that code for proteins with sequence homology to the GluR1 glutamate receptor have been identified, GluR2, GluR3, GluR4, GluR5, and GluR6 (2, 3, 4). The functional and structural properties of the cloned glutamate receptor subunits and their distribution in the brain will be discussed. Evidence will be presented indicating that glutamate receptors with very different properties can be made by combining different subunits.

1. Hollmann, M., O'Shea-Greenfield, A., Rogers, S.W., and Heinemann, S., Nature **342**:643-648 (1989).

2. Boulter, J., Hollmann, M., O'Shea-Greenfield, A., Hartley, M., Deneris, E., Maron, C., and Heinemann, S., Science **249**:1033-1037 (1990).

3. Bettler, B., Boulter, J., Hermans-Borgmeyer, I., O'Shea-Greenfield, A., Deneris, E., Moll, C., Borgmeyer, U., Hollmann, M., and Heinemann, S., Neuron **5**:583-595 (1990).

4. Edgebjerg, J., Bettler, B., Hermans-Borgmeyer, I., and Heinemann, S., Nature *in press* (1991).

*Molecular Neurobiology Laboratory, **The Howard Hughes Medical Institute, The Salk Institute P.O. Box 85800, San Diego, CA 92138, USA.
***Department of Neuroscience, University of California, San Diego, CA 92093, USA.

S4

PROPERTIES OF RECONSTITUTED GABA$_A$/BENZODIAZPINE RECEPTOR SUBTYPES P.H. Seeburg, H. Lüddens, H. Wieland, D.B. Pritchett

It is recognized that central benzodiazepine receptors are intrinsic parts of the GABA$_A$ receptor and exhibit diversity generated by assembly of different GABA$_A$ receptor subunit combinations. Currently, 13 subunits have been molecularly characterized and can be grouped into four different sequence classes, termed α, β, γ and δ. Within these classes, the α subunit class is particularly heterogeneous consisting of six variants. Recombinant studies show that receptors reconstituted from α, β and γ variants bind benzodiazepines and the benzodiazepine pharmacology is similar to that of central benzodiazepine receptors. Of note, different α variants generate disparate pharmacologies. Thus, $\alpha_1\beta_2\gamma_2$ receptors show BZI pharmacology, $\alpha_2\beta_2\gamma_2$, $\alpha_3\beta_2\gamma_2$ and $\alpha_5\beta_2\gamma_2$ receptors show BZII pharmacologies. However, these latter receptors display a pronounced difference in their affinities to zolpidem. Thus, $\alpha_2\beta_2\gamma_2$ receptors and $\alpha_3\beta_2\gamma_2$ receptors bind zolpidem with moderate affinities whereas $\alpha_5\beta_2\gamma_2$ receptors do not bind zolpidem at all. These results on reconstituted GABA$_A$ receptors indicate that zolpidem has highest affinity for $\alpha_1\beta_x\gamma_2$ receptors and can distinguish between $\alpha_2\beta_x\gamma_2$ or $\alpha_3\beta_x\gamma_2$ receptors on one hand and $\alpha_5\beta_x\gamma_2$ receptors on the other.

ZMBH, Im Neuenheimer Feld 282, 6900 Heidelberg, Germany

S5

ATP-SENSITIVE K$^+$ CHANNELS : MOLECULAR PHARMACOLOGY, REGULATION AND ROLE IN DISEASED STATES. M. Lazdunski*, M. Fosset, J. De Weille, E. Honoré, C. Mourre

ATP-dependent K$^+$ (K$_{ATP}$) channels have now been identified in many tissues including β-cells, cardiac cells, skeletal muscle cells and neurons. They are the targets of 2 important classes of drugs, the antidiabetic sulfonylureas, which block the channel, and a series of compounds called K$^+$ channel openers and which include cromakalim, pinacidil, nicorandil, minoxidil sulfate, and RP 49356, which tend to maintain the channel in an open conformation. The activity of K$_{ATP}$ channels is regulated by the ATP/ADP ratio. The K$_{ATP}$ channel is an excellent reporter of intracellular variations of the ATP/ADP ratio and has been used to demonstrate the presence of Cl$^-$ channels essential for oxydative phosphorylation in mitochondria. K$_{ATP}$ channels are regulated by hormones in the absence of any variation of the ATP/ADP ratio. Another class of K$^+$ permeable channels which are inhibited by ATP has been identified. However, this channel unlike the K$_{ATP}$ channel is a non selective cationic channel and is not sensitive to sulfonylureas.

K$_{ATP}$ channels are present in cardiac cells where they are also inhibited by antidiabetic sulfonylureas. ATP depletion, such as the one that can occur during cardiac ischemia, activates K$_{ATP}$ channels and this results in a drastic action potential shortening similar to the shortening which occurs during ischemia and which is believed to be responsible for ischemia-induced fibrillations. The shortening produced by ATP depletion is suppressed by sulfonylureas such as glibenclamide. K$^+$ channel openers which, like ATP depletion, activate cardiac K$_{ATP}$ channels also shorten the cardiac action potential and seem to be good protectors of the cardiac cell integrity.

ATP-sensitive K$^+$ channel and sulfonylurea receptors are present in the brain from which they have been purified. Sulfonylurea receptors are in large quantity in substantia nigra and globus pallidus, they are also present in good amounts in hippocampus and cerebellum. K$_{ATP}$ channels are present both pre- and post-synaptically. Presynaptic K$_{ATP}$ channels are involved in GABA secretion. Treatments which induce K$_{ATP}$ channel closure such as increased glucose or sulfonylureas include GABA secretion. Conversely, treatments that produce K$_{ATP}$ channel opening treatments such as anoxia that changes the ATP/ADP level or K$^+$ channel openers such as nicorandil, pinacil or cromakalim tend to decrease GABA secretion. K$_{ATP}$ channels are also present in hyppocampus, they are situated in mossy fibers and are apparently involved in glutamate release. The presence of glucose-sensitive K$_{ATP}$ channels in substantia nigra synapses has probably important implications to explain disease states associated with hypo- or hyperglycemia.

Sulfonylurea sensitive K$^+$ channels are present in follicular cells associated to oocyte in follicle enclosed oocytes. These channels are activated by cAMP by hormones that stimulate cAMP and by K$^+$ channel openers.

* Present address : Institut de Pharmacologie Moléculaire, Université de Nice-Sophia Antipolis, 660 route des lucioles Sophia Antipolis 06560 Valbonne, FRANCE

S6

STRUCTURE AND REGULATION OF CALCIUM CHANNELS
Franz Hofmann

The "L-type" calcium channels are activated at a high membrane potential, are inhibited by the calcium channel blockers (CaCB) and are modulated by cAMP-dependent protein kinase and the α subunit of G proteins. The drug binding protein is the α_1 subunit of the CaCB-receptor which has been purified from rabbit skeletal muscle. The purified CaCB-receptor contains up to five proteins; the 165 kDa α_1 subunit, the 132/28 kDa α_2/δ disulfide linked subunit, the 55 kDa β subunit and the 32 kDa y subunit. The primary structure of these proteins has been deduced by cloning their cDNAs. The structure of the α_1 subunit is similar to that of other voltage-dependent ion channels and is the calcium conducting pore. The α_2/δ and the y subunits are membrane spaning, glycosylated proteins whereas the β subunit may be of cytoskeletal origin. The α_1 subunit contains several putative phosphorylation sites among which Ser-687 is phosphorylated rapidly in vitro by cAMP kinase. cGMP-kinase and protein kinase C incorporate stoichiometric amounts of phosphate into the β subunit. The α_1 subunit binds the dihydropyridines and phenylalkylamines to a region which contains the last transmembrane α-helix (IV S6) and a putative calcium binding EF hand.

α_1 like cDNAs have been isolated from heart, lung and brain and β like cDNAs from heart on the basis of sequence homology with the skeletal muscle proteins. Injection of the α_1 cRNAs into Xenopus oocytes leads to the expression of high voltage activated calcium channels which are either modulated by dihydropyridines (heart, smooth muscle) or not affected by these compounds (brain). The α_1 subunits from heart and smooth muscle are over 95% identical, but are expressed in a tissue specific manner. The cloned sequences suggest the existance of at least 3 genes for the α_1 subunit. Expression of the smooth muscle α_1 subunit in CHO cells results in a regular "L-type" high voltage activated calcium channel which appears not to be regulated by hormones or kinases. Coexpression of the cardiac α_1 subunit with the other subunits from skeletal muscle in Xenopus oocytes alters the electrophysiological properties of the channel, i.e. regular inactivation and activation is only seen in the presence of the other subunits. Coexpression of the β subunit increases 10- to 100-fold the density of the calcium current in oocytes and CHO cells. These results suggest that the α_1 subunit does not contain all the properties of a cardiac L-type calcium channel. Other proteins, probably subunits of the calcium channel are necessary for normal electrophysiological properties.

Institut für Pharmakologie und Toxikologie der Technischen Universität München, Biedersteiner Str. 29, W-8000 München 40, Germany

S7

ION CHANNELS AS G PROTEIN EFFECTORS, A.M. Brown

Ion channels are targets for the α subunits of heterotrimeric G proteins through pathways that may be cytoplasmic or membrane-delimited. Two hypotheses are possible: 1. the membrane pathway may have the ion channel as a G protein effector or 2. an intermediary produced by a phospholipase may be interposed. To distinguish between them we used a defined system consisting of purified skeletal muscle Ca^{2+} channel protein and purified $G\alpha$ protein reconstituted in planar lipid bilayeres formed from purified phospholipids. We tested numerous $G\alpha s$ preactivated with GTPγS but only $G\alpha_s$ had any effect. The effect only occurred when $G\alpha_s$ was applied to the cytoplasmic side of the channel and consisted of a large increase in opening probability. Since no intermediaries were possible, hypothesis 1 is confirmed. We have also analyzed another G protein effect on Ca^{2+} channels, namely the inhibitory effect via G_0 on neuronal Ca^{2+} channels. The inhibition was relieved by strong depolarization and the rate of reinhibition was directly correlated with the extent of G protein activation. An explanatory hypothesis would be that a blocking particle possibly $G_0\alpha$ is dissociated from the Ca^{2+} channel by depolarization and reassociates in a concentration-dependent manner. Muscarinic atrial K^+ channels are effectors for the small G protein ras p21 via the ras effector GAP. The mechanism of ras-GAP action will also be presented.

Present address: Department of Molecular Physiology and Biophysics, Baylor College of Medicine, One Baylor Plaza, Houston, Texas 77030, USA

S8

THE CENTRAL ROLE OF THE IGF-1 RECEPTOR IN THE REGULATION OF CELL GROWTH. R. Baserga, Z. Pietrzkowski*, and A. Ullrich°.

BALB/c3T3 cells are exquisitely growth regulated and require both PDGF and IGF-1 for optimal proliferation. BALB/c3T3 cells that constitutively express elevated levels of IGF-1 and IGF-1 receptor (IGF-1R) are capable of growth in serum-free medium without the addition of exogenous growth factors. BALB/c3T3 cells transfected with only the IGF-1R plasmid required IGF-1 (or insulin) for serum-free growth. Antisense oligonucleotides complementary to IGF-1R mRNA reduced this potential. The levels of IGF-1 and IGF-1R mRNA (as well as the number of IGF-1 binding sites on cellular membranes) are also increased by PDGF, EGF, the proto-oncogenes c-myc and c-myb, and the SV40 T antigen. These and other results in fibroblasts and hemopoietic cells indicate that the IGF-1R plays a crucial role in the control of cellular proliferation, at least in these two types of cells.

*Present address: Jefferson Cancer Institute, Thomas Jefferson University, Bluemle Life Sciences Building, 233 S. 10th Street, Philadelphia, PA 19107-5541, USA.
°Max-Planck-Institut für Biochemie, Department of Molecular Biology, Am Klopferspitz 18A, 8033 Martinsried, Germany.

S9

MUSCLE DETERMINATION GENES: A GENETIC FRAMEWORK FOR DIFFERENTIATION AND GROWTH CONTROL.
H.H. Arnold

Myogenesis is a particularly useful experimental system to study the molecular mechanisms underlying development and differentiation of highly specialized cell types. Four muscle-specific protein factors (Myf3-Myf6) which constitute a subgroup of the large family of helix-loop-helix (H-L-H) DNA binding proteins, provide the genetic framework which controls developmental decision that lead to the establishment of the myogenic lineage within the mesodermal compartment (1-3). This view is based on the observation that forced expression of any one of the four Myf proteins converts embryonic mouse 10T1/2 fibroblasts to the muscle phenotype. Furthermore it is supported by the fact that Myf proteins are expressed in early somites, myotomes and skeletal muscle tissue where each protein follows a defined temporal and spatial pattern during prenatal and postnatal development (4-6). We and others have shown that the muscle H-L-H regulatory proteins act as transcription factors which activate the expression of muscle-specific genes (3,7). To acquire the capacity to bind to DNA with high affinity, Myf proteins heterodimerize with various ubiquitously expressed H-L-H proteins, a property that increases the complexity of transcription factors and generates a potential for regulation (8,9).

Differentiation of skeletal muscle cells _in vivo_ and _in vitro_ is generally incompatible with proliferation. To investigate this relationship, we have employed growth factors and serum mitogens and analyzed their effects on muscle cell differentiation and on the expression of the regulatory gene Myf4 (myogenin) which is normally activated only at the onset of terminal differentiation when growth is arrested. Basic fibroblastic growth factor (bFGF), transforming growth factor (TGF-β) and agents which increase intracellular levels of cAMP (forskolin, cholera toxin) inhibit the expression of myogenin and prevent cellular differentiation which suggests that myogenin is critically involved in the final steps of differentiation (10).

In order to study the antagonism of malignant cell transformation and differentiation, model systems were utilized. A dimethylbenzanthracene (DMBA) induced rat rhabdomyosarcoma cell line which normally fails to form muscle cells _in vitro_, can be triggered to differentiate by a brief treatment with retinoic acid (RA) (11). RA activates the expression of the myogenin gene which is otherwise silent in these cells. Activation of the myogenin gene requires protein and DNA synthesis suggesting that the block of myogenin gene transcription that is alleviated by RA involves both cis- and trans-acting elements (Arnold, unpublished).

In an alternative approach, differentiation of the rat muscle cell line L6 was blocked by the expression of the transforming protein E1a, an early transcriptional factor of adenovirus. This protein interferes with the transactivator domain of the muscle protein Myf5 without affecting its synthesis or ability to bind to DNA. The inhibitory activity of E1a protein resides in its transforming domains (CR1 and CR2) and does not involve its transactivator function (CR3). As a result of Myf5 inactivation, the expression of myogenin, the other muscle-specific H-L-H protein normally expressed in L6 cells, is completely abolished. This may be the cause for the failure of E1a transformed cells to differentiate (12). Taken together, our results suggest that myogenic factor proteins function as a network to establish and maintain the muscle phenotype. Interference with the expression of myogenin either in the context of an isolated tumor cell or by the expression of a transforming viral protein results in the loss of the differentiated phenotype.

Department of Toxicology, Medical School, University of Hamburg, Grindelallee 117, 2000 Hamburg 13, Germany

References

1)	Braun et al.	1989	EMBO J. 8, 3617-3625
2)	Braun et al.	1989	EMBO J. 8, 701-831
3)	Braun et al.	1990	EMBO J. 9, 821-831
4)	Sassoon et al.	1989	Nature 341, 303-307
5)	Ott et al.	1991	Development 111
6)	Bober et al.	1991	J.Cell.Biol.112
7)	Braun et al.	1990	Nature 346, 663-665
8)	Murre et al.	1989	Cell 56, 777-783
9)	Braun and Arnold	1991	J.Biol.Chem.(in press)
10)	Salminen et al.	1991	J.Cell.Biol.(in press)
11)	Gerherz et al.	1989	Br.J.Cancer 59, 61-67
12)	Braun et al.	1991	Cell (in press)

TRANSGENIC ANIMALS IN STUDIES OF CHEMICAL CARCINOGENESIS

A Balmain, K Brown, P Burns, C J Kemp, A B Stoler

Carcinogenesis proceeds in a series of steps involving sequential activation of oncogenes and the inactivation of tumour-suppressor genes. These alterations in gene structure can be observed during multistep carcinogenesis in mouse skin. Treatment with an initiating chemical frequently involves mutation of the cellular H-*ras* gene (1) but further changes are observed during the formation of benign papillomas and progression to malignancy (2). These include amplification of the mutant *ras* gene and/or loss of the normal *ras* allele on mouse chromosome 7 predominantly in tumours classified as high grade or spindle cell carcinomas. The spindle cell phenotype can be reversed in fusions between spindle cell carcinomas and immortalised or benign keratinocytes, indicating that this late stage of carcinogenesis is caused by loss of a putative tumour suppressor function controlling the epidermal differentiation phenotype.

Functional loss of tumour suppressor genes is an important feature of neoplastic progression in humans. We have developed an *in vivo* model system to study loss of tumour suppressor genes in chemically induced skin tumours of F1 hybrid mice. Hybrid mice can be produced which are highly polymorphic at multiple chromosomal loci. Loss of heterozygosity, indicating the presence of putative tumour suppressor loci can be detected by Southern blotting or by the use of microsatellite polymorphisms amenable to analysis by the polymerase chain reaction. Such studies have shown that loci on mouse chromosomes 7 and 11 are frequently lost during skin tumour progression. The crucial gene on chromosone 11 is the p53 tumour suppressor gene, which is mutated in a substantial proportion of carcinomas. Sequencing of mutant p53 alleles has revealed a number of mutations in positions similar to those altered in human tumours. A different tumour suppressor locus on mouse chromosome 7, located at or close to the H-*ras* gene itself, is involved in the transition from squamous to spindle cell carcinomas.

Transgenic mice offer an ideal system to test the causal role of oncogene activation in carcinogenesis. We have introduced a mutant *ras* gene into the germline of mice under the control of a keratin promoter (3). The promoter region of the suprabasal keratin 10 gene has been used to direct expression of a mutant human Harvey-*ras* oncogene to the differentiating cells of the mouse epedermis. Transgenic animals develop hyperkeratosis of the skin and forestomach - the two sites known to express high levels of the keratin 10 polypeptide in vivo. Papillomas subsequently develop on the skin surface, initially at sites subject to biting or scratching such as the base of the tail or behind the ears. The results suggest that the "second event" involved in tumour development in these transgenic animals is the loc 1 induction of a mild wounding stimulus. Furthermore, because the H-*ras* transgene is expressed in suprabasal cells, it appears that cells which have left the stem cell compartment can be induced form at last benign tumors in vivo. The localisation and identification of the cells which constitute the main target for transformation by chemical carcinogens remains to be determined. However, the results obtained using these transgenic animals have shown that at least the initiation and promotion stages can be reproduced by expression of the mutant *ras* gene in the skin, together with induction of a mild wounding stimulus.

References
1. Balmain, A and Brown, K. Adv Cancer Res. *51*, 147 - 182 (1988).
2. Bremner, R and Balmain, A. Cell *61* 407-417 (1990).
3. Bailleul, B, Surani, M A, White, S, Barton, S C, Brown, K, Blessing, M, Jorcano, J and Balmain, A. Cell *62*, 697-708 (1990).

Address: A Balmain, Beatson Institute for Cancer Research, Garscube Estate, Switchback Road, Bearsden, Glasgow G61 1BD, UK.

S11

VARIOUS SEBACEOUS TISSUES EXPRESS A NOVEL CYTOCHROME P450IIB GENE: ISOLATION AND CHARACTER-IZATION OF THE FULL LENGTH cDNA FOR EXPRESSION IN CELL CULTURE. T. Friedberg, F. Oesch, and M.A.G. Grassow.

Cytochromes P450 metabolize a wide variety of endogenous and exogenous compounds. The genes coding for cytochromes P450 can be classified into various gene families according to their sequence homology (eg. P450IA, P450IIB, P450IIIA etc.). Most of these gene families contain several closely related members. The P450IIB family contains members which encode the major phenobarbital inducible hepatic cytochromes P450. Within the P450IIB family we have detected the expression of a novel P450IIB gene by oligonucleotide hybridization to mRNA of the preputial gland which is a large sebaceous gland being highly active in the metabolism of steroids. The expression of this protein was age and sex independent. Moreover immunohistochemistry revealed that the corresponding P450IIB protein is also localized in the meibomian gland of the eyelids which secretes a protective lipid into the tear film. The P450IIB protein was also found to be expressed in the hair shafts. The full-length cDNA of this P450IIB protein was isolated and sequenced. This sequence revealed that the cDNA should encode a functionally active cytochrome P450 which is most likely active in the metabolism of cyclo-phosphamide. The presence of this specific cytochrome P450 isoform in hair follicles might explain the phenomenon of allopecia (loss of hair) observed after treatment of cancer patients with cyclo-phosphamide. We are currently in the process of expressing this cDNA in cell cultures to define the role of this novel cytochrome P450 in the metabolism of endogenous and exogenous compounds.

Institute of Toxicology, University of Mainz, Obere Zahlbacherstr.67, DW 65 Mainz, Germany.

S12

ENDOGENOUS MECHANISMS IN CARCINOGENESIS
H.W. Rüdiger

Cancer is produced by carcinogens. This statement is not trivial. It implicates, that cancer must be preventable if carcinogenic exposure is prevented or at least mini-mized. To prevent carcinogenic exposure, however, makes it a condition that

- carcinogens can be identified
- carcinogenicity can be defined as a property of an agent
- carcinogens are of exogenous origin

The identification of carcinogenic agents is either based on epidemiologic observa-tions, or on in vitro tests or on animal studies. The results of all these approaches are unsatisfying for different reasons: Epidemiology has a poor sensitivity, in vitro tests - being based largely on the detection of genotoxicity - have a poor specifi-city, and animal studies suffer from an enormous interspecies variability with respect to the cancerogenicity of any agent tested so far. Animals are treated with very high doses up to LD$_{50}$ even parenterally in order to obtain unequivocal results. This further limits their use for human risk assessment.

Moreover, the large interspecies variability illustrates the importance of the indivi-dual response in the process of carcinogenicity. Many agents like oxygen and UV-light, though clearly having genotoxic and cancerogenic properties, are well tolera-ted because of highly effective defense mechanisms. Others which themselves may be not genotoxic at all may interfere with individual defense and repair mechanisms and hereby may alter the response to ubiquitous genotoxicants. The latter may also arise from endogenous sources since every living cell is containing thousands of reactive substances being needed to maintain its metabolism. Many of these will certainly be able to react with DNA. DNA itself is an unstable molecule and needs continous preservation and repair. This maintenance is provided by processes which in return are protecting living cells against adverse exogenous influences as well.

Cancer prevention may thus not focus solely on exogenous agents which could be eliminated, but must take into consideration endogenous factors as well and the many defense and protective mechanisms. From driving a naked man into a swarm of bees we could well conclude, that bee-keeping is a very dangerous job, though it is not in reality.

*Present address: Arbeitsgruppe Toxikogenetik, Ordinariat für Arbeitsmedizin, University of Hamburg, Adolph-Schönfelder-Str. 5, D-2000 Hamburg 76, FRG

S13

SIGNAL TRANSDUCTION BY RECEPTOR TYROSINE KINASES
A. Ullrich

Cell-cell interaction is an essential requirement for the integrated function of a multicellular organism during development and mature life. Molecules secreted by one cell type and their specific plasma membrane receptors on the target cell are key components of this cellular communication network. Ligand-receptor interaction on the cell surface is translated into activation of intracellular signal transduction pathways, initiating a sequence of events that eventually results in specific cellular responses. Currently, two general mechanisms of cellular signal transduction are relatively well understood: coupling of receptors to various effectors by means of G proteins or coupling through the activation of a tyrosine-specific protein kinase activity that is intrinsic to the receptor molecule. Signaling by tyrosine kinase (TK) activation is shared by at least nine known hormones and growth factors and their corresponding receptors. These receptor tyrosine kinases (RTKs) constitute a family of structurally related receptor polypeptides with a rapidly increasing number of members.

In recent years it has become clear that the study of receptor function and particularly RTK-activated signaling pathways will provide a better understanding of fundamental processes in the areas of cell biology, endocrinology, and development. Furthermore, one can expect that under-standing receptor-mediated signal transduction will provide insights into the molecular basis of important human diseases, such as cancer and Type II diabetes, and open new avenues for diagnosis and therapy.

Two advances have brought us substantially closer to an elucidation of RTK function. The primary structures of a number of RTKs have become available from cloned cDNA sequences, and comparative analysis has offered clues to receptor domain function. This family of cell surface glyco-proteins can now be classified into several distinct structural subclasses that may reflect unique molecular pathways of cellular activation. In combination with classical biochemical approaches, the availability of cloned cDNAs for RTKs and their respective ligands opened the way for detailed dissection of the mechanism(s) of growth signal generation.

Partial amino acid sequence determination of peptides derived from purified receptors enabled determination of the nucleotide sequences of mRNA molecules encoding the receptors for epidermal growth factor (EGF), insulin, platelet-derived growth factor (PDGF), and insulin-like growth factor 1 (IGF-1). The structure of the putative receptor for the macrophage growth factor (CSF-1) was determined on the basis of its homology to the viral *fms* oncogene. A similar approach yielded the structure of a receptor-like molecule encoded by the cellular homologue of the viral *kit* oncogene. Another putative receptor encoded by the HER2/*neu* protooncogene (also called c-*erb*B-2) exhibits extensive sequence homology with EGFR. A common structural organization emerged from the analysis of the deduced primary structures. The presence of an amino-terminal signal peptide and a single internal hydrophobic sequence confers the same transmembrane orien-tation for all RTKs. The extracellular ligand binding domain resides in the amino-terminal half of the molecule, whereas the catalytic function, a tyrosine-specific kinase, is contained in the cytoplasmic, carboxy-terminal portion of the receptor. This topology provides a common overall structural basis for signal transduction. Closer primary sequence examination reveals the existence of subdomains which are distinct between structural subgroups of the RTK family.

New members of the family of transmembrane tyrosine kinases are being discovered at a rapid pace. In addition to the already characterized PDGF receptor, a related human receptor was identified that binds the A-chain homodimer of PDGF, and similarly two receptors for acidic and basic fibroblast growth factors have been identified. Furthermore, the cellular homologues of the viral oncogenes *sea* and *ros*, the fusion genes *trk* and *ret*, the protooncogene *met*, the *sevenless* and *torso* genes of *Drosophila*, and the *Xmrk* gene product, which is involved in the development of melanoma in fish, have been characterized as receptor-like tyrosine kinases.

Basic aspects of receptor domain characteristics, organization, and function will be discussed.

Complementary DNA (cDNA) clones encoding RTKs allowed the construction of structurally altered receptors, which provided insights into the molecular mechanism of signal transduction. Such studies employed a large variety of receptor mutants to address the role of structural domains and subdomains in diverse functions, such as ligand binding, affinity definition and modulation, transmembrane activation, ATP binding, kinase activity, endocytosis, degradation, recycling, Ca^{2+} release, auto/transphospho-rylation, substrate phosphorylation, and signal generation. These studies, as well as the current state of knowledge with respect to the characteristics of RTK-mediated cellular signals, will be discussed.

An important conceptual breakthrough occurred when it was realized that polypeptides that are known to play important roles in the control and transmission of cellular growth and differentiation signals are identical or closely related to oncogene products. The B chain of platelet-derived growth factor is the cellular homolog of the v-*sis* oncogene of the simian sarcoma virus. The receptors for epidermal growth factor, and colony stimulating factor I were found to be protooncogene counterparts of v-*erb*B and v-*fms*, and HER2, the human homolog of the chemically-induced rat *neu* oncogene, is likely to be a growth factor receptor whose ligand has yet to be identified. Moreover, *Xmrk*, a gene that had been shown to be causally involved in the development of melanoma in fish, was shown to encode another EGFR-like RTK. Recently, phospholipase C, a key component of the intracellular signal transduction network, was described to be structurally related to *crk*, a newly discovered oncogene product of CT10 avian sarcoma virus, as well as regulatory regions of *src*.

While retroviral oncogenes serve largely as important animal model systems for the investigation of molecular mechanisms involved in oncogenesis, the important role of HER2/*neu* and EGFR in human cancer is strongly supported. p185$^{HER2/neu}$ has been found to be amplified and overexpressed in a number of human cancers, including breast carcinoma, stomach adeno-carcinoma, salivary gland adenocarcinoma, endometrial cancer, and ovarian adenocarcinoma. About 30% of human breast cancer patients exhibit a two-fold or greater amplification of the HER2 gene, and patients with >5-fold gene amplification have a statistically significant reduction in disease-free and overall survival.

Current studies are aimed at understanding which alterations in receptor structure and expression lead to transformation of cells in culture, formation of tumors in animals, and oncogenesis in humans. Furthermore, initial attempts towards new approaches for cancer therapy will be discussed.

Relevant references can be found in the recent review by A. Ullrich and J. Schlessinger (1990) *Cell* 61, 203-212 (copy attached).

Present address: Max-Planck-Institut für Biochemie, Am Klopferspitz 18A, D-8033 Martinsried

HETEROGENEITY OF DOPAMINE RECEPTORS.

Marc G. Caron, Depts. of Cell Biology and Medicine, Duke University Medical Center, Durham, NC 27710

Dopamine mediates several important functions in the body. In the central nervous system (CNS), dopamine is involved in the control of motor, cognitive, affective, and neuroendocrine functions. Peripherally, dopamine regulates hormone synthesis and secretion, vascular tone, and renal function. Dopaminergic systems are of particular interest because of their role in the etiology and management of various disorders, such as Parkinson's disease, schizophrenia, tardive dyskinesia, hyperprolactinemia and pituitary adenomas, and hypertension. For a long time, these effects of dopamine were thought to be mediated by only two distinct G protein-coupled receptor subtypes, D_1 and D_2, coupled respectively to stimulation and inhibition of the effector enzyme adenylyl cyclase, which produces the second messenger cAMP. Our original approach toward the characterization of these receptors was to develop specific photoaffinity ligands and affinity chromatography procedures, which led to the purification and characterization of both D_1 and D_2 dopamine receptors from striatum and anterior pituitary. These studies contributed significantly to the biochemical definition of these systems.

Recent developments from several experimental approaches, but in particular from molecular biology, now demonstrate that the family of dopamine receptors is much larger than previously thought. The cDNA's and/or genes of six distinct dopamine receptor subtypes have already been isolated. Further, additional evidence suggests that still other members of this family remain to be isolated.

Three distinct subtypes of D_1-like receptors have been characterized. All 3 subtypes bind dopaminergic ligands with a pharmacological profile which is similar to the classical D_1 dopamine receptor. These three receptors have all the characteristic properties of G protein-coupled receptors, in particular 7 transmembrane domains (TM) and show high amino acid identity (75-80%) between each other within these 7 TM segments. These D_1 receptor subtypes have distinct properties. Whereas the mRNA for the D_{1A} dopamine receptor is distributed mostly within the striatum, nucleus accumbens and olfactory tubercule, the mRNA for the D_{1B} receptor is restricted to the hippocampus, the anterior pretectal nuclei and the mammilary nucles (Tiberi et al., Proc. Natl. Acad. Sci. in press). The other D_1-like subtype (D_5, Sunabara et al., Nature 350, 614, 1991) displays an mRNA distribution similar to the D_{1A} receptor but binds dopamine with roughly 10-fold higher affinity than either the D_{1A} or D_{1B} receptor.

Three distinct D_2-related subtypes have been characterized. The D_2 dopamine receptor, which displays two alternatively spliced forms (Bunzow et al. Nature 336, 783, 1989; Grandy et al., Proc. Natl. Acad. Sci. 86, 9762, 1989); the D_3 receptor, which has a restricted limbic distribution (Sokoloff et al., Nature 347, 146, 1990); and the D_4 receptor, which has high affinity for the atypical antipsychotic clozapine (Van Tol et al., Nature 350, 610, 1991).

Despite this growing number of receptor subtypes for dopamine, several additional subtypes must exist, based on existing evidence: a brain and/or kidney D_1 receptor subtype coupled to phospholipase C hydrolysis of phosphatidylinositol; a D_1 receptor subtype present in amygdala not coupled to adenylyl cyclase; D_2 receptors in kidney and in posterior pituitary that are pharmacologically distinct from the brain D_2 receptor; a D_2 receptor with high affinity for both sulpiride and clozapine; and a D_2 receptor in the frontal cortex pharmacologically distinct from the classical D_2 receptor (Andersen et al., Trends in Pharmacol. Sci. 11, 231, 1990). The multiplicity of the receptors for dopamine and the availability of molecular biology probes for these receptors represent a unique opportunity to understand more thoroughly in molecular terms the actions of dopamine and its potential implications in various disorders. This wealth of information also provides a excellent framework for the development of more specific drugs for the management of various disorders.

S15

FUNCTIONAL ASPECTS OF RECEPTOR-G-PROTEIN COUPLING

T. Wieland, G. Hilf*, P. Gierschik* and K.H. Jakobs

Membrane-associated signal-transducing guanine nucleotide-binding proteins (G proteins) are composed of an α-subunit carrying the binding site for guanine nucleotides (GDP, GTP and their analogs) and a dimer of β- and γ-subunits. It is generally assumed that under resting conditions GDP is bound to the α-subunit and that the GDP-liganded α-subunit is associated with the $\beta\gamma$-dimer, thus forming the inactive, holotrimeric G protein complex $\alpha_{GDP}\beta\gamma$.

In the activated state, the α-subunit is liganded with the nucleoside triphosphate GTP and apparently is dissociated from the $\beta\gamma$-dimer. GTP-liganded G protein α-subunits as well as free $\beta\gamma$-dimers are reported to modulate activities of effector moieties (e.g. enzymes, channels), being finally responsible for alteration in intracellular second messenger concentration. This active state of G proteins is terminated by hydrolysis of bound GTP to GDP by the α-subunit-inherent GTPase activity, leading to a GDP-liganded α-subunit capable of reassociating with $\beta\gamma$-dimers.

The transition of G proteins from the inactive, $\alpha_{GDP}\beta\gamma$ state to the active, free α_{GTP} plus $\beta\gamma$ state is catalyzed by a large number of membrane receptors, which, as known so far, all exhibit a typical seven transmembrane-spanning pattern. With some G proteins, the transition from the inactive to the active state, i.e. the GDP-GTP exchange reaction, can be observed even in the absence of receptors and appears to be additionally dependent on the membrane environment. Furthermore, both reconstitution experiments with purified receptors and G proteins as well as studies on various intact membrane systems strongly suggest that agonist-free receptors (e.g. β-adrenoceptors, muscarinic acetylcholine receptors, opiate receptors and formyl peptide receptors) can exhibit some distinct activity in catalyzing the GDP-GTP exchange reaction at G proteins. This agonist-independent but receptor-mediated activation of G proteins can be inhibited by specific receptor antagonists. Furthermore, sodium ions known to affect ligand binding to receptors apparently also interfere with the coupling to and activation of G proteins by agonist-free receptors. Agonist binding causes a large increase in the catalytic activity of receptors in G protein activation. Data from various receptors, G proteins and intact membrane systems suggest that one agonist-liganded receptor can activate up to ten or even hundred G proteins. Thus, there is a large variation possible in G protein activity, depending on whether being activated even without receptors, with agonist-free or agonist-activated receptors.

Although available evidence strongly suggests that the GDP-liganded and the GTP-liganded states are the inactive and active configurations, respectively, of G proteins, the mechanisms by which bound GDP is exchanged by GTP are only poorly described and resolved. With only some systems, it has indeed been shown that agonist-liganded receptors can cause a dissociation of apparently G protein-bound GDP. However, quantitative data with regard to receptor and affected G protein number are missing. Furthermore, receptor-stimulated release of G protein-bound GppNHp, a GTPase-resistant GTP analog, has been reported and taken as evidence for receptor-induced release of G-protein-bound GDP, although it is generally assumed that GTP- or GppNHp-liganded G protein α-subunits are dissociated from and thus do not interact with receptors. Similar data as with GppNHp were recently reported for G proteins liganded with the hydrolysis-resistent GTP analog GTP[γS].

In addition to the "classical" direct GDP-GTP exchange reaction, two alternatives were recently proposed to be involved in the activation of G proteins, i.e. the transition from the GDP- to the GTP-bound state. First, there is circumstantial evidence that G proteins are associated with nucleoside diphosphokinase (NDP kinase), an enzyme capable of converting GDP to GTP (or GTP[γS]) using ATP (or ATP[γS]) as (thio)phosphate donator. Furthermore, under some conditions, activated receptors appear to be capable to increase the formation of GTP (or GTP[γS]) by the NDP kinase. Finally, preliminary evidence suggests that the conversion of GDP to GTP (or GTP[γS]) catalyzed by NDP kinase may even occur with the GDP bound to G protein α-subunits. A second, additional mechanism involved in G protein activation appears to be mediated by the G protein βγ-dimers, known to be absolutely required for receptor-catalyzed G protein activation. As recently reported, β-subunits of the G protein G_t (transducin) can be intermediately (thio)phosphorylated by GTP (or GTP[γS]). Preliminary data suggest that for both the (thio)phosphorylation of β-subunits as well as for the (thio)phosphate group transfer to GDP G protein α–subunits are required. These data suggest that this type of reaction may not initiate G protein activation but is involved in propagation of the signal cascade, i.e. the amplification reaction. Thus, it appears that the transition from the GDP-bound to the GTP-bound state, i.e. the activation of G proteins and thus the initial step in transmembrane signalling by G protein-coupled receptors, involves various different mechanisms, which may even act in concert. None of these mechanisms is understood in detail as well as the possible interplay of these reactions, particularly considering the receptor-mediated activation of G proteins in intact cells.

Institut für Pharmakologie, Universität-GHS-Essen, Hufelandstr. 55, D-4300 Essen, FRG, and *Pharmakologisches Institut, Universität Heidelberg, D-6900 Heidelberg, FRG

STRUCTURE AND DIVERSITY OF G-PROTEINS. M. I. Simon

The heterotrimeric G-proteins act as switches that regulated information processing circuits connecting cell surface receptors to a variety of effectors. There are more than 100 different receptors and effectors, including dozens of different adenylcyclases, phospholipases, phosphodiesterases, and ion channels. In order to explore the specificity of the interactions between G proteins and different receptor-effector systems we have been characterizing the extent of diversity in the genes that encode the components of the G protein heterotrimers.

Thus far, we have characterized seven novel alpha subunits. We have been able to subdivide the sixteen different alpha subunit isotypes into four distinct classes based on amino acid sequence comparisons. The Gq class in mouse includes four different isotypes, $G_{\alpha q}$, $G_{\alpha 11}$, $G_{\alpha 14}$ and $G_{\alpha 15}$ and the G_{12} class includes $G_{\alpha 12}$ and $G_{\alpha 13}$. The relative distribution of the Gq class gene products has been studied. $G_{\alpha 11}$ mRNA is found to be expressed in every cell type that was examined and while $G_{\alpha q}$ is ubiquitously expressed, its level varies widely in different cell and tissue types. The $G_{\alpha 14}$ and $G_{\alpha 15}$ gene products are expressed in a limited number of cells; $G_{\alpha 15}$ appears to be restricted to myeloid and lymphoid cells while $G_{\alpha 14}$ is found in a variety of stromol cells. Work by P. Sternweis (University of Texas, Dallas) and J. Exton (Vanderbilt University, Tennessee) has suggested that $G_{\alpha q}$ activates the phospholipase C beta isotype (PLC). In an effort to further explore the function of the Gq proteins we have expressed them by transfection of the appropriate cDNA clones into Cos cells together with cDNA clones of PLC. In this system activation of $G_{\alpha 11}$ and $G_{\alpha q}$ led to marked increases in phospholipase activity while $G_{\alpha OA}$, $G_{\alpha Z}$, and $G_{\alpha T}$ had no effect on phospholipase activity. The relative ability of different members of the Gq class to activate specific phospholipase isotypes was studied. The Gq class of alpha subunits appears to be coupled to PLC. Little is currently known about the function of the G_{12} class of alpha subunits.

In addition to the diverse α subunits, beta and gamma subunits show marked diversity and tissue specific expression. The role of beta-gamma diversity in G-protein function will be reviewed.

The different G_α subunit classes are found to be conserved in a variety of species. We have studied cell type specific expression of G proteins in nerve cells in the worm, *C. elegans*, in order to understand the molecular basis for signaling.

Strathmann, M., T. M. Wilkie and M. I. Simon. Diversity of the G-protein family: Sequences from five additional α subunits in the mouse. *Proc. Natl. Acad. Sci. USA* **86**, 7407-7409, 1989.

Strathmann, M., T. M. Wilkie and M. I. Simon. Alternative splicing produces transcripts encoding two forms of the α subunit of GTP-binding protein G$_O$. *Proc. Natl. Acad. Sci. USA* **87**, 6477-6481, 1990.

Strathmann, M. and M. I. Simon. G protein diversity: A distinct class of α subunits is present in vertebrates and invertebrates. *Proc. Natl. Acad. Sci. USA* **87**, 9113-9117, 1990.

Strathmann, M., B. A. Hamilton, C. A. Mayeda, M. I. Simon, E. M. Meyerowitz and M. J. Palazzolo. Transposon-facilitated DNA sequencing. *Proc. Natl. Acad. Sci. USA*, **88**, 1247-1250 (1991).

Simon, M. I., M. P. Strathmann and N. Gautam. Diversity of G proteins in signal transduction. *Science* **252**, 802-808 (1991).

Amatruda, T. T., III, D. A. Steele, V. Z. Slepak and M. I. Simon. Gα16, a novel G-protein alpha subunit specifically expressed in hematopoietic cells. *Proc. Natl. Acad. Sci. USA*, in press.

Strathmann, M. P. and M. I. Simon. Gα12 and Gα13 define a fourth class of G protein alpha subunits. *Proc. Natl. Acad. Sci. USA*, in press.

Division of Biology, California Institute of Technology, Pasadena, California, 91125, U. S. A.

REGULATION OF PHOSPHOINOSITIDE PHOSPHOLIPASE C BY G-PROTEINS J. H. Exton

Many hormones, neurotransmitters and growth factors stimulate the hydrolysis of phosphatidylinositol 4,5-bisphosphate (PIP_2) in the plasma membrane of their target cells to produce two signalling molecules: inositol 1,4,5-trisphosphate (IP_3) which releases intracellular Ca^{2+} and 1,2-diacylglycerol (DAG) which activates protein kinase C. There is much evidence that G-proteins are involved in the activation of the phospholipase C that hydrolyzes PIP_2, but their nature has only recently been elucidated.

Ca^{2+}-mobilizing agonists induce a rapid, large decrease in PIP_2 in many cells. This is associated with a parallel increase in IP_3, and slower changes in other inositol phosphates due to the further metabolism of IP_3. In experiments utilizing isolated plasma membranes, submicromolar concentrations of GTP and its stable analogues activate a PIP_2-selective phospholipase C. This activation is not produced by other nucleotides, requires millimolar Mg^{2+} and is competitively inhibited by a stable GDP analogue. The phospholipase is also activated by Ca^{2+}-mobilizing agonists in the presence of low concentrations of GTP analogues. Further evidence that Ca^{2+}-mobilizing receptors are linked to a G-protein(s) is provided by the observations that GTP and its analogues reduce the binding of agonists to these receptors, that Ca^{2+}-mobilizing agonists stimulate a low K_m GTPase activity in plasma membranes and that AlF_4^- stimulates IP_3 formation and Ca^{2+} mobilization in cells.

There are several phosphoinositide phospholipase C isozymes (α-ϵ) which have different molecular weights and sequences, and can be distinguished immunologically. These all hydrolyze PI, PIP and PIP_2 in a Ca^{2+}-dependent manner, but PIP_2 is preferred at low Ca^{2+} concentrations. The phospholipase C isozyme responsible for growth factor-stimulated PIP_2 hydrolysis in several tissues has been identified as the γ_1 isozyme.

Recent work in our laboratory has purified to homogeneity the G-proteins that regulate PIP_2 phospholipase C in bovine liver plasma membranes. Silver-stained gels of the final preparations revealed proteins of 42, 43 and 35 kDa. The 42 and 43 kDa proteins were recognized by an antiserum raised to a peptide common to many α-subunits, and the 35 kDa protein by an antiserum to a β-subunit peptide. In recent work, it has been possible to resolve the two α-subunits sufficiently to demonstrate that both activate purified phospholipase equally well.

To test which phospholipase isozyme is specifically stimulated, the α-subunits were reconstituted with the β_1, γ_1 and δ_1 isozymes purified from bovine brain and supplied by Dr. Sue Goo Rhee, National Institutes of Health. The results showed unequivocally that only the β_1 isozyme was activated. Furthermore, only antibodies to the β_1 isozyme inhibited the activation of the endogenous phospholipase of liver plasma membranes by a GTP analogue.

The 42 and 43 kDa α-subunits have been shown to be members of the newly discovered G_q class of G-proteins (G_q and G_{11}) identified as cDNAs in a mouse brain library by M. Simon and associates at the California Institute for Technology. Polyclonal antisera (WO82, WO83, X384) raised to peptides corresponding to unique regions in the deduced amino acid sequence of α_q and supplied by Dr. P. C. Sternweis, University of Texas Southwestern Medical School, reacted strongly with the 42 kDa protein, whereas the 43 kDa protein was recognized by WO83, X384 and E976 raised to peptides corresponding to unique regions in α_{11}. In parallel studies in Dr. Sternweis' laboratory, two 42 kDa α-subunits prepared from rat or bovine brain by affinity chromatography on $\beta\gamma$ agarose have been partially sequenced and the tryptic peptides shown to correspond to sequences in α_q and α_{11}. In more recent work, Sternweis and his collaborators have demonstrated that activation of the proteins by AlF_4^-, but not guanine nucleotides stimulated phosphoinositide phospholipase C. The G-proteins that regulate phosphoinositide phospholipase C have also been purified in the heterotrimeric ($\alpha\beta\gamma$) form. The final preparation contained two 42 and 43 kDa α-subunits and a 35 kDa β-subunit. Rapid activation of the phospholipase in the presence of the G-proteins was observed with GTPγS and other poorly hydrolyzable GTP analogues, but relatively high concentrations of the nucleotides (1-100 μM) were needed. The activation was inhibited by high concentrations of GDPβS and by excess G-protein $\beta\gamma$ subunits. AlF_4^- also activated the phospholipase in the presence of the G-proteins. Like the purified α-subunits, the G-proteins were not substrates for pertussis toxin-stimulated ADP-ribosylation.

There is evidence that the G-proteins are regulated by Ca^{2+}-mobilizing agonists in rat liver plasma membranes. For example, two proteins of 42 and 43 kDa bound a photoreactive GTP analogue, [^{32}P]γ-azidoanilido GTP, in response to vasopressin and other Ca^{2+}-mobilizing agonists, but not glucagon. The labeling required Mg^{2+} and was inhibited specifically by GTP and its analogues. Vasopressin-stimulated labeling was selectively inhibited by a V_1-vasopressin receptor antagonist and required vasopressin concentrations similar to those which activate PIP_2 phospholipase C. Immunodetection or immunoprecipitation of the photo-labeled 42 and 43 kDa proteins with antisera WO82, WO83 and X384 confirmed that these proteins are members of the G_q class of G-proteins.

In collaboration with Dr. E. Ross at the University of Texas Southwestern Medical School, the heterotrimeric G-proteins purified as described above have been reconstituted with expressed M1 and M2 muscarinic cholinergic receptors in phospholipid vesicles. Reconstitution with the M1 receptor, but not the M2 receptor, resulted in a very large stimulation of GTPγS binding and GTPase activity by carbachol, but not atropine.

In summary, two pertussis toxin-insensitive G-proteins that regulate phosphoinositide phospholipase C have been purified. These are both members of the G_q class of G-proteins and have the properties of heterotrimeric G-proteins, although their affinity for GTP and its analogues is very low in the unactivated state. Their selectivity for phosphoinositide phospholipase isozymes is extremely high, with only the β_1 form being activated. Their selectivity for activation by receptors is also very high, with only Ca^{2+}-mobilizing receptors being effective.

Howard Hughes Medical Institute, Department of Molecular Physiology and Biophysics and Department of Pharmacology, Vanderbilt University School of Medicine, Nashville, TN 37232-0295 USA

S18

REGULATORY FUNCTIONS OF SMALL MOLECULAR WEIGHT GTP-BINDING PROTEINS D. Gallwitz

Both in unicellular and multicellular organisms, a large number of structurally related, small GTP-binding proteins, collectively known as ras superfamily of proteins, has been identified within the past few years. These proteins share similar size and biochemical properties. According to characteristic features of their primary structure, members of the ras superfamily of proteins can be further subdivided into ras, rho and ypt(rab) proteins. Common to all of these proteins is a conformational change that occurs during the transition from the GDP- to the GTP-bound form and allows the interaction with specific targets, resulting in the activation of diverse cellular reactions. The action of the regulatory proteins is temporally limited by the hydrolysis of the bound GTP, brought about by an intrinsic GTPase which is accelerated by interacting GTPase-activating proteins (1, 2).

Despite their common biochemical features and their ubiquitous occurrence in eukaryotic organisms, different members of the ras superfamily of proteins appear to be required for a variety of cellular functions, including the transmission and amplification of extracellular signals, the intracellular vectorial transport of membrane-enclosed vesicles and the maintenance of the cytoskeletal architecture (3).

Ras proteins which are associated with the plasma membrane through C-terminal lipidation, are thought to function as signal amplifiers. Although they are functionally interchangeable between yeast and mammals, Ras proteins interact with different targets in uni- and multicellular eukaryotes. Mostly from studies with yeast mutants, evidence is accumulating for a role of members of the ypt (rab) subfamily of proteins in vesicular transport of the secretory pathway (4, 5). Localization of mammalian ypt/rab proteins to defined compartments of the exocytic and endocytic pathway points to an analogous function of these proteins in multicellular organisms (6).

Comparative studies on small molecular weight GTP-binding proteins in yeast and mammalian cells, employing classical genetics, molecular genetic and biochemical analyses, are currently pursued in many laboratories to unravel the functional specificity of the more than 30 ras-like proteins that are presently known.

1. Bourne, H.R., Sanders, D.A. and McCormick, F. (1990) Nature 348, 125-132.
2. Bourne, H.R., Sanders, D.A. and McCormick, F. (1991) Nature 349, 117-127.
3. Hall, A. (1990) Science 249, 635-640.
4. Walworth, N.C., Goud, B., Kabcenell, A.K. and Novick, P.J. (1989) EMBO J. 8, 1685-1693.
5. Becker, J., Tan, T.J., Trepte, H.-H. and Gallwitz, D. (1991) EMBO J. 10, 785-792.
6. Chavrier, P., Parton, R.G., Hauri, H.P., Simons, K. and Zerial, M. (1990) Cell 62, 317-329.

Department of Molecular Genetics, Max Planck Institute for Biophysical Chemistry, P.O. Box 2841, D-3400 Göttingen, Germany

S19

MOLECULAR STUDIES OF THE STRESS AXIS, H.Akil* and S.Watson

The hypothalamus-pituitary adrenal (HPA) axis is a neuroendocrine system for sensing and responding to environmental and physiological stressors, and as such, is critical for survival of the organism. Its ultimate function is the production of glucocorticoids which bind to specific receptors and cause them to translocate and activate or inhibit numerous target genes. Thus, glucocorticoids are extremely potent hormones, with widespread effects which need to be maintained at optimal basal levels and are needed to respond rapidly, but also to terminate rapidly. Insufficient levels, as well as exceedingly high levels of glucocorticoids are detrimental to the organism. Thus, the HPA axis has to a) maintain an ideal level of readiness to respond to stress. b) Produce efficient well-orchestrated responses which are proportional to the intensity and duration of the stressful stimulus. c) Terminate stress responses promptly, to prevent untoward side effects and avoid possible desensitization events. These requirements are met via an exquisite orchestration between the secretory drive which leads to release of key stress hormones, and multiple negative feedback mechanisms, which "read" the level of circulating steroids and stop secretion, as well as limiting the expression of genes involved in the activation of the axis.

The "activating" elements of the axis involve several neuropeptides and neurohormones in key structures. In particular, the paraventricular nucleus of the hypothalamus (PVN) serves as a final common path for various neuronal inputs which stimulate the axis - within the PVN, neurons express the gene for corticotropin releasing hormone (CRH) and for vasopressin (AVP). Both serve as secretagogues which trigger secretion of the stress hormone ACTH (Adreno-corticotropic hormone) from the anterior pituitary. ACTH, in turn, activates the adrenal cortex which results in the synthesis and release of corticosteroids.

Two classes of receptors recognize glucocorticoids and are present throughout the body and in brain. These are termed the glucocorticoid receptor (GR) and the mineralocorticoid receptor (MR). They belong to the steroid receptor gene family. They are essentially transacting factors which bind steroids, translocate to the nucleus, and bind specific DNA sequences termed glucocorticoid responsive elements or GRE's. Both GR and MR are expressed in brain, with highest levels of expression in the hippocampus as determined by both receptor binding and mRNA quantitation. Based on this anatomy and on a number of physiological studies, the hippocampus is thought to play a key role in steroid feedback upon the axis.

Given this background, and the fact that all the key proteins in this system have been cloned and all the neuropeptides genes have been mapped, it is possible to study the regulation of this system at a molecular level, in the context of the integration of stress responsiveness. Our studies have focused on the following:

a) **Understanding gene expression and regulation of the key genes of the stress axis** including POMC (pro-opiomelanocortin, the ACTH precursor) CRH and vasopressin, as well as the effect of glucocorticoids on this expression. For example, we have shown that POMC can be regulated by repeated stress both at the pre- and post-translational level. Activation-induced cellular events include increased transcription, as evidenced by higher levels of primary transcript (heteronuclear RNA or hnRNA), increased message pools, increased peptides stores and increased rates of post-translational maturation of the precursor. Conversely, glucocorticoids reduce secretion as well as biosynthesis of POMC. Similarly, gene expression of CRH and vasopressin in the brain is sensitive to levels of glucocorticoids. In particular, vasopressin can become co-expressed within CRH neurons when glucocorticoid levels are low, but this expression is dramatically suppressed with elevated steroid levels. Since the co-expressed secretagogues - AVP and CRH - act synergistically to dramatically enhance ACTH secretion, inhibition of AVP/CRH co-expression by cortisol can have a profound effect in limiting release of POMC products.

b) **Studying the expression and cell biology of GR and MR.** These receptors are associated with heat-shock protein (HSP-90) which is critical in insuring their ability to bind, to translocate and interact with genes. The exact points of interaction between GR and HSP-90 are being examined using peptide competition and site-directed mutagenesis.

In addition, the MR gene is complex and exhibits multiple splicing pathways, leading to multiple forms of the MR

receptor which vary at their 5' UT. These multiple forms are differentially expressed in various tissues.
c) **At a more integrative level, investigating the mechanisms which control the HPA axis across the circadian rhythm.** In particular, the gene expression of CRH across the daily rhythm will be described, and the role of glucocorticoids in shaping this rhythm will be delineated. Our findings suggest that circulating glucocorticoids affect the overall level of CRH mRNA but do not dictate the pattern of the circadian rhythm.
d) **Developing sensitive molecular tools for studying the effects of stressors on the brain.** The rapid activation of the key points of this axis by stressors can be monitored by looking at gene expression with two methods -- the examination of immediate early genes, such as c-fos, and the quantitation of primary transcripts by looking with intronic probes. Measurement of heteronuclear RNA provides an index of novel transcription, and thus reflects rapid changes in gene expression. We have succeeded in measuring CRH hnRNA following acute activation of secretion using *in situ* hybridization. Changes are evident within 10 minutes.
e) **Finally, all these elements from molecular to circuits can become altered with aging,** leading to subtle but important changes in the stress axis, which will be briefly summarized.
In sum, the work being presented offers an overview of the interplay between various genes located in precise anatomical structures, which work in unison to insure a rapid and well-tuned response of the organism to impinging stressors.

*Present address: Mental Health Research Institute, University of Michigan, Ann Arbor, Michigan 48109-0720

PEPTIDES AND TRANSMITTERS IN NEURONS AND NON-NEURONAL TISSUES

T. Hökfelt, A. Bean, S. Ceccatelli, Å. Dagerlind, R. P. Elde, B. Meister, A. P. Nicholas, M. Pelto-Huikko, V. Pieribone, M. Schalling, V. Verge, Zhang Xu, T. Bartfai[1] and Z. Wiesenfeld-Hallin[2].

In addition to amino acids, such as GABA and glutamate, and biogenic amines, such as dopamine and noradrenaline, neurons produce and release peptides. In fact, there is evidence that a single neuron may contain several types of messenger molecules, sometimes both an amino acid, a biogenic amine and a peptide. Our understanding of the functional significance of such coexistence of multiple signal substances is not clear. Particularly with regard to the peptides, their role and physiological function still remain to be analyzed in many cases. In spite of these uncertainties, some general findings have been obtained concerning the coexistence phenomenon. They may be summarized as follows. (1) Classical transmitter systems, for example the bulbospinal 5-hydroxytryptamine (5-HT) neurons can be subdivided on the basis of specific peptides. Thus, the 5-HT neurons projecting to the ventral horn contain substance P and thyrotropin releasing hormone (TRH), whereas those projecting to the dorsal horn seem to lack these peptides. (2) Classical transmitters and peptides have a different subcellular distribution and are presumably localized in different types of storage vesicles. (3) At least in certain systems the release of peptides and classical transmitters is frequency coded, that is whereas classical transmitters are released already at low firing rates, peptides may only be released when neurons are firing at high activity or exhibit bursting activity. The above mentioned storage in two types of vesicles may form the structural basis for the differential release. Recent evidence suggests that peptides often are released extrasynaptically. (4) Classical transmitters and neuropeptides may interact in different fashions. Thus, peptides may have actions which are synergistic or antagonistic to the classical transmitter, in the latter case for example by inhibiting the release of the classical transmitter. (5) In several instances, peptides have been shown to exert trophic-like actions, especially in peripheral tissues and this is perhaps particularly common for peptides released from the peripheral branches of sensory neurons. For example, substance P is known to affect mitotic activity of smooth muscle cells, and calcitonin gene related peptide (CGRP), which is present in motoneurons and thus coexists with acetylcholine in these neurons, has been shown to increase biosynthesis of cholinergic receptors in striated muscle.

Coexistence situations can be found in all parts of the peripheral and central nervous system. In the present lecture we would like to focus on a limited number of such systems. (1) Coexistence of dopamine and cholecystokinin (CCK) in mesencephalic neurons projecting to the forebrain is found in many species including rat, cat, monkey and also in the human brain. In man, using in situ hybridization, brains from subjects with the diagnosis of schizophrenia treated with neuroleptics seem to express higher levels of CCK mRNA than control brains. No CCK or CCK mRNA has been observed in dopamine neurons in the guinea pig and hamster. Many types of intricate interactions between CCK and dopamine have been observed in rat, for example effects of

Department of Histology and Neurobiology, Karolinska Institute, [1]Department of Biochemistry, Arrhenius Laboratory, University of Stockholm and [2]Department of Clinical Physiology, Section of Clinical Neurophysiology, Karolinska Institute, Stockholm, Sweden.

CCK on dopamine release. (2) The 29 amino acid peptide galanin is present in basal cholinergic forebrain neurons. These neurons project in the rat to the ventral hippocampus. Under normal circumstances, levels of galanin peptide and galanin mRNA are very low in these neurons, but after hippocampal lesions or after impairment of axonal transport, there is a dramatic upregulation of both peptide and mRNA levels. Functionally it has been shown that galanin can inhibit acetylcholine release in the ventral hippocampus. Possible implications of these findings in relation to Alzheimer's disease will be discussed. (3) Galanin is also present in primary sensory neurons. Again, in these neurons galanin levels are under normal circumstances low, but peripheral axotomy causes a dramatic upregulation both of galanin mRNA and galanin peptide. Also other sensory peptides such as vasoactive intestinal polypeptide (VIP), cholecystokinin and neuropeptide Y are upregulated after such a lesion, whereas substance P, CGRP and somatostatin are downregulated. Functionally, after axotomy, VIP seems to replace substance P and CGRP as mediators in this reflex. Galanin has been shown to suppress the nociceptive flexor reflex, probably by antagonizing substance P and CGRP under normal circumstances, and VIP after peripheral axotomy. Galanin may therefore represent an endogenous analgesic compound, a hypothesis further supported by studies on the effect of administration of exogenous galanin on the nociceptive flexor reflex. Thus, galanin attenuates this reflex, an effect which is markedly potentiated by concomitant administration of morphine and a CCK B receptor antagonist. Such findings may open up new possibilities to approach treatment of pain.

Peptides have more recently been shown also to occur in non-neuronal systems. We have focused on the testes. Thus, CCK/gastrin is present in the acrosome of mature sperms. The possible involvement of this peptide and other messenger molecules in the fertilization process will be discussed.

The findings discussed here provide evidence that peptides are present in multiple systems and are involved in a wide variety of functions. The recent cloning of several peptide receptors by Japanese and American groups represent further evidence for a physiological role of peptides in neuronal function. The elucidation of such functions will also be greatly facilitated by the recent development of novel non-peptide antagonists which pass the blood brain barrier. In this way it will be possible to further substantiate the present view that peptides are particularly important under conditions of increased neuronal activity and under pathological conditions.

Supported by the Swedish MRC (04X.2887) and NIMH (MH-43230).

S21

NEUROPEPTIDE RECEPTORS: STRUCTURE AND FUNCTION
V. Höllt

During the last few years an increasing number of neuropeptides has been found in central and peripheral neurones. These peptides exhibit a high degree of functional diversity. Within a neuropeptide system, such as the endogenous opioids, the expression of three genes and the proteolytic processing and modification of the translated propeptides result in a multiplicity of peptide products. In addition, these peptides interact with variety of pharmacologically distinct receptors (μ, δ, κ and ϵ; Höllt , *Ann. Rev. Pharmacol.* **26**, 59 (1986)). Moreover, there exists a variety of non-peptide and peptide antagonists which show high selectivity for the receptor subtypes. A putative binding protein with the characteristics of a μ opiate receptor has been cloned (Schofield *et al.*, *EMBO J.* **8**, 489 (1989). This protein has been termed OBCAM (opioid-binding protein-cell adhesion molecule) in view of its homology to neural cell adhesion and related molecules. OBCAM has a putative phosphatidylinositol (PI)-linked site for membrane attachment, but does not belong to the seven membrane-spanning G protein-coupled receptor superfamily. This is somewhat surprising, since there is evidence that δ and also μ opioid receptors associate with G proteins. Recent data suggest that opioids inhibit adenylyl cyclase via $G_{i\alpha}$ whereas they block voltage-dependent Ca^{2+} channels and stimulate K^{+} channels via G_o. In addition, all neuropeptide receptors cloned so far have the characteristic structure of proteins with seven membrane-spanning segments. Therefore, the question whether or not OBCAM is a member of a novel family of peptide receptors remains to be answered.

The tachykinin system comprises multiple peptides (substance P, neurokinin A (=substance K) and neurokinin B (=neuromedin K) which derive from two precursor genes (preprotachykinin A and B). Usage of different promoters and/or alternative splicing results in the generation of different mRNAs which are translated in different precursor proteins from which the tachykinins are liberated by proteolytic processing. The three tachykinin peptides interact with pharmacologically distinct receptors (NK_1, NK_2, NK_3) which bind selectively substance P, neurokinin A or neurokinin B respectively. Recently, a specific non-peptide antagonist (CP-96,345) for the NK_1 receptor has been found (Snider *et al.*, *Science* **251**, 435 (1991). The structure of the three tachykinin receptors has been identified by molecular cloning in combination with electrophysiology (for a review see Nakanishi, *Ann. Rev. Neurosci.*, **14**, 123 (1991). The tachykinin receptors can be expressed in *xenopus* oocytes via their action through a G protein which induces IP_3 production. The latter mediator is thought to elevate cytoplasmic Ca^{2+} which , in turn, activates Ca^{2+} dependent chloride channels in the oocyte. The tachykinin receptors belong to the G protein-coupled family of receptors with seven putative membrane-spanning domains. They share significant sequence homology with adrenergic, dopamine, serotonin, and muscarinic receptors.

A variety of additional neuropeptide receptors which all belong to the seven membrane-spanning protein superfamily have been cloned recently.

There is evidence for multiple receptor subtypes for angiotensin II (AT_1, AT_2) which can be distinguished by their sensitivity to non-peptide antagonists (Chu *et al.*, *Biochem. biophys. Res. Commun.* **165**, 196 (1989). The vascular type-1 angiotensin (AT_1) receptor has been cloned (Sasaki *et al.*, *Nature* **351**, 320 (1991); Murphy *et al.*, *Nature* **325**, 233 (1991). In addition, the *mas* oncogene has been shown to encode a "neuronal" type of an angiotensin receptor (Jackson *et al.*, *Nature* **335**, 437 (1988). The subtype of angiotensin receptor that is encoded by the *mas* oncogene remains to be determined.

A diversity at the level of peptide recognition also exists for the endothelin peptide families. An endothelin receptor whith a high specifity for endothelin 1 (ET-1) has recently be cloned (Arai *et al.*, *Nature* **348**, 730 (1990). This receptor (ET_A) is crucial in the regulation of vascular smooth muscle tone. In addition, the structure of a non-selective subtype of endothelin receptor (ET_B) which does not distinquish between ET-1, ET-2 and ET3 has been identified (Sakurai *et al.*, *Nature* **348**, 732 (1990). The ET_A and ET_B receptors are highly expressed in the brain, indicating that the endothelins may function as neuropeptides.

Recently, also the receptors for neurotensin (Tanaka *et al.*, *Neuron* **4**, 847 (1990), bombesin/gastrin-releasing peptide ((Battey *et al.*, *Proc. Natl. Acad. Sci. USA* **88**, 395 (1991) and thyrotropin-releasing hromone (TRH; Straub *et al.*, *Proc. Natl. Acad. Sci. USA* **87**, 9514 (1990) have been cloned. Moreover, the receptors for vasopressin and vasoactive intestinal peptide have been sequenced and their structures will be published soon. Finally, a putative receptor with structural similarity to the tachykinin receptors has been cloned. However, no ligand could be assigned to this orphan receptor (FC5; Eva *et al.*, *FEBS Lett.* **271**, 81 (1990)).

All the neuropeptide receptor cloned so far have the transmembrane topology of G protein-coupled receptors. Interestingly, these receptors have been shown to be coupled to a G protein which activates phospholipase C. No neuropeptide receptor cloned so far has been shown to be positively or negatively coupled to adenlylyl cyclase. The reason for this might be that the majority of the peptide receptors have been cloned using the oocyte expression system which selects for PI-linked receptors.

The structural features of the neuropeptide receptors are very similar to those of the aminergic and muscarinic receptors. However, with the exception of the neurotensin receptor, the third membranous domain of the neuropeptide receptors does not contain aspartic acid which is present in adrenergic, muscarinic, serotonin, dopamine and histamine receptors. The binding of adrenergic and muscarinic substances has been suggested to involve hydrogen bonding bewteen the carboxylate group of the aspartate and the protonated amino group of the ligands (Strader *et al.*, *Proc. Natl. Acad. Sci. USA* **84**, 4384 (1987). This suggest that the interaction of the neuropeptides with their receptor is different from that of the neurotransmitters. The long N-terminal portion of the endothelin receptors preceeding transmembrane segment I has been suggested to be involved in the binding of the relatively large endothelin peptides, since receptors for large peptide hormones, such as thyrotropin and luteotropin-choriongonadotropin also possess large N-terminal sequences preceding the first transmembrane segment (Loosfelt *et al.*, *Science* **245**, 525 (1989). The structural homology among the G protein-coupled receptors would suggest that the ligand binding sites for the neuropeptides may also involve regions within the transmembrane cores of the receptors. The precise location of the ligand-binding sites for the neuropeptides, however, is not known yet.

Sequences at the N and C termini of the third intracellular loop and sequences in the proximal cytoplasmic tail have been reported to be critical for the G_i and/or G_s protein binding specificity among G protein-coupled receptors (Liggett *et al.*, *J. Biol. Chem.* **266**, 4816 (1990). There is, however, no extreme homology in these portions between the neuropeptide receptors, although they are all coupled to a G protein activating phospholipase C. The precise sequences of the receptor G protein coupling for the PI-linked neuropeptide receptors remain to be determined by mutagenesis studies.

All neuropeptide receptors have several serine and/or threonine residues in the third cytoplasmic loop and in the carboxy-terminal cytoplasmic region. Studies of the adrenergic and muscarinic receptors indicated that these receptors are desensitized as a result of phosphorylations of serine and threonine residues at the carboxyl termini and/or the third cytoplasmic loops of these proteins (O´Dowd *et al.*, *Ann. Rev. Neurosci.* **12**, 67 (1989). When expressed in oocytes, a clear desensitization to their respective ligands was observed for the three tachykinin and the neurotensin receptors The degree of desensitization to repeated agonist application, however, was different amongst the three tachykinin receptors. It has been suggested that a different distribution of threonine and/or serine residues in the above cytoplasmic regions, resulting in a different phosphorylation, may be responsible for this effect (Nakanishi, *Ann. Rev. Neurosci.* **14**, 123 (1991).

In conclusion, an increasing number of neuropeptides show diversification at the levels of peptide production and peptide recognition. For a given neuropeptide system, a multiplicity of receptors can be identified. The development of an increasing number of peptide and non-peptide antagonists allows the pharmacological distinction of multiple neuropeptide receptors. In addition, the structure of a variety of neuropeptide receptors has been identified by molecular cloning. These receptors belong to the seven membrane-spanning superfamily of receptors and are coupled to a G protein activating phospholipase C. The precise analysis of the structure of neuropeptide receptors and the location of the ligand-binding sites will aid the design of novel therapeutic agents that specifically act at these reseptor proteins.

Department of Physiology, University of Munich
Pettenkoferstrasse 12, D-8000 München, FRG

S22

NEUROPEPTIDE - NEUROTRANSMITTER INTERACTIONS
T. Ott

Over the years many neuropeptides has been found to occur both in peripheral organs and in the central nervous system. Although the physiological and functional meaning is largely unknown, it is clear that many of these neuropeptides are able to potently modulate the function of several neurotransmitter systems.

With respect to the mechanisms underlying the modulatory effect of neuropeptides the concept of the co-called cotransmission (Hökfelt et al., Nature 285, 476-478, 1980) has received much attention during the last years. The morphological basis of the cotransmission, which rests largely on the co-localization of defined neuropeptides with defined neuro-transmitters in the same nerve endings (e. g. CCK/dopamine, neurotensin/dopamine, substance P/serotonin) is well documented. However, in many regions of the brain the situation is more complex. Beside coexisting neuropeptide/neurotransmitters both classes of signal molecules are found in close vicinity, yet in different nerve endings. This "local circuits" (Fuxe and Agnati, Medicinal Res. Rev. 5, 441-482, 1985) may be regarded as the morphological basis of neuropeptide-neurotransmitter interaction.

In the presentation special attention will be given to the mutual interaction of neuropeptides/neurotransmitters at the synaptic level. Evidence showing that neuropeptides are able to act presynaptically on neurotransmitter release mechanisms in a complex manner will be presented. Additionally, the mutual interaction of neuropeptides/neurotransmitters at the level of receptors (receptor cross-talk) will be discussed. Taking the modulation of dopamine (DA2) and serotonin (5-HT2) receptors by cholecystokinin as an example, it will be shown that neurotransmitter receptors can be changed in different ways with different effects by neuropeptides.

In spite of the rapid progress in this field, there are still serious open questions. Among them, the problem of receptor-dependent vs. receptor-independent effects of neuropeptides will be discussed. Since for some neuropeptides fairly specific antagonists are now available the view is emerging that at last cationic amphiphilic neuropeptides may act by using both modes of action.

Finally it well be emphasized that the functional meaning of the synaptic interaction of neuropeptides/neurotransmitters is still poorly understood.

Institut für Pharmakologie und Toxikologie, Medizinische Fakultät (Charité) der Humboldt-Universität zu Berlin, Clara-Zetkin-Str. 94, O - 1040 Berlin, FRG

S23

COMPLEX BRAIN FUNCTIONS OF NEUROPEPTIDES
D. de Wied

A cascade of processes evolves in peptidergic neurons in order to express the genetic information into biologically active neuropeptides. These processes determine the quantities of neuropeptides synthetized and their biological activity through size, form and derivatization. In this way sets of neuropeptides with different opposite and more selective properties are formed from the same precursor. An example of a cell specific gene expression is the formation of calcitonin in thyroid tissue and that of calcitonin gene related peptide in the brain by different mRNA from a single gene. The processing of neuropeptide precursors also is a cell specific phenomenon. Thus, pro-opiomelanocortin (POMC) is processed by corticotrophs of the anterior pituitary to ACTH-(1-39) and a 16-N-terminal fragment, while the melanotrophs in the intermediate lobe convert ACTH-(1-39) to α-MSH, ACTH-(18-39), γ-LPH and β-endorphin (βE). Posttranslational modifications as a result of acetylation, sulphation, amidation, glycosylation and phosphorylation again is cell specific and causes marked alterations in the biological activity of neuropeptides. Thus, acetylation of ACTH-(1-13) to α-MSH markedly enhances the melanotrophic and behavioral effects while reducing their anti-opiate effects. Acetylation of endorphins eliminates their analgesic effects but not their neuroleptic-like effects while acetylation of vasopressin blocks its peripheral endocrine and central nervous system effects. Neuropeptides and the fragments which they generate in the brain exert presynaptic actions that affect the release of the neurotransmitter and affect the sensitivity of the postsynaptic element. Such influences are the basis of the behavioral manifestations of neuropeptides. Early studies with ACTH on shuttle box avoidance learning in hypophysectomized rats showed that the influence of ACTH on their deficient avoidance learning was not the result of the corticotrophic effect of this polypeptide hormone, but resided in the heptapeptide ACTH-(4-10). This appeared to be a common feature of peptide hormones found in the brain; their CNS effects are dissociated from their classical endocrine influence. Evidence was found that ACTH-(1-39) in the brain is converted into fragments (ACTH-(1-16), α-MSH, ACTH-(4-16), ACTH-(7-16)) which may be responsible for the behavioral effects. More recent studies focus on the neurotrophic effect of these neuropeptides. Various ACTH neuropeptides enhance development (Van der Helm-Hylkema H & De Wied D, Life Sci. 18: 1099, 1976) accelerate functional recovery from peripheral nerve damage (Gispen WH et al., Progr. Brain Res. 72: 319, 1987) as well as following brain damage. More potent analogues as the ACTH-(4-9) analogue (Org 2766) and related compounds accelerate recovery from 6-OHDA lesions in the nucleus accumbens following chronic systemic as well as intracranial administration (Wolterink G et al., Life Sci. 48: 155, 1991). Chronic treatment with Org 2766 also prevents the occurrence of cognitive dysfunction and reduction in sociability of aged rats (Spruijt BM et al., in: Neuropeptides: Basics and Perspectives (D. de Wied, ed.) Elsevier, Amsterdam, 353, 1990).

Vasopressin exerts a long term effect on active and passive avoidance behavior. This effect is time-dependent. These and the antiamnesic effects of vasopressin and related peptides were interpreted as memory effects Oxytocin possesses amnesic effects. Many other CNS effects of the neurohypophyseal hormones have been found which have been discussed elsewhere (De Wied D et al., in Peptide Hormones: Effects and Mechanisms of Action (A. Negro-Villar & P.M. Conn, eds.), CRC Press, Boca Raton, 97, 1988). As with ACTH, vasopressin and oxytocin are converted to behaviorally active fragments such as [pGlu⁴,Cyt⁶]AVP-(4-9): OXT-(4-9) e.o. (Burbach JPH et al., Science 221: 1310, 1983) which have lost their classical endocrine effect but act in a much more selective manner than the parent molecules on memory processes. These peptides also lack certain CNS effects of vasopressin such as those on thermoregulation, barrel rotation, and epilepsy. The memory effect of vasopressin and related peptides has long been debated and several authors felt that the influence may be secondary to changes in attention and arousal mediated by effects on blood pressure or other peripheral effects. The results of a recent behavioral study with [Desglycinamide⁹-Arg⁸]vasopressin (DGAVP) show both an immediate and a long term effect of vasopressin on behavior. The immediate effect is caused by its arousal properties and results in a shift in the bell shaped curve which is known to exist between arousal and performance (Skopkova J et al., Peptides, in press, 1991). Electrophysiological effects also indicate acute arousal influences of vasopressin and related peptides (Urban IJA & De Wied D, in: Proceedings 27th DRG Seminar Sleep and Its Implications for the Military, ACEML, Lyon, 161, 1988) and a long term i.e. enhancement of glutamate activity in lateral septum neurons (Joëls M and Urban IJA, Brain Res. 311: 201, 1984). ACTH/MSH and vasopressin and related neuropeptides which have a positive effect on avoidance behavior, act in an opposite manner on pilocarpine induced epilepsy. ACTH-(4-10), but not ACTH-(1-24) attenuates, while vasopressin but not the fragment [pGlu⁴,Cyt⁶]AVP-(4-9)

potentiates pilocarpine induced epilepsia. The effect of vasopressin could be blocked by a V₂ antagonist only, suggesting that the effect is mediated by V₂ receptors. These however, are not identical to the V₂ receptor found in the kidney (Wamil A et al., Neurosci. Res. Commun. 4: 109, 1989; Croiset G & De Wied D, Eur. J. Pharmacol. 183: 506, 1990).

A larger part of the vasopressin receptor in the brain resembles the peripheral V₁ type receptor. V₂ type receptors have not been found as yet. Also oxytocin receptors have been found in the brain. In addition, binding sites for such fragments as [pGlu⁴,Cyt⁶]AVP-(4-9) have been detected. This peptide has a low affinity for the V₁ receptor and binds specifically to brain regions, distinctly different from the distribution of V₁ and oxytocin binding sites (Burbach JPH and Wiegant VM, in: Neuropeptides: Basics and Perspectives (D. de Wied, ed.), Elsevier, Amsterdam, 45, 1991). Interestingly, V₁, V₂ and oxytocin antagonist can block the behavioral effect of vasopressin, oxytocin and their more selective fragments. These findings suggest the existence of a separate neurohypophyseal hormone receptor complex in the brain which differs from the peripheral V₁, V₂ and oxytocin receptor (De Wied D et al., Proc. Natl. Acad. Sci USA 88: 1494, 1991). Another example of a peptide hormone which generates neuropeptides with differential effects is cholecystokinin (CCK), a 33 amino acid peptide hormone found in the gut. It is a precursor for the octapeptide CCK-8 in the brain, found either in the sulphated or non-sulphated form. CCK-8-S and NS neuropeptides possess neuroleptic-like activity as judged from studies on avoidance behavior, grasping responses and their interaction with apomorphine and amphetamine (Van Ree JM et al., Eur. J. Pharmacol. 93: 63, 1983). CCK-4 has anxiogenic effects while antagonists have anxiolytic activity (Crawley JN, TIPS 12: 233, 1991). Two receptors have been identified for CCK. A peripheral type CCK-A which has high affinity for CCK-(1-33) and CCK-8-S, and less for CCK-8-NS and CCK-4, and a central type CCK-B receptor which binds all four peptides with the same affinity (Hughes J et al., Proc. Natl. Acad. Sci. USA 87: 6728, 1990). CCK stimulates the release of dopamine in the posterior and inhibits the release of dopamine in the anterior nucleus accumbens. The former effect is mediated by the CCK-A while the latter is mediated by the CCK-B receptors. The CCK-B effect may be related to its neuroleptic-like effect (Crawley JN, TIPS 12: 233, 1991). In 1978 we found that γ-type endorphins also possess neuroleptic-like effects. γ-Type endorphins facilitate extinction of active and attenuate passive avoidance behavior as also found with neuroleptic drugs. Other effects were a positive grasping response and attenuation of apomorphine induced hypolocomotion (Van Ree JM et al., in: Neuropeptides: Basics and Perspectives (D. de Wied, ed.), Elsevier, Amsterdam, 255, 1990). Intra-accumbal injection of apomorphine induced hypolocomotion which could be blocked by neuroleptic drugs and γ-type endorphins. These effects are presumably mediated by presynaptically located dopamine receptors. The non-opioid γ-type endorphins (DTγE, DEγE) could not block the effects of high doses of apomorphine and amphetamine injected into the accumbens. However, these effects could be inhibited by the opioid peptide γ-endorphin. Recently, binding sites for DEγE have been found. High affinity binding using [³⁵S]-Met-DEγE was found in mesocorticolimbic structures involved in the neuroleptic-like effect of the peptide. Endorphins sharing the C-terminus completely displaced the labelled compound. An antiidiotypic antibody raised against DEγE could be displaced by excess non-labelled DEγE suggesting that the binding sites for the antibody and the ligand are identical. Evidence was obtained for an effect of the peptide on catecholamine uptake in the nucleus accumbens. This may be related to its neuroleptic-like effects (Ronken, thesis, Utrecht, 1991). Neuropeptide Y (NPY), a 36 amino acid peptide, increases feeding and improves retention of avoidance behavior in a T-maze following intracranial administration. (Flood JF & Morley JE, Peptides 10: 963, 1989). The influence on feeding is caused by the intact peptide while the effect on retention is elicited by the intact peptide and the fragment NPY-(20-36). NPY effects on feeding seem to be mediated by NPY-(1-36) through postsynaptic (Y₁) NPY receptors while effects on memory are mediated by NPY-(20-36) through presynaptic (Y₂) NPY receptors. βE-(1-31) possesses opiate-like effects while βE-(1-27) is an opiate antagonistic neuropeptide. It also generates non-opiate fragments which possess neuroleptic-like (γ-type endorphins), amphetamine-like (α-type endorphins) or serotonin-like effects (βE-(10-16) (Van Ree JM et al., Progr Brain Res 72: 249, 1987). Intra-accumbal injection of Substance P (SP-(1-11) inhibits extinction of pole-jumping avoidance behavior while the fragment SP-(7-11) has the opposite effect (Gaffori O et al., Experientia 40: 89, 1984). A few words of caution may be due here. Identical CNS effects of different neuropeptides may be caused by their structural relationship. Thus ACTH-(4-10), LHRH and TRH may affect avoidance behavior as a result of the presence of a number of similar amino acid residues (Flood JF and Morley JE, Peptides 10: 963, 1989). Many behavioral studies are performed with neuropeptides in relatively high amounts. Effects induced by the massive flooding of the brain through the ventricular system may be mediated also by the simultaneous release of endogenous ligands with profound behavioral effects. Thus the administration of behaviorally effective amounts of vasopressin either following intraventricular or systemic administration causes a measurable increase in IRβE in the CSF (Wiegant VM & Sweep CGJ, in: Endorphins in Reproduction (W. Distler and L. Beck, eds.), Springer-Verlag, Berlin, 81, 1990). It has been suggested that neuropeptides come into play only following intense stimulation but not under normal stimulatory conditions. Peptides as such or fragments appear to influence the release of the neurotransmitter with which they are colocalized. NPY is colocalized with noradrenaline in sympathetic nerve endings. NPY modulates the release of noradrenaline but only following intense stimulation and not under normal stimulatory conditions. CRH is a powerful stimulant of the sympathetic nervous system. This influence is of central origin and is induced in supraphysiological amounts. This suggests that CRH affects the sympathetic nervous system only in situations of stress (Diamant M & De Wied D, Endocrinology, in press, 1991). Besides these effects, CRH has CNS effects independent of the influence on the autonomic nervous system. In doses as low as 0.1 ng i.c.v. which do not affect heart rate, core temperature, grooming, locomotion and digging in free moving rats, CRH attenuates passive avoidance behavior. The antagonist α-CRH-(9-41) blocks the attenuating influence of CRH on passive avoidance behavior.

More than 40 neuropeptides have been found sofar in the brain which generate a multitude of biologically active principles, many of which have not yet been discovered. As yet we do not understand the need for such diversity of regulatory molecules in the brain. The long fiber systems which carry POMC, or the precursor molecules of vasopressin and oxytocin from the sites of production in the hypothalamus to extrahypothalamic brain sites seem to modulate the whole spectrum of central nervous system functions. Neuropeptides generated from these precursors affect learning and memory processes, pain, mood, aggression, social, sexual and maternal behavior, drug seeking behavior, maintenance behavior (grooming), stretching and yawning. These neuropeptides are involved in the regulation of the autonomic nervous, the cardiovascular, and the respiratory system, body temperature, cerebral blood flow, brain metabolism, and sleep-waking cycle. The limbic system plays an important role in learning and memory processes. The system is richly innervated by fibres containing the classical neurotransmitters as the monoamines, acetylcholine and serotonin as well as the excitatory (glutamate) and inhibitory amino acid neurotransmitter (γ-aminobutyric acid (GABA)). Besides it is innervated by POMC, vasopressin, oxytocin, and CRH containing nerve fibres. Behavioral studies have shown that neuropeptides related to ACTH/MSH peptides, the endorphins, vasopressin and oxytocin and CRH and other stress hormones modulate learning and memory processes.

Many other neuropeptides affect learning and memory processes. Interestingly, the gut hormones (CCK, Bombesin, Gastrin releasing peptide, pancreastatin) exhibit U-shaped dose-dependent and time-dependent effects on retention of avoidance behavior and prevent amnesia induced by protein synthesis inhibition or scopolamine. Such peptides may mediate the memory effects of feeding and act probably through the vagus nerve (Flood JF et al., Science 236: 832, 1987).

Department of Pharmacology, Rudolf Magnus Institute, University of Utrecht, Vondellaan 6, 3521 GD Utrecht, The Netherlands

S24

THE PLASMA MEMBRANE AND CALCIUM PUMP
Ernesto Carafoli

The plasma membrane calcium pump (1-2) is an ATPase of the P-type, present in all eucaryotic cells examined so far. It is a target of calmodulin regulation: the interaction with calmodulin has permitted its isolation using calmodulin columns (3). Its primary structure has been elucidated in rat brain and in several human cells (4-5). Several isoforms are known: 4 are products of different genes, others are formed by alternative mRNA splicing. The gene for human isoform 4 has been located on chromosome 1, that for human isoform 1 on chromosome 12. (6). The human teratoma cell isoform has been studied in particular detail and is shown in the figure below, which outlines its suggested secondary structure organization and indicates some of the important functional domains described below.

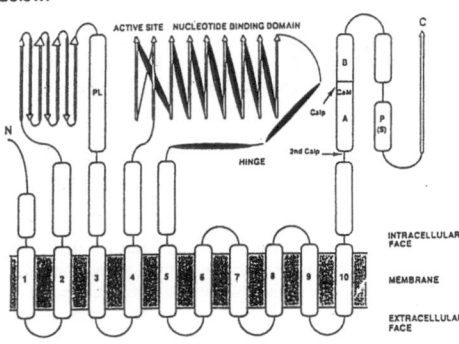

It contains 1220 amino acids (Mr 134683) and ten putative hydrophobic domains spanning the membrane. 4 are located in the N-terminal portion of the pump, 6 in the C-terminal portion. The mid-portion of the pump (about 500 residues) contains no transmembrane stretches and contains the active site, the nucleotide binding domain and a flexible "hinge" that permits the two to come close in space during the catalytic cycle. The calmodulin (CaM) binding domain, which can be subdivided into 2 subdomains, A and B, has been identified next to the C-terminus (residues 1100-1127) as a highly basic sequence which has propensity to form an amphiphilic helix. The calcium-dependent protease calpain (calpin the scheme) attacks the domain, removing it from the pump in two steps. Trypsin also attacks the calmodulin-binding domain, gradually removing the calmodulin sensitivity of the pump. In the absence of calmodulin, the pump is activated by a number of acidic phospholipids (PL) including (and especially) the phosphorylated derivatives of phosphatidyl-inositol (7). Trypsin degradation has permitted to locate the site of interaction of PL between transmembrane domains two and three in a highly charged sequence of about 50 amino acids which is typical of the plasma membrane calcium pump, i.e., not found in other P-type ion pumps. However, acidic phospholipids apparently also interact with the positively charged calmodulin-binding domain. Work with synthetic peptides has shown that two aromatic residues (a Trp and a Phe) located in the N-terminal portion of the calmodulin-binding domain may be important in the interaction of the domain with calmodulin. It has also shown that the domain or a highly charged sequence N-terminal to it, could be involved in the dimerization of the pump. The high affinity calcium binding site of the reaction cycle has not been identified as yet, but is probably located in the intramembrane portion of the pump. A serine (1178) (P (s) in the scheme), located on the C-terminal side of the calmodulin-binding domain is phosphorylated by the cAMP-dependent kinase, but only in one of the human isoforms of the pump. This isoform is expressed in human erythrocytes together with another isoform which is much more abundant and does not contain the cAMP-responsive site. The phosphorylation increases the Ca-affinity of the pump. Most of the pump isoforms have been found to differ in the C-terminal portion, which contains the calmodulin-binding domain and the cAMP-dependent phosphorylation site, and could thus display different regulation properties. The calmodulin-binding domain acts as a natural inhibitor of the pump. In the resting state, it binds to a domain of the pump next to the active site (residues 500-560), repressing activity. Calmodulin "removes" the autoinhibitory sequence, permitting full expression of activity.

1. Schatzmann, H.J. The calcium pump of erythrocytes and other animal cells. Membrane Transport of Calcium. (Ed. E. Carafoli), Acad. Press, London, p. 41-108, 1982.

2. Carafoli, E. Calcium Pump of the Plasma Membrane, Physiol. Rev., 71, p.129-153, 1991.

3. Niggli, V., Penniston, J.T. and Carafoli, E. Purification of the (Ca^{2+} + Mg^{2+})-ATPase from human erythrocyte membranes using a calmodulin affinity column. J. Biol. Chem. 254, p. 9955-9958, 1979.

4. Verma, A.K., A.G. Filoteo, D.R. Stanford, E.D. Wieben, J.T. Penniston, E.E. Strehler, R. Fischer, R. Heim, G. Vogel, S. Mathews, M.A. Strehler-Page, P. James, T. Vorherr, J. Krebs and E. Carafoli. Complete primary structure of a human plasma membrane Ca^{2+} pump. J. Biol. Chem. 263: p. 14152-14149, 1988.

5. Shull, G.E. and J. Greeb. Molecular cloning of two isoforms of the plasma membrane Ca2+ transporting ATPase from rat brain. Structural and functional domains exhibit similarity to Na+, K+- and other cation transport ATPases. J. Biol. Chem. 263: p. 8646-8657, 1988.

6. Olson, S., M.G. Wang, E. Carafoli, E.E. Strehler and O.W. McBride. Localization of two genes encoding plasma membrane Ca^{2+}-transporting ATPases to human chromosomes 1q25-32 and 12q21-23. Genomics 9: 629-641, 1991.

7. Niggli, V., E.S. Adunyah, J.T. Penniston and E. Carafoli. Purified Ca^{2+} + Mg^{2+}) ATPase of the erythrocyte membrane: reconstitution and effect of calmodulin and phospholipids. J. Biol. Chem. 256: p. 395-401, 1981.

Institute of Biochemistry, Swiss Federal Institute of Technology (ETH) 8092 Zürich, Switzerland.

S25

Modulatory Domains on L-Type Ca2+-Channels

Jörg Striessnig, Hartmut Glossmann* and William A. Catterall

Voltage-gated L-type Ca2+-channels mediate the increase of the plasma membrane permeability for Ca2+ ions upon depolarization in excitable cells. Biochemical studies have shown that they exist as hetero-oligomeric complexes, in which pore-forming α1 subunits (apparent molecular masses ≈ 200 kDa) are non-covalently associated with α2-δ (brain, muscle), β (brain, skeletal muscle) and γ (skeletal muscle) subunits (for review see [1,2,3,4]).

L-type Ca2+-channel activity is physiologically modulated by cAMP-dependent phosphorylation, GTP-binding proteins (Gs activates skeletal muscle and cardiac L-type channels, [5]) and putative endogenous ligands (e.g. an acidic peptide, which modulates brain and cardiac L-type channel activity [6], and heparin [7]) . Pharmacological probes are available in the form of organic Ca2+-channel blockers and activators (e.g. dihydropyridines, phenylalkylamines and benzothiazepines), cations (e.g. Cd2+, Co2+) and peptide toxins (e.g. omega-agatoxin IIIA [8]). Although the effects of GTP-binding proteins, putative endogenous ligands and toxins have been characterized in functional and/or ligand binding studies, the location of their interaction sites on the channel complex has not been investigated in detail. In contrast, recent biochemical studies identified regions within the channel protein which are involved in the modulation of channel function by phosphorylation and drugs.

Activation of the cAMP-dependent protein kinase (c-PK) leads to an enhanced channel activity in cardiac as well as skeletal muscle cells. Activation of purified skeletal muscle Ca2+-channels is accompanied by a stoichiometric phosphorylation of the beta and two size forms of the α1 subunits [9,10]. The two forms differ in the length of their C-terminal domain, the shorter and more abundant one (175 kDa in SDS-PAGE, "$\alpha1_{175}$") being derived from the full length form ("$\alpha1_{212}$") by proteolytic cleavage within the long C-terminus [10,11]. Both forms are rapidly phosphorylated on a consensus sequence (Ser-687) located between the transmembrane domains II and III [12]. Only the full length form is phosphorylated at several additional sites which are removed from $\alpha1_{175}$ upon proteolytic processing [11]. Therefore the regulation of the functional properties of $\alpha1_{175}$ and $\alpha1_{212}$ may differ. It has been proposed that the two forms, which are also present *in vivo* [11] may serve different roles, as ion conducting channels ($\alpha1_{212}$) and as voltage-sensors ($\alpha1_{175}$), respectively [2,10].

α1 subunits of L-type Ca2+-channels in neuronal and muscle cells also carry the binding domains for organic Ca2+-channel drugs. as shown by photoaffinity labeling [4]. Distinct binding domains, selective for the different chemical classes of Ca2+-channel blockers, are allosterically coupled to one another and to divalent cation binding sites on the channel [4,13]. The biochemically best characterized domains are those for phenylalkylamines (e.g. verapamil, desmethoxyverapamil), dihydropyridines (e.g. nifedipine, PN200-110) and benzothiazepines (e.g. (+)-cis-diltiazem). Using photoaffinity labeling and an antibody mapping technique we have identified the regions of the skeletal muscle α1 subunit involved in the formation of the phenylalkylamine and dihydropyridine binding domains. Partially purified skeletal muscle Ca2+-channels were specifically photolabeled with domain-selective photoaffinity ligands ([N-methyl-3H]LU49888 for the phenylalkylamine binding domain, [3H]azidopine and (+)-[3H]PN200-110 for the dihydropyridine binding domain). The α1 subunits were digested with various enzymes and labeled fragments localized within its primary structure by probing them with several sequence directed antibodies against putative extra- and intracellular regions. The smallest [N-methyl-3H]LU49888-labeled peptide (4.8 kDa, obtained by V8-protease treatment), which contained about two thirds of the specific labeling [14], comprised the transmembrane segment S6 of domain IV and some of the adjacent extracellular and intracellular amino acid residues. This region must therefore be involved in the formation of the intracellular binding domain of phenylalkylamines [14]. The same fragment was also labeled with the dihydropyridines and contained about 25% and 10% of the [3H]azidopine and (+)-[3H]PN200-110 labeling, respectively.

However, the major site of dihydropyridine labeling (about half of the specific labeling) occurred in an endoproteinase lys-C fragment comprising the connecting loop between the transmembrane segments S5 and S6 of domain III and segment IIIS6 itself. Half of the [3H]azidopine labeling in this fragment could further be restricted to the tryptic fragment between Arg-988 and Ala-1023. This region corresponds to the proposed short segments SS1 and SS2, which have been shown to fold into the membrane in a non-helical structure in voltage-gated Na+- and K+-channels [15,16]. We conclude that the two photolabeled regions close to segments IIIS6 and IVS6 are in close proximity to one another in the folded structure of the α1 subunit as predicted by current folding models [15] and participate in the formation of the dihydropyridine binding domain.

References:
[1] Campbell KP, Leung AT, Sharp AH (1988) Trends Neurosci. 11: 425-430
[2] Catterall WA (1991) Cell 64: 871-874
[3] Hofmann F, Nastainczyk W, Röhrkasten A, Schneider T, Sieber M (1987) Trends Pharmacol. Sci. 8: 393-398
[4] Glossmann H, Striessnig J (1990) Rev. Physiol. Biochem. Pharmacol. 114: 1-105
[5] Brown AM, Birnbaumer L (1990) Annu. Rev. Physiol. 52: 197-213
[6] Callewaert G, Hanbauer I, Morad M (1989) Science 243: 663-666
[7] Knaus HG, Scheffauer F, Romanin C., Schindler HG, Glossmann H (1990) J. Biol. Chem. 265: 11156-11166
[8] Mintz IM, Venema VJ, Adams ME, Bean BP (1990) Neurosci. Abstr. 16: 956
[9] Nunoki K, Florio V, Catterall WA (1989) Proc. Natl. Acad. Sci. (USA) 86: 6816-6820
[10] De Jongh KS, Merrick DK, Catterall WA (1989) Proc. Natl. Acad. Sci. (USA) 86: 8585-8589
[11] Lai Y, Seagar MJ, Takahashi M, Catterall WA (1990) J. Biol. Chem. 265: 20839-20848
[12] Röhrkasten A, Meyer HE, Nastainczyk W, Sieber M, Hofmann F (1988) J. Biol. Chem. 263: 15325-15329
[13] Staudinger R, Knaus HG, Glossmann H (1991) J. Biol. Chem.: in press
[14] Striessnig J, Glossmann H, Catterall WA (1990) Proc. Natl. Acad. Sci. (USA) 87: 9108-9112
[15] Guy HR, Conti F (1990) Trends Neurosci. 13: 201-206
[16] Miller C (1991) Science 252: 1092-1096

Department of Pharmacology, University of Washington, Seattle, WA 98195 and *Institut für Biochemische Pharmakologie, Universität Innsbruck, A-6020 Innsbruck.

S26

REGULATION OF cAMP HYDROLYSIS BY c GMP

J.A. Beavo, W.K. Sonnenburg, and R.T. MacFarland*

It is generally accepted that the steady state levels of cAMP and cGMP are controlled not only by their rates of synthesis but also by their rates of degradation. In the last few years it has become obvious that cyclic nucleotide hydrolysis is regulated in most tissues by the concerted effects of a series of different cyclic nucleotide phosphodiesterases (PDEs) (see reference 1 for a review). We now know that there exists a rather large family of related but different genes that code for PDEs, a "supergene family" if you will. Moreover, additional diversity is created by differential processing of the mRNAs for many of these genes. According to our current understanding a minimum of 5 different families of PDEs are present in mammalian tissues. Moreover each family often contains several closely related genes and many of these are alternatively spliced in a cell type specific manner. Furthermore, it is clear that several of the isozymes are differentially regulated at both the transcriptional and post translational level. What is only beginning to be clarified are answers to the questions of exactly how many different PDEs are expressed in an individual tissue or cell type, how they interact to control cyclic nucleotide mediated function, which isozymes are present in what cellular and subcellular locations and how they are regulated by other processes in the cell.

Over the past few years we have determined complete or partial amino acid sequence for 5 different PDE isozymes and used this information to isolate partial cDNA clones for seven representatives of three PDE families. In addition, other laboratories have described partial or complete cDNA clones for members of the, the low km, cAMP-specific and photoreceptor cGMP-specific PDEs. Finally, very recently Manganiello and colleagues have presented predicted sequence data for one member of the cGMP-inhibited PDE family.

In the talk today I will present data on the structure, regulation and physiological function of one of these isozymes, the cGMP-stimulated PDE of bovine adrenal cortex. This enzyme was originally described in particulate fractions of liver and thymus and since has been purified to homogeneity from heart and adrenal. The enzyme is a 230 k Da dimer in its native state which dissociates into two identical monomers of 105 k Da in the presence of denaturing agents. The enzyme exhibits highly positively cooperative kinetics with either cAMP or cGMP as substrate. This property conveys the ability of cGMP to stimulate cAMP hydrolysis up to 50 fold at physiological concentrations of cyclic nucleotide. The enzyme also has high affinity binding site(s) which are different from the catalytic sites. The cGS PDE is by far the major isozyme in adrenal and hepatic tissues.

Recently, we have completed the complete amino acid sequence of this isozyme [2]. Using a combination of limited proteolysis and direct photolabeling we have obtained direct evidence for the location of the catalytic and allosteric cyclic nucleotide binding domains on the cGMP-stimulated PDE[3]. Taken together, this has allowed the general domain structure of the isozyme to be identified. Localization studies utilizing isozyme specific probes indicates that very high concentrations are present in the glomerulosa layer of the adrenal cortex. Since the glomerulosa cells make up a relatively small percentage of the total adrenal, the PDE concentration may approach or exceed the steady state level of cAMP in these cells. Moreover, a series of studies utilizing cyclic nucleotide analogs strongly suggests an important and novel regulatory role for ANP and the cGMP-stimulated PDE in adrenal steroidogenesis [4]. It also provides a good example of how cell type specific expression of a particular isozyme of PDE has been adapted by the body to provide a unique and specific regulatory function. Recently, Manganiello and colleagues [5] have shown that the major form of cGS PDE in brain is particulate and not soluble as it is in heart and adrenal. Very recently we have obtained a full length cDNA for two different cGS PDEs [6]. These data provide a structural basis for the distinct properties of the cGS PDE isozymes present in adrenal and brain.

* Present address: Department of Pharmacology, University of Texas Southwestern Med. Ctr., Dallas, TX 75235
Department of Pharmacology, SJ-30, University of Washington, Seattle, WA 98195   USA

Selected references

1. Beavo, J. A. and D. H. Reifsnyder. (1990). Primary sequence of cyclic nucleotide phosphodiesterase isozymes and the design of selective inhibitors. *Trends Pharmacol Sci.* 11(4): 150-5.

2. Le Trong, H, Beier, N, Sonnenburg, W.K., Stroop, S.D., Walsh, K.A., Beavo, J.A. and Charbonneau, H. (1990) Amino acid sequence of the cyclic GMP simulated cyclic nucleotide phosphodiesterase from bovine heart. *Biochemistry* 29:10280-10288.

3. Stroop, S.D., Charbonneau, H., and Beavo, J.A. (1989) Direct photolabeling of allosteric and catalytic domains of the cGMP-stimulated cyclic nucleotide phosphodiesterase. *J. Biol. Chem.* 264:13718-13725.

4. MacFarland, R.T., Zelus, B., and Beavo, J.A. (1991) High concentrations of a cyclic GMP-stimulated PDE mediate ANP-induced decreases in cAMP and steroidogenesis in adrenal glomerulosa cells. *J. Biol. Chem.* 266:136-142.

5. Murashima, S., Tanaka, T., Hockman, S., and Manganiello, V. C. (1990). Characterization of a particulate cyclic nucleotide phosphodiesterase from bovine brain: purification of a distinct cGMP-stimulated isoenzyme. *Biochemistry* 29: 5285-5292.

6. Sonnenburg, W.K., Mullaney, P.J., and Beavo, J.A. (1991) Molecular cloning of a cyclic GMP-stimulated cyclic nucleotide phosphodiesterase cDNA: identification and distribution of isozyme variants. *J. Biol. Chem.* 266: Sept/Oct (in press).

* Present address: Department of Pharmacology, University of Texas Southwestern Med. Ctr., Dallas, TX 75235
Department of Pharmacology, SJ-30, University of Washington, Seattle, WA 98195   USA

S27

THE GUANYLYL CYCLASE RECEPTOR FAMILY D.L. Garbers

Guanylyl cyclase activity is found in both the soluble and particulate fractions of most tissue homogenates. The particulate enzymes can be further divided into those that are easily solubilized and those that are relatively resistant to non-ionic detergent solubilization. Cloning of the mRNA of vaious guanylyl cyclases has revealed two general enzyme structures: heterodimeric structures, one member of which is a soluble form of guanylyl cyclase (Koesling D, Herz J, Gausepohl H, Niroomand F, Hinsch KD, Mulsch A, Bohme E, Schultz G, Frank R, FEBS Letters 239:29, 1988; Nakane M, Saheki S, Kuno T, Ishii K, Murad, F, Biochem Biophs Res Commun 156:1000, 1988), and single chain forms, all of which appear to exist on membranes. The cell membrane forms may normally exist as higher ordered structures such as homodimers, but this has not yet been determined. The first heterodimeric form cloned from rat or bovine lung contains an α and β subunit, both of which appear required for expression of guanylyl cyclase activity(Harteneck C, Koesling D, Soling A, Schultz G, Bohme E FEBS Letters 272:221, 1990; Nakane M, Arai K, Saheki S, Kuno T, Buechler W, Murad F J Biol Chem 265: 16841, 1990). When both subunits are coexpressed, the enzyme is also markedly stimulated by nitroprusside. Both the α and β subunits contain a region near the carboxyl tail that is homologous to the the catalytic domain of a plasma membrane form of guanylyl cyclase, suggesting that this is also a catalytic domain within the heterodimeric form of the enzyme. Recently, we have isolated a second β subunit for a presumed heterodimeric form of guanylyl cyclase from kidney RNA(Yuen PST, Potter LR, Garbers DL Biochemistry 29: 10872, 1990). The β_2 subunit(isolated from kidney) was expressed principally in liver and kidney of various tissues analyzed by Northern hybridization. Unlike the β_1 subunit of lung, the β_2 subunit contained an addition 86 amino acids at the carboxyl terminus; the final four amino acids of Cys-Val-Val-Leu coincided with the consensus site for isoprenylation. If the protein is modified, it could result in heterodimeric forms of guanylyl cyclase also being associated with membranes.

There have been three forms of plasma membrane guanylyl cyclase cloned from various tissues. GC-A, for guanylyl cyclase A, encodes a protein that contains one apparent transmembrane domain; this divides the protein in about one-half. Just within the predicted transmembrane domain exists a protein kinase-like region that is followed by the cyclase catalytic domain. When GC-A is expressed in various cultured mammalian cells, high expression of both atrial natriuretic peptide (ANP) binding and guanylyl cyclase activity are observed. Radiolabeled ANP also can be specifically crosslinked to the expressed protein. It is also possible to express GC-A in insect cells (Sf-9), and under these conditions both high ANP binding activity and guanylyl cyclase activity also are obtained.

From these and other studies, it is apparent that GC-A serves as an ANP cell surface receptor. Studies on the mechanism of signal transduction are still incomplete, but the protein kinase domain appears to play a prominent role. In the Sf-9 cells, both ATP and ANP are required for transduction of the ANP binding signal to the cyclase catalytic domain. Presumably, ATP binds to the protein kinase-like domain, although this is not yet proven. When the protein kinase-like domain is deleted from GC-A, high, but unregulated, guanylyl cyclase activity is obtained. In neither broken cells nor intact cells is ANP able to stimulate cyclic GMP production, even though it continues to bind to the extracellular region of GC-A. Whether or not the protein kinase-like domain is capable of transferring the γ-phosphoryl group of ATP to another protein or to water is not yet known, but since ATPγS and AMPPNP replace ATP for signal transduction, clearly phosphorylation is not a requirement for activation of the guanylyl cyclase catalytic domain by ANP.

The other member of the natriuretic peptide receptor family that has been identified is known as GC-B; it appears to bind C-type natriuretic peptide in preference to ANP or brain natriuretic peptide (Koller KJ, Lowe DG, Bennett GL, Minamino N, Kangawa K, Matsuo H, Goeddel DV Science 252:120, 1991). GC-B is about 43% identical with GC-A within the extracellular domain at the amino acid level. Whether or not C-type natriuretic peptide is the natural ligand for GC-B remains to be determined since the tissue distribution of GC-B at the protein level has not yet been determined. C-type natriuretic peptide appears to be brain specific.

After the discovery of GC-A and GC-B, a third member of the plasma membrane guanylyl cyclase family was cloned from the mRNA of rat small intestine(Schulz S, Green CK, Yuen PST, Garbers DL Cell 63:941, 1990). The predicted protein (GC-C) was homologous with GC-A and GC-B within the intracellular regions, but was only 10% identical within the putative extraceullar ligand binding domain. After expression of this cDNA in cultured mammalian cells, both high heat-stable enterotoxin binding and guanylyl cyclase activity were observed. It appears, therefore, that GC-C binds the heat-stable enterotoxins of bacteria and that subsequent rises in cyclic GMP mediate the acute secretory diarrhea. Whether an endogenous ligand for this receptor exists is not yet known.

University of Texas Southwestern Medical Center, 5323 Harry Hines Boulevard, Dallas, TX 75235-9050 USA

S28

SYNTHESIS AND ACTIONS OF NITRIC OXIDE IN THE CARDIOVASCULAR SYSTEM

R.M.J. Palmer and S. Moncada, Wellcome Research Laboratories, Beckenham, Kent BR3 3BS U.K.

The synthesis of nitric oxide (NO) from the amino acid L-arginine has, in recent years, been shown to be a widespread mechanism for regulating cell function and communication (for review see 1). Vascular endothelial cells synthesise NO (2) from the amino-acid L-arginine (3) by the action of a calcium-calmodulin-dependent enzyme present constitutively in these cells (4,5). The NO thus formed accounts for the vasodilator action of endothelium-derived relaxing factor (6). This effect is mediated through the stimulation of the soluble guanylate cyclase in vascular smooth muscle to cause relaxation. Since nitrovasodilators also exert their effect through stimulation of the soluble guanylate cyclase (7), and are known to be converted to NO (8), the L-arginine:NO pathway in vascular endothelium can be considered as the endogenous nitrovasodilator.

Nitric oxide is synthesised continuously by vascular endothelial cells (2) and this release can be enhanced by endothelium-dependent vasodilators (3b) such as acetylcholine, and by flow and shear force (9). The synthesis of NO is inhibited by L-arginine analogues, such as N^G-monomethyl-L-arginine (L-NMMA; 10). These compounds causes an increase in the tone of aortic rings and inhibit the relaxation induced by acetylcholine (11). Furthermore, administration of these compounds to anaesthetised rabbits cause a substantial rise in blood pressure and inhibits the hypotensive effect of acetylcholine (12). Thus, the continuous release of NO by the vascular endothelium maintains the cardiovascular system in a state of active vasodilatation.

The evidence implicating changes in the activity of this endogenous vasodilator in the aetiology of cardiovascular diseases is only circumstantial. However, it is likely that such a fundamental local regulatory mechanism will be important in some clinical conditions. Indeed, we have recently shown that removal of basal NO synthesis in aortic rings, either by endothelium removal or by inhibition of NO synthesis, leads to a supersensitivity to nitrovasodilators at the level of their receptor, the soluble guanylate cyclase (13). It is tempting to speculate that this mechanism may account for the effectiveness of these compounds in angina where a reduced synthesis of NO by the coronary vascular endothelium, and the consequent up-regulation of their receptor, may confer some selectivity of nitrovasodilators on this vascular bed. Endotoxin shock is characterised by hypotension and a reduced response to vasoconstrictors. Vascular rings from endotoxin-treated rats or from control rats treated with endotoxin in vitro also show a time-dependent loss of tone, accompanied by a reduced response to vasoconstrictors and a direct relaxation induced by L-arginine (14). Vascular endothelial cells (15) and vascular smooth muscle (14,16,17) express a calcium-independent NO synthase when activated with endotoxin alone or in combination with interferon-γ. This enzyme is distinct from that present constitutively in vascular endothelium and is similar to that induced in cytotoxic macrophages, Kupffer cells, hepatocytes and neutrophils following activation by endotoxin and cytokines. The expression of this enzyme is these cells is associated with cytotoxicity (18). The expression of the inducible NO synthase in vascular tissue requires de novo protein synthesis and correlates with the appearance of the functional changes that follow exposure to endotoxin (14).

We have recently shown that vascular endothelial cells incubated with endotoxin show a significant reduction in viability, which is prevented by L-NMMA. This indicates that the induction of NO synthase in these cells provides a mechanism for local endothelial damage. Therefore, the induction of an NO synthase in the vessel wall contributes to the aetiology of endotoxin shock and may also be the mechanism underlying the hyperdynamic circulation characteristic of cirrhosis (19).

The expression of the inducible calcium-independent NO synthase in vascular endothelium and smooth muscle is inhibited by glucocorticoids such as dexamethasone and hydrocortisone (14,15). These compounds also inhibit the induction of this enzyme in macrophages (20) and neutrophils and abolish the functional effects of endotoxin on vascular endothelium and smooth muscle (14). The inhibition by glucocorticoids of the induction of this NO synthase may play a role in the diverse therapeutic actions of these compounds.

In addition to its effects on vascular tone, NO also inhibits platelet aggregation and adhesion (21,22). Recently, platelets have been shown to possess a calcium-dependent-constitutive NO synthase (23). This enzyme synthesises NO to elevate platelet cyclic GMP levels and down-regulate their response to agonists such as collagen. Thus, in platelets the L-arginine:NO pathway acts as an autocrine mechanism to down-regulate their activation.

The discovery of the L-arginine:NO pathway in the vessel wall and its role as the endogenous nitrovasodilator and as a pathological mechanism will have a significant effect on our understanding of the cardiovascular system and its regulation in health and disease (for review see 24).

REFERENCES

1. Moncada S., Palmer R.M.J. and Higgs E.A. (1989). Biochem. Pharmacol., 38: 1709-1715.
2. Palmer R.M.J., Ferrige A.G. and Moncada S. (1987). Nature, 327: 524-526.
3. Palmer R.M.J., Ashton D.S. and Moncada S. (1988). Nature, 333: 664-666.
4. Palmer R.M.J. and Moncada S. (1989). Biochem. Biophys. Res. Commun., 158: 348-352.
5. Busse R. and Mulsch A. (1990). FEBS Lett., 265: 133-136.
6. Furchgott R.F. and Zawadzki J.V. (1980). Nature, 288: 373-376.
7. Schultz K.D., Schultz K. and Schultz G. (1977). Nature, 265: 750-751.
8. Feelisch M. and Noack E.A. (1987). Eur. J. Pharmacol., 139: 19-30.
9. Inoue T., Tomoike H., Hisano K. and Nakamura M. (1988). J. Am. Coll. Cardiol., 11: 187-191.
10. Palmer R.M.J., Rees D.D., Ashton D.S. and Moncada S. (1988). Biochem. Biophys. Res. Commun. 153: 1251-1256.
11. Rees D.D., Palmer R.M.J., Hodson H.F. and Moncada S. (1989). Br. J. Pharmacol., 96: 418-424.
12. Rees D.D., Palmer R.M.J. and Moncada S. (1989). Proc. Natl. Acad. Sci. USA. 86: 3375-3378.
13. Moncada S., Rees D.D., Schulz R. and Palmer R.M.J. (1991). Proc. Natl. Acad. Sci. USA. 88: 2166-2170.
14. Rees D.D., Cellek S., Palmer R.M.J. and Moncada S. (1990). Biochem. Biophys. Res. Commun. 173: 541-547.
15. Radomski M.W., Palmer R.M.J. and Moncada S (1990). Proc. Natl. Acad. Sci. USA., 87: 10043-10047.
16. Busse R. and Mulsch A. (1990). FEBS Lett., 275: 87-90.
17. Knowles R.G., Salter M., Brooks S.L. and Moncada S. (1990). Biochem. Biophys. Res. Commun., 172: 1042-1048.
18. Hibbs J.B. Jr., Taintor R.R., Vavrin Z., Granger D.L., Drapier J-C., Amber I.J. and Lancaster J.R. Jr. (1990). In: Nitric oxide from L-arginine. A bioregulatory system. ed. Moncada S. and Higgs E.A. 189-223. Elsevier.
19. Vallance P. and Moncada S (1991). Lancet, 337: 776-778.
20. Di Rosa M., Radomski M.W., Carnuccio R. and Moncada S. (1990). Biochem. Biophys. Res. Commun., 172: 1246-1252.
21. Radomski M.W., Palmer R.M.J. and Moncada S. (1987). Br. J. Pharmacol., 92: 181-187.
22. Radomski M.W., Palmer R.M.J. and Moncada S. (1987). Biochem. Biophys. Res. Commun., 148: 1482-1489.
23. Radomski M.W., Palmer R.M.J. and Moncada S. (1990). Proc. Natl. Acad. Sci. USA., 87: 5193-5197.
24. Moncada S., Palmer R.M.J. and Higgs E.A. (1991). Pharm. Res., 43: 109-142.

S29

ROLE OF CYCLIC GMP AND CYCLIC GMP-DEPENDENT PROTEIN KINASE FOR THE SIGNAL TRANSDUCTION MECHANISM OF VASODILATORS

U. Walter, E. Butt, J. Geiger, M. Halbrügge, S.M. Lohmann, and C. Nolte

Elevation of the intracellular level of cGMP by certain direct vasodilators results in the inhibition of smooth muscle contraction and platelet activation (1-4). Elevated cGMP levels are due to the stimulation of either the particulate guanylyl cyclase (e.g. by ANF and related peptides) or the soluble, heme-containing guanylyl cyclase (e.g. by nitroprusside, EDRF and other NO-generating nitrovasodilators) [1-4]. In contrast to cAMP which achieves most of its physiological effects [with the possible exception of regulation of cAMP-gated ion channels (5,6)] by activating cAMP-dependent protein kinases (7,8), cGMP appears to regulate several different signal transduction pathways (4). In vertebrate photoreceptors and certain sensory neurons, cation channels are directly gated by cGMP (5). cGMP is also capable of antagonizing or potentiating cAMP-mediated effects via its effects on cGMP-stimulated (cGS-PDE) or cGMP-inhibited (cGI-PDE) cAMP-phosphodiesterases, respectively (9,10). The family of cGMP-dependent protein kinases (cGK) is known to consist of an exclusively membrane-bound form (type II) present in brush border membranes and two types of soluble and membrane-associated forms (types I alpha and beta) present in cerebellar Purkinje cells, smooth muscle cells, platelets, and at very low concentrations in cardiac myocytes (4,11). Interestingly, many cells of the cardiovascular system (including vascular smooth muscle cells, platelets and cardiac myocytes) contain the two types of cGMP-regulated phosphodiesterases (cGI-PDE, cGS-PDE) as well as cGMP-dependent protein kinases (4,10,11) and perhaps cyclic nucleotide-gated channels (6). Often, it is therefore difficult to determine the precise contribution of these diverse cGMP-regulated proteins to the control of complex cellular functions such as contraction and platelet activation. One of our interests, the development of specific activators or inhibitors for these cGMP-regulated proteins, will be reviewed.

There is increasing evidence that one major functional effect of cGMP and cGK in cardiovascular cells is the lowering of cytosolic calcium (3,4). In whole cell patch clamp experiments with cardiac myocytes, cGK was shown to inhibit the cAMP-activated L-type calcium channel (11), suggesting that cGK mediates some of the negative inotropic effects of cGMP-elevating hormones and drugs. In smooth muscle cells and human platelets, cGK appears to mediate effects of cGMP-elevating vasodilators and to inhibit agonist-induced elevation of cytosolic calcium levels (4,12 - 14). For platelets, considerable evidence exists that cGMP-mediated inhibition of cytosolic calcium is due to cGK-mediated inhibition of intracellular calcium mobilization and possibly also to inhibition of receptor-regulated calcium channels, although the molecular details are not yet completely understood (4,14). We have recently identified and purified a 46/50 kDa protein which is rapidly and efficiently phosphorylated in intact human platelets in response to cGMP- and cAMP-elevating vasodilators acting via cGMP- and cAMP-dependent protein kinases, respectively (15,16). In addition, rapid EDRF- and cGMP/cGK-mediated phosphorylation of this platelet protein was also demonstrated in coincubations of human endothelial cells and platelets (17). Some current concepts concerning the possible structure and function of this vasodilator-regulated phosphoprotein and its role in the possible mechanism(s) of nitrovasodilator inhibition of smooth muscle contraction and platelet activation will be discussed.

References

1) Waldmann SA, Murad F (1987) Cyclic GMP synthesis and function. Pharmacol Rev 39: 163 - 196
2) Tremblay J, Gerzer R, Hamet P (1988) Cyclic GMP in cell function. Adv Second Messenger Phosphoprotein Res 22: 319 - 383
3) Lincoln TM (1989) Cyclic GMP and mechanisms of vasodilation. Pharmacol Ther 41: 479 - 502
4) Walter U (1989) Physiological role of cGMP and cGMP-dependent protein kinase in the cardiovascular system. Rev Physiol Biochem Pharmacol 113: 41 - 88
5) Kaupp UB (1991) The cyclic nucleotide-gated channels of vertebrate photpreceptors and olfactory epithelium. Trends in Neuroscience 14: 150 - 157

6) DiFrancesco D, Tortora P (1991) Direct activation of cardiac pacemaker channels by intracellular cyclic AMP. Nature 351: 145 - 147

7) Meinecke M, Büchler W, Fischer L, Lohmann SM, Walter U (1990) cAMP-dependent protein kinase: subunit diversity and functional role in gene expression. In: Cellular and molecular biology of myelination (eds. Jeserich G, Althaus HH, Waehneldt TV), NATO ASI Series H, Vol.43, Springer Verlag, Heidelberg, pp 201 - 215

8) Taylor SS, Buechler JA, Yonemoto W (1990) cAMP-dependent protein kinase: framework for a diverse family of regulator enzymes. Annu Rev Biochem 59: 971 - 1005.

9) Beavo JA (1988) Multiple isoenzymes of cyclic nucleotide phosphodiesterase. Adv Second Messenger and Phosphoprotein Res 22: 1 - 38

10) Beavo JA, Reifsnyder DH (1990) Primary sequence of cyclic nucleotide phosphodiesterase isozymes and the design of selective inhibitors. Trends Pharmacol Sci 11: 150 - 155

11) Mery P-F, Lohmann SM, Walter U, Fischmeister R (1991) Ca^{++}-current is regulated by cGMP-dependent protein kinase in cardiac myocytes. Proc Natl Acad Sci USA 88: 1197 - 1201

12) Felbel J, Trockur B, Ecker T, Landgraf W, Hofmann F (1988) Regulation of cytosolic calcium by cAMP and cGMP in freshly isolated smooth muscle cells from bovine trachea. J Biol Chem 263: 16764 - 16771

13) Cornwell TL, Lincoln TM (1989) Regulation of intracellular Ca^{++} levels in cultured vascular smooth muscle cells: reduction of Ca^{++} by atriopeptin and 8-Br-cGMP is mediated by cGMP-dependent protein kinase. J Biol Chem 264: 1146 - 1155

14) Walter U, Nolte C, Geiger J, Schanzenbächer P, Kochsiek K (1991) Inhibition of platelet function by cyclic nucleotides and cyclic nucleotide-dependent protein kinases.
In "Antithrombotics: Pathophysiological rationale for pharmacological interventions" (Herman AG, Moncada S, eds.), Kluwer Academic Publishers, In Press

15) Halbrügge M, Walter U (1989) Purification of a vasodilator-regulated phosphoprotein from human platelets. Eur J Biochem 185: 41 - 50

16) Halbrügge M, Friedrich C, Eigenthaler M, Schanzenbächer P, Walter U (1990) Stoichiometric and reversible phosphorylation of a 46 kDa protein in human platelets in response to cGMP- and cAMP-elevating vasodilators. J Biol Chem 265: 3088 - 3093

17) Nolte C, Eigenthaler M, Schanzenbächer P, Walter U (1991) Endothelial cell-dependent phosphorylation of a platelet protein mediated by cAMP- and cGMP-elevating factors. J Biol Chem 266: In press

Medizinische Universitätsklinik, Klinische Forschergruppe, Josef-Schneider-Str.2, 8700 Würzburg, F.R.G.

MOLECULAR BIOLOGY, PATHOPHYSIOLOGY AND PHARMACOLOGY OF THE RENIN-ANGIOTENSIN SYSTEM

Detlev Ganten, Michael Kaling, Michael Bader, Martin Paul, Jörg Peters

The development of potent inhibitors of the renin-angiotensin axis, such as renin and CE-inhibitors as well as angiotensin II antagonists has fostered a rapid expansion of our understanding of its pathophysiological significance and clinical relevance. This has gained additional interest due to the discovery of local tissue renin-angiotensin systems in addition to the classical hormonal system. The existence of such local renin-angiotensin systems has now been confirmed by a number of recent studies demonstrating unequivocally expression of the genes for renin and angiotensinogen in a variety of tissues e.g. brain, adrenal gland, heart, arterial wall, testis, ovary and kidney. To study the tissue-specific expression of components of the RAS we have used molecular biological and transgenic techniques. The use of specific gene constructs permits the localisation of expression in specific tissues and cell types and to study molecular mechanisms of gene regulation.

1) The liver is the predominant site of production of angiotensinogen (Aogen). Expression of the angiotensinogen gene in liver responds to a wide range of hormonal modulators such as thyroxine, glucocorticoids, estrogen and angiotensin II. Steroid induced hypertension and hypertension in connection with pregnancy may be mediated through the influence of hormones on angiotensinogen synthesis. The molecular mechanism are largely unknown. We investigated the 5'-flanking region of the rat angiotensinogen gene to define DNA elements conferring inducibility by glucocorticoids and estrogens. Two putative glucocorticoid responsive elements (GREs) based on sequence comparison were identified. Here we report the functional importance of these sequences. We constructed several deletion mutants of the 5'-region in front of the bacterial reporter gene for chloramphenicol acetyltransferase (CAT). The angiotensinogen-CAT-reporter plasmids (pRagCAT) were transiently transfected into the rat hepatoma cells FTO 2B and Fe 33. All pRag CAT-constructs containing at least one of the two GRE consensus sequences were stimulated by dexamethasone. On the other hand deletion mutants lacking GRE sequences were not inducible by dexamethasone. In additional experiments the transcriptional functions of the two putative GREs were assessed by cloning synthetic oligonucleotides encompassing the GRE sequences directly in front of the heterologous HSV thymidine-kinase (tk) promotor. Our results showed that each synthetic GRE was capable of stimulating the tk-promotor after administration of dexamethasone and that both GREs together act synergistically. We also investigated the transcriptional control of angiotensinogen by estrogen. Although no estrogen responsive element (ERE) consensus sequences were detectable by sequence comparison we have identified sequences between -60 to -92 which conferred estrogen inducibility to the rat angiotensinogen gene. In this region a so called half-palindromic ERE is localized at position -91 to -87. These studies provide a molecular basis for a better understanding of steroid regulation of the angiotensinogen gene and possibly steroid induced hypertension.

2) The transgenic animal methodology was used to identify promoter sequences which mediate cell specific expression of the rat Aogen gene.
Several deletion mutants of the wild type rat Aogen promoter (1.6 kb of 5'flanking sequences) were constructed, in which sequences known to participate in gene regulation were successively removed. Wild type promoter and deletions of it were cloned in front of the E. coli lac Z gene which codes for the enzyme ß-galactosidase (ß-gal). The expression of this reporter gene can be monitored by histochemical staining. A nuclear translocation signal was included in all constructs to direct the transport of the gene product ß-gal into the nucleus, thus providing a more intense staining signal. All constructs have been tested for expression in tissue culture. When transiently transfected into the rat hepatoma cell line Fe 33, known to express the estrogen receptor, all Aogen-lac Z fusion genes were expressed when stimulated with estrogen. The protein product accumulated in the nucleus as evidenced by histochemical staining for ß-galactosidase.

3) To define promoter sequences which direct correct expression of the gene in transgenic animals we injected the entire wild type rat Aogen gene including 1.6 kb of 5'flanking sequences into the germline of NMRI mice. We obtained three different lines of transgene positive mice which were screened for expression of the transgene by in situ hybridization and RNAse protection assay. One line showed an aberrant expression pattern which is most probably due to integration artifacts. The expression pattern of the transgene in the other two lines was similar to that of the endogenous gene in the rat with high expression of the gene in specific brain regions (hypothalamus, thalamus, subfornical organ, pons).
These studies demonstrate that defined promoter-lacZ fusion genes are expressed correctly in tissue culture and that tissue specific expression in transgenic animals can be obtained with 1.6 kb of 5'flanking sequences of the rat Aogen gene.

4) In order to study the role of tissue specific gene expression of the renin gene for the development of hypertension, we have also established transgenic rats by introducing the mouse renM-2 gene. Several independent lines of transgenic rats have been established. Those animals which possess the mouse gene exhibit extreme hypertension. The segregation of the hypertensive phenotype with the

presence of the transgene in independent lines, indicates that expression of the mouse renin gene is responsible for the hypertension. Interestingly, these rats do not have abnormal levels of renin, angiotensin I or angiotensin II in their plasma and therefore overexpression of renin in the kidney does not account for the phenotype. The transgene is highly expressed in several tissues with especially high levels in the adrenal gland. Steroid hormones are stimulated in these animals. These transgenic rats provide an attractive new experimental model for pharmacological and pathophysiological cardiovascular studies on the tissue RAS. We submit that different roles with respect to blood pressure regulation are realized by the plasma RAS and by the tissue RAS. The plasma RAS may be an acute regulator of vascular tone and electrolyte and volume homeostasis while the tissue RAS probably carries out more long-term functions on an autocrine or paracrine level. The inhibiton of the tissue RAS may well be more important to the long-term therapeutic effects than interference with the hormonal plasma RAS.

Hypertension is a chronic disease and treatment of mild to moderate hypertension does not warrant acute lowering of blood pressure. Thus, inhibition of the long-term effects of tissue angiotensin may be more desirable and important than the acute inhibitory effetcs on the plasma RAS. As we learn more about the RAS and unravel an increasingly complex picture, we are presented with ever new questions and challenges to be addressed by both basic scientists and clinical investigators.

1. Wagner D, Metzger R, Paul M, Ludwig G, Suzuki F, Takahashi S, Murakami K, Ganten D. Androgen dependence and tissue specificity of renin messenger RNA expression in mice. J Hypertens 1990;8:45-52

2. Mullins JJ, Peters J, Ganten D. Fulminant hypertension in transgenic rats harbouring the mouse Ren-2 gene. Nature 1990;344:541-544

3. Lindpaintner K, Takahashi S, Ganten D. Structural alterations of the renin gene in stroke-prone spontaneously hypertensive rats: examination of genotype-phenotype correlations. J Hypertens 1990;8:763-773

4. Schelling P, Fischer H, Ganten D. Angiotensin and cell growth: a link to cardio-vascular hypertrophy? J Hypertens 1991;9:3-15

5. Lindpaintner K, Jin M, Niedermeier N, Wilhelm MJ, Ganten D. Cardiac angiotensinogen and its local activation in the isolated perfused beating heart. Circ Res 1990;67/3:564-573

German Institute for High Blood Pressure Research and Department of Pharmacology, University of Heidelberg, Im Neuenheimer Feld 366, D-6900 Heidelberg, FRG

S31

THE THERAPEUTIC VALUE OF POSITIVE INOTROPIC DRUGS.
G. Hasenfuss

In the search for therapeutic alternatives in treating heart failure, during the last decade new inotropic drugs with different modes of action have been developed (1). On a subcellular level, positive inotropism can be achieved by increased calcium availability to contractile proteins or by increased sensitivity of troponin C for calcium ions. This results in activation of additional units of contractile proteins. Accordingly, positive inotropic drugs either increase intracellular calcium concentration and/or augment calcium sensitivity of troponin C. For clinical use, three different groups of inotropic drugs are available: 1) agents which increase intracellular calcium by increasing intracellular cyclic AMP concentration, 2) agents which increase intracellular calcium without altering cyclic AMP levels, and 3) agents which increase calcium sensitivity of contractile proteins.

Intracellular cyclic AMP levels are increased by two types of inotropic agents. 1) Beta-receptor agonists increase cyclic AMP by activation of adenylate cyclase resulting in increased cyclic AMP production. 2) Phosphodiesterase inhibitors increase cyclic AMP by preventing its degradation by phosphodiesterases; these agents, in addition have vasodilating properties. Most beta-receptor agonists and phosphodiesterase inhibitors produce short-term hemodynamic improvement in patients with acute and chronic heart failure. Therefore, these drugs are used for intravenous treatment of acute heart failure and cardiogenic shock. However, long-term treatment of congestive heart failure with beta-receptor agonists or phosphodiesterase inhibitors appears to be accompanied by accelerated disease progression, worsening of ventricular tachycardia and adverse effects on survival (2). Increased mortality also seems to be present with intermittent administration of the beta-receptor agonist dobutamine (3). Unfavorable effects of beta-receptor agonists and phosphodiesterase inhibitors, which may result from increased heart rate, increased intracellular calcium, or increased myocardial oxygen consumption, contrast markedly with reports that beta-adrenergic antagonists may exert beneficial effects on exercise tolerance and survival of patients with chronic heart failure (4). Beneficial long-term effects of dopamine analogues on exercise tolerance and clinical symptoms in patients with congestive heart failure may primarily result form vasodilating properties of these agents, in particular from renal artery vasodilation (5).

Cardiac glycosides exert positive inotropic effects by increased calcium availability without aleration of the cyclic AMP level. While beneficial effects of digitalis was unquestioned in patients with heart failure and atrial fibrillation, the efficacy of digitalis in the management of heart failure with normal sinus rhyhtm was controversial. In recent studies, however, digoxin has proved to have a favorable effect on left ventricular ejection fraction, exercise tolerance and thus the clinical syndrome of heart failure (6,7). Efficacy of digitalis appears to be most clearly demonstrable in patients with more severe symptoms and more dilated left ventricles. Whether digitalis has beneficial effects on prognosis of these patients is still questionable.

Most inotropic drugs which augment calcium sensitivity of troponin C also increase cyclic AMP levels by phosphodiesterase inhibition. Of this group of agents, pimobendan is currently under long-term clinical investigation. Preliminary data suggest beneficial effects of this drug on exercise tolerance and clinical symptoms in patients with congestive heart failure.

Recent findings on force-frequency relation in isolated human myocardium may indicate a new therapeutic approach in the treatment of congestive heart failure (8). While in nonfailing human myocardium isometric contractile force increases with increasing stimulation frequency (maximum force at 166 ± 9 beats per minute), in failing human myocardium maximum force is developed at a significant lower frequency (36 ± 2/min) and decreases continuously over the whole physiological frequency range. The inverse force-frequency relation in the failing human myocardium suggests that the beneficial effects of beta-receptor antagonists in patients with heart failure may result from increased contractile force following reduction in heart rate, despite negative inotropic properties of these agents. In view of the inverse force-frequency relation in failing human myocardium, negative chronotropic drugs without direct effects on myocardial contractility may represent a new class of "positive inotropic" agents.

REFERENCES
1) Colucci WS, et al. N Engl J Med 1986;314:290
2) Cohn JN. N Engl J Med 1989;320:729
3) Dies F, et al. Circulation 1986; 74,II:39
4) Waagstein F, et al. Br Heart J 1975;137:1022
5) Hasenfuss G, et al. Basic Res Cardiol 1989;84,I:191
6) The Captopril-Digoxin Multicenter Research Group. JAMA 1988;259:539
7) DiBianco R, et al. N Engl J Med 1989;320:677
8) Hasenfuss G, et al. Klin Wochenschr 1991;69,XXIII:120

Present address: Department of Medicine, Cardiology, University of Freiburg, Hugstetter Strasse 55, 7800 Freiburg, FRG

ANTIARRHYTHMIC THERAPY AFTER CAST

T. Meinertz

The Cardiac Arrhythmia Suppression Trial (CAST) was designed to test the hypothesis that suppression of ventricular arrhythmias in survivors of acute myocardial infarction would reduce the risk of arrhythmic death. During a routine interim analysis an unsuspected increase in arrhythmic death in the encainide/flecainide group compared to placebo was discovered (relative risk = 3,6). These unfortunate results were surprising in that the CAST population represented patients in whom the risk of arrhythmic death was only moderate and the risk of proarrhythmia was thought to be low.

The excessive arrhythmic death rate in patients taking encainide or flecainide occured over the duration of the study, implying early as well as late deleterious cardiac effects of these antiarrhythmic agents. It remains open whether this excess antiarrhythmic death rate as a consequence of a new type of proarrhythmia ("late proarrhythmia" as compared to "classic proarrhythmia" occuring early after administration of an antiarrhythmic agent). Alternatively, the deleterious effects of these agents might be the consequence of drug induced asystole or deterioration of preexisting left ventricular dysfunction. A detailed analysis of the CAST-database supports the view that these arrhythmic deaths represent a new type of proarrhythmia, perhaps suggesting a unique mechanism. It may involve the interaction of ischemia, ventricular arrhythmias and antiarrhythmic agents with specific electrophysiological properties. Such a phenomenon has been recently demonstrated in animal infarct models.

Another fascinating issue of the CAST-results is the extraordinary low mortality rate in the placebo group, approximately one-third of the arrhythmic death rate seen in the Cardiac Arrhythmia Pilot study. This low mortality in the placebo group and the excess mortality in patients treated with encainide/flecainide have resulted in a re-evaluation of our traditional concepts regarding the appropriate use of antiarrhythmic agents. The most important questions being whether the CAST results can be extrapolated to other antiarrhythmic agents and to other patients populations.

References:

1. CAST investigators. Prelimnary report: effect of encainide and flecainide on mortality in a randomized trial of arrhythmia suppression after myocardial infarction. N. Engl. J. Med. 1989. 321; 406-412

2. Ruskin JN. The Cardiac Arrhythmia Suppression Trial (CAST) (editorial). N. Engl. J. Med. 1989. 321; 386-388

3. The CAPS Investigators. The Cardiac Arrhythmia Pilot Study. Am. J. Cardiol. 1986. 57; 91-95

Present address: II. Medizinische Klinik, AK St. Georg, 2000 Hamburg, Lohmühlenstr. 5

S33

DOSE AND CONCENTRATION INTENSITY RELATIONSHIPS FOR CANCER CHEMOTHERAPY

William E. Evans, Pharmaceutical Division, St. Jude Children's Research Hospital and Center for Pediatric Pharmacokinetics and Therapeutics, University of Tennessee, Memphis, USA 38101

Cytotoxic anticancer drugs usually have a narrow therapeutic index, typically producing acute toxicity at dosages similar to those required for therapeutic efficacy. These toxicities can be severe and life threatening (e.g., neutropenia, thrombopenia), while the consequences of underdosing these drugs may be equally life threatening (i.e. lack of efficacy). For drug-sensitive cancers where it is important to avoid underdosing cancer chemotherapy, more precise methods are needed to determine the optimal dosage in individual patients.

Several clinical trials of drug-sensitive cancers (e.g., breast cancer, leukemia, Hodgkin lymphoma, testicular cancer) have demonstrated a dose-response relationship for various anticancer drugs, thus providing an impetus to investigate the relation between therapeutic response and the pharmacokinetics of these drugs. Steep dose-response relationships for many anticancer drugs, coupled with numerous studies describing large inter-patient variability in their pharmacokinetics, provide a strong rationale for systematically investigating the clinical pharmacodynamics of cancer chemotherapy. Over the last 5-10 years, several clinical pharmacodynamic studies of anticancer drugs have been published and representative studies will be reviewed in this presentation. The major purpose of this presentation is to heighten awareness of pharmacokinetic and pharmacodynamic strategies for investigating the clinical activity of antineoplastic agents and for adjusting the dosage of certain anticancer drugs in individual patients.

Methotrexate, carboplatin, etoposide, teniposide and 5-fluorouracil will be discussed as examples of anticancer drugs for which plasma concentrations correlate with gastrointestinal and/or hematologic toxicity, as well as with the risk of relapse (for high-dose methotrexate in acute lymphocytic leukemia) or with the degree of hepatic metastatic involvement (for colorectal cancer treated with 5-fluorouracil). Mercaptopurine will be discussed as an example of intracellular (RBC) concentrations of active metabolites (6TGNs) correlating with the risk of toxicity (neutropenia) and the risk of treatment failure (relapse) for children with acute lymphocytic leukemia.

There are also pharmacogenetic considerations for some anticancer drugs. For both mercaptopurine and 5-fluorouracil, the risk of toxicity is associated with a genetic polymorphism in a specific drug metabolizing enzyme. With mercaptopurine, low activity of thiopurine methyltransferase (TPMT) is associated with increased intracellular concentrations of thioguanine nucleotides (TGN), the active metabolites of mercaptopurine. One in 300 Caucasians is deficient in TPMT activity, inherited as an autosomal co-dominant trait, and such patients typically experience extensive toxicity (e.g., neutropenia) unless their mercaptopurine dosage is substantially reduced (e.g., 15-fold dosage reduction). Likewise, patients with dihydropyrimidine dehydrogenase deficiency, inherited as an autosomal recessive trait, have aberrant metabolism of 5-FU and experience excessive neurotoxicity.

The principles of pharmacodynamics are also proving useful as refinements of the dose escalation process in the evaluation of newer anticancer drugs in Phase I and II studies. A Phase I-II study of teniposide is discussed as an example in which systemic exposure (measured as area-under-the-curve or as steady-state plasma concentration) correlated better with both oncolytic response and gastrointestinal toxicity than did the administered dose.

Examples in which pharmacodynamic relationships have been tested and demonstrated not to hold, will also be mentioned, for completeness. In essentially all cases where significant concentration-effect relationships have been demonstrated, prospective randomized trials are needed to rigorously assess the clinical importance of using pharmacokinetic and pharmacodynamic principles to individualize the dosages of anticancer drugs. An ongoing, randomized, prospective trial of individualized versus conventional dosages of chemotherapy for childhood ALL will be described to exemplify one strategy for testing pharmacodynamic hypotheses at the clinical level.

SELECTED REFERENCES:

Evans WE, Relling, MV. Clinical pharmacokinetics-pharmacodynamics of anticancer drugs. Clinical Pharmacokinetics 16: 327-336, 1989.

Evans WE, Crom WR, Stewart CF, et al. Clinical pharmacodynamics of high-dose methotrexate in acute lymphocytic leukemia, New England Journal of Medicine 314:471-477, 1986.

Egorin MJ, Van Echo DA, Olman EA, et al. Prospective validation of a pharmacologically based dosing scheme for carboplatin. Cancer Research 45:5432-5438, 1985.

Rodman JH, Abromowitch M, Sinkule JA, Rivera GK, Evans WE. Clinical pharmacodynamics of continuous infusion teniposide: systemic exposure as a determinant of response in a Phase I trial. Journal of Clinical Oncology 5: 1007-1014, 1987.

Stoller RG, Hande KR, et al. Use of plasma pharmacokinetics to predict and prevent methotrexate toxicity. New England Journal of Medicine 297: 630-634, 1977.

Milano G, Namer M, Boublil JL, et al. Relationship between systemic 5-FU passage and response in colorectal cancer patients treated with intrahepatic chemotherapy. Cancer Chemotherapy and Pharmacology 20: 71-74, 1987.

Lennard L, Lilleyman JS. Variable mercaptopurine metabolism and treatment outcome in childhood lymphoblastic leukemia. Journal of Clinical Oncology 7:1816-1823, 1989.

Lennard L, Lilleyman JS, Van Loon J, Weinshilboum RM. Genetic variation in response to 6-mercaptopurine for childhood acute lymphoblastic leukaemia. Lancet 336:225-29, 1990.

Supported in part by NIH grants R37 CA36401, PO1 CA20180, PO1 CA23099, P30 CA21765, a Center of Excellence grant from the state of Tennessee, and by ALSAC.

S34

P-170 GLYCOPROTEIN AS A TUMOR RESISTANCE MARKER
M. Volm

A number of biochemical mechanisms have been postulated to account for resistance to antineoplastic drugs. At present, of major investigational and therapeutic interest is the characterization of the multidrug-resistant phenotype and its clinical relevance (for review see Riordan and Ling, Pharmac. Ther. 28:51, 1985; Bradley et al., Biochim. Biophys. Acta 948:87, 1988; Volm et al., Tumordiagn. u. Ther. 11:189, 1990). Multidrug resistance (MDR) is characterized by the simultaneous acquisition of cross-resistance to structurally and functionally unrelated anticancer drugs (anthracylines, alkaloids, antibiotics). Over-production of a 170 kDA protein (P-glycoprotein) in the plasma membrane is the most consistent change detected in independently derived MDR cell lines. The level of P-glycoprotein correlates well with the level of drug resistance and the decrease in intracellular drug accumulation. Genomic and cDNA sequences encoding P-glycoprotein have been isolated and characterized. From the DNA sequence encoding P-glycoprotein from mouse, hamster and human a model of P-glycoprotein as an energy-dependent, drug efflux pump has been postulated. The predicted structure of P-glycoprotein (1280 amino acids) is a highly conserved tandemly duplicated molecule. Each half of the molecule consists of six transmembrane regions and two putative nucleotide-binding regions. There exists a remarkable similarity to bacterial transport proteins. P-glycoprotein is encoded by a multigene family but genomic analysis established that only the mdr1-gene has been linked to multidrug resistance.
While MDR has been extensively studied in animal and human tissue cultures, information about invivo tumor models with inherent or acquired MDR is sparse. Therefore, we developed and analyzed various in vivo tumor models with different resistant phenotypes including MDR (Sarcoma 180-, L1210-ascites tumor lines, human tumor xenografts). As detection systems for P-glycoprotein-expression we used the streptavidin-biotin-peroxidase and the streptavidin-biotin-phycoerythrin method using different monoclonal antibodies. Expression of mdr1 RNA and gene-amplification was assayed by Northern- and Southern-blotting. For instance, using a panel of human epidermoid lung cancer xenografts grown in nude mice with different degrees of intrinsic MDR, we demonstrated that these tumors exhibited a similar pattern of cross-resistance to that observed in cell lines with acquired MDR. The xenografts revealed immunoreactivity with different monoclonal antibodies to P-glycoprotein according to the degree of resistance. The level of expression of mdr1-RNA could be correlated with the degree of drug resistance. Moreover, we have developed drug-resistant sublines in vivo. Elevated mdr1 RNA levels and overexpression of P-glycoprotein were detected.
To date, the most comprehensive study of MDR in human tumors is that of Goldstein et al. (J. Natl. Cancer Inst. 81:116,1989) who analyzed over 400 tumor samples from a broad range of human malignancies. They found that many tumors from untreated cancer patients had relatively high mdr1 RNA expression. These tumors arose in organs with MDR as a normal component, including the liver, colon, and kidney. Such tumors are generally resistant to chemotherapy. In contrast, mdr1 RNA was not detected in a large number of tumors, particulary in carcinomas arising in organs without MDR expression.In cooperation with several hospitals we investigated the expression of P-glycoprotein in more than 100 human tumors of different origin using immunohistochemical methods. We found an increase of P-glycoprotein expression in tumors

where patients had been treated with drugs implicated in the development of MDR. These studies suggested that P-glycoprotein over-expression might be related to clinical resistance to chemotherapy (Volm et al. Eur. J. Cancer. Clin. Oncol. 25:743, 1989). There are currently only a few reports involving only small numbers of patients relating P-glycoprotein expression in human tumors to clinical response to antineoplastic drugs (Chan et al., J. Clin. Oncol. 8: 689, 1990; Verelle et al., J. Natl. Cancer Inst. 83: 111, 1991). Therefore, the significance of P-glycoprotein as a prognostic factor remains to be evaluated in controlled prospective clinical studies.
Interestingly, there exists a remarkable parallel between the biochemical changes with multidrug resistance and carcinogen resistance. The most frequently reported alteration in multidrug resistant cells, the overexpression of P-glycoprotein, is also found in both pre-neoplastic and neoplastic lesions produced by carcinogens (Thorgeirsson et al., Science 236:1120,1987). We induced rat hepatocellular carcinomas with N-nitrosomorpholine. After treatment with the carcinogen for several weeks, administration was stopped and the animals were maintained without carcinogen for a further one and half years. In our experiment, specific carcinogen-induced alterations could be separated from non-specific, toxic changes. P-glycoprotein was increased in hepatocellular carcinoma and these results were confirmed by immunoblotting. A significant increase in mdr1-gene transcripts was also found in hepatocellular carcinomas as compared to normal liver (Volm et al. Carcinogenesis 11:169, 1990).
Since human lung cancers are predominantly caused by combined action of multiple carcinogens (cigarette smoking), we investigated firstly whether lung tumors of smokers tend to be chemoresistant more frequently than tumors occuring in non-smokers and secondly whether there exists a correlation between expression of P-glycoprotein and smoking habits of the patients. Overall carcinomas of smokers tended to be resistant more frequently (81%) than carcinomas of non-smokers (52%). When the analysis was restricted only to those patients with epidermoid lung carcinomas 91% of the tumors of smokers were resistant compared to 50% of non-smokers tumors (p<0.001). In addition, in the analyses for the presence of P-glycoprotein a significant relationship was found between smoking habits of the patients and P-glycoprotein-expression. Furthermore, a significant relationship exists between resistance and expression of P-glycoprotein.
Modulation of P-glycoprotein expression offers new strategies to improve treatment and different reports have shown that a variety of compounds are capable of reversing multidrug resistance (e.g. calcium channel blockers, calmodulin inhibitors, local anesthetics, synthetic isoprenoids) (for review see Ford and Hait, Pharmacol. Rev. 42:155, 1990). The most compelling evidence suggests that reversing substances act by directly affecting the function of P-glycoprotein. Certain "chemosensitizers" have been shown to bind directly to membranes enriched for P-glycoprotein, and this binding was inhibited by other chemosensitizers and by chemotherapeutic drugs. We have analyzed a panel of substances which are capable of overcoming MDR and which share common structural features, namely, a tertiary nitrogen and an aromatic ring system. In this context we were able to identify two new chemosensitizers whose resistance-modifying capability has not been described so far: Hycanthone and chlorophenoxamine. By flow cytometry we were able to show that the reversal of both of these substances is caused by an increase of drug-accumulation in resistant

cells. In spite of the apparent successes in overcoming multidrug resistance in vitro, the question remains open as to which of this potentially wide assortment of chemicals might be the most suitable candidate(s) for use in patients. Pilot studies with some of these substances have shown severe side effects in patients. The presence of P-glycoprotein in normal tissues such as liver, colon and kidney raises the question whether P-glycoprotein expressing normal cells might also show enhanced toxicity (e.g. in liver, kidney) when they are treated by combination of cytostatics and reversing substances. We examined, therefore, whether "chemosensitizers" can also enhance the cytotoxicity of anticancer drugs to P-glycoprotein-positive primary human kidney cells as it does to human kidney carcinoma cells (Volm et al., Cancer 67:2484, 1991). Indeed, the resistance of both P-glycoprotein expressing normal and malignant kidney cells could be reversed by "chemosensitizers". In contrast, the cytostatic effect of anticancer drugs was not enhanced in P-glycoprotein-negative normal kidney and kidney carcinomas. Thus, reversal of primary resistance is not limited to tumor cells. These findings could have important implications for the use of resistance modifiers in the clinical setting.
In an effort to devise an effective treatment for drug-resistant tumors we have evaluated the therapeutic potential of monoclonal antibodies against P-glycoprotein with regard to its ability to inhibit growth of MDR cells. Furthermore, we have constructed an immunotoxin by coupling ricin-α-chain to antibodies. We have shown that only resistant cells are inhibited by antibodies and antibody-toxin conjugates. Future experiments must investigate whether antibodies and immunotoxins also inhibit P-glycoprotein in resistant normal cells.
In response to toxic insults P-glycoprotein expression can be induced within a few hours. In spite of an increase in the level of P-glycoprotein, cells sometimes did not reveal increased resistance to drugs or decreased accumulation of drugs (Mickley et al., J. Biol. Chem. 264: 18031, 1989). Similar results were also found in our laboratory. Whether this has any clinical significance remains to be determined.
Multidrug resistance is a phenotype most commonly associated with the overexpression of P-glycoprotein but other genes may contribute to this phenotype (e.g. glutathione-S-transferase, topoisomerase II). Therefore, the significance of P-glycoprotein as a prognostic factor remains to be evaluated in controlled prognostic clinical studies.

German Cancer Research Center, Institute of Experimental Pathology, Im Neuenheimer Feld 280, W-6900 Heidelberg

S35

IMMUNOPHARMACOLOGY AND IMMUNOTOXICOLOGY: INTRODUCTION
K. Resch, and M. Szamel

Immunopharmacology possesses two sides of the same coin.
Firstly it comprises all pharmacological maneuvers   to
interfere with the function of the immune system. Among
these immunosuppressive drugs have gained great importance
in the treatment of autoimmune diseases or chronic inflammatory disorders, as well as in allowing succesful transplantation of allogeneic organs or cells. Until recently,
immunosuppressive drugs were mostly cytotoxic such as
cyclophosphamid. Because of the large diversity of lymphocytes (10^6-10^8) competitive antigen receptor antagonists
are not feasible. With cyclosporin A drugs have been introduced which like glucocorticoids, but rather selectively,
inhibit the activation of predominantly T-lymphocytes, by
suppressing the synthesis of lymphokines such as inter-
leukin-2 (IL-2) involved in the activation cascade.
The molecular mechanisms whereby cyclosporin A (CyA) or
FK 506 affect IL-2 gene expression will be subsequently
discussed by E. Serfling. Both drugs also inhibit signal
transduction of the antigen receptor of T-lymphocytes. The
induction of IL-2 requires as crucial event a long lasting
activation of a protein kinase C (PKC) isoenzyme, whereas
for the expression of IL-2 receptors a short term activation
is sufficient (1,2). Both, CyA and FK 506, suppress selectively the long lasting PKC activation, and concomitantly
IL-2 synthesis; whereas both IL-2 receptor expression and
short term PKC activation are resistant to both immunosuppressive drugs. CyA inhibits an increase of polyunsaturated
fatty acids in membrane phosphatidylcholine (PC) of stimulated T-lymphocytes, which becomes substrate for a PC
specific phospholipase C generating diglycerides in a
sustained fashion (3).
Cytokines such as IL-2 bind to specific membrane receptors.
Interestingly, truncated soluble receptors containing only
the extracellular binding domain have been found, which
compete with cellular receptors for the binding of their
cytokine. Molecular cloning has allowed to exploit these
receptors as immunosuppressive drugs which will be reviewed
by S. Gillis.
Secondly, products of the immune system may be used as drugs.
This possibility has long been known in the case of immuno-
globulin preparations, which can substitute in deficiency
diseases, but, more recently, have also proven useful to
control some autoimmune diseases by putatively their content
of anti-idiotypic antibodies which block autoantibodies.
Monoclonal antibodies are used increasingly as drugs; ranging
from those affecting cells of the immune system and thus
being immunosuppressive to others used for cell specific
targetting of e.g. cytostatic drugs.
Immune reactions require the participation of several cells,
including T- and B-lymphocytes, macrophages, granulocytes or
even platelets. A plethora of protein factors, termed cytokines, control the differentiation and activation of these
cells, or mediate important effector functions. Some of these
including interferons, IL-2, tumor necrosis factor, or the
colony stimulating factors (CSF) are increasingly used as
drugs in a number of clinical situations, ranging from
immunodeficiency diseases to treatment of malignant tumors.
As an example the prospects of the powerful CSFs will be
discussed in the presentation of K. Welte.
The interaction of xenobiotics with target organs such as
liver, generally results in loss of function, if these xenobiotics reach toxic concentrations. With the immune system
- and thus immunotoxicology - again reactions can be am-
biguous. Like with other organs, cells can be destroyed, resulting in immunodeficiency. For some environmental toxins,
the developing immune system appears to be exquisitely sensitive. As an example, the effectiveness of dioxin on the
human immune system will be discussed by W.F. Greenlee. As,
however, regulatory cells may be the predominant target of
toxic xenobiotics, the outcome can be the opposite such as
the induction of autoimmune disorders.
The function of the immune system is the recognition and
subsequent elimination of foreign substances. Thus the
immune system not only can be disturbed by xenobiotics but
- in contrast to other organ systems - it can actively

react to those as antigens, which are the by far predominant
consequences of immunotoxicants. This can lead to allergy or
autoimmune diseases. The mechanisms involved will be analyzed by E. Gleichmann.

1) M. Szamel, B. Rehermann, B. Krebs, R. Kurrle, and
K. Resch
Activation signals in human lymphocytes. Incorporation
of polyunsaturated fatty acids into plasma membrane
phospholipids regulates interleukin-2 synthesis via
sustained activation of protein kinase C.
J. Immunol. 143, 2806-2813 (1989)
2) M. Szamel, M. Kracht, B. Krebs, J. Hübner, and K. Resch
Interleukin 2 synthesis and expression of high affinity
interleukin 2 receptors require different signalling for
the activation of protein kinase C.
Cellular Immunol. 126, 117-128 (1990)
3) M. Szamel, B. Rehermann, U. Hübner, and K. Resch
Inhibition of T-cell activation by cyclosporin A: inhibition of IL-2 Synthesis via prevention of sustained activation of protein kinase C by interference with the plasma
membrane phospholipid metabolism.
J. Immunol., submitted

Institute of Molecular Pharmacology, Medical School Hannover,
D-3000 Hannover 61, Germany

Department of Pharmacology and Toxicology, Institute of
Molecular Pharmacology, Medical School Hannover,
D-3000 Hannover 61, FRG

S36

THE ACTION OF IMMUNOSUPPRESSIVES CYCLOSPORIN A AND FK 506 ON THE EXPRESSION OF LYMPHOKINE GENES IN T LYMPHOCYTES

E. Serfling, I. Pfeuffer and T. Brabletz

Cyclosporin A (CsA), a product of the fungus Tolypocladium inflatum, is a cyclic oligopeptide that is widely used in transplantation medicine. Due to its selective inhibitory effect on the synthesis of lymphokines it suppresses adaptive immune responses after organ transplantation, thus preventing graft rejections (Ref. 1). FK 506, a macrolide isolated from Streptomyces tsukubaensis, exhibits an immunosuppressive activity similar to CsA, though it is structurally unrelated to CsA. Since FK 506 is about 100fold more potent in its immunosuppressive action than CsA, it will probably be used in place of CsA in transplantation medicine (2). Detailed experimental studies have shown that CsA and FK 506 inhibit the transcription of the same set of genes involved in the early activation of T lymphocytes. Among these genes are the lymphokine genes Interleukin 2 (Il−2), Il−3 and Il−4, the gamma interferon, GM−CSF and TNF−α genes (3).

The inducible, T lymphocyte−restricted transcription of the murine Il−2 gene is controlled by a 275 base pair long transriptional enhancer element located within its immediate upstream region (4). This enhancer spans the majority of DNA sequences necessary for the T lymphocyte−specific induction of the Il−2 gene by mitogens. As shown in Fig. 1, the Il−2 enhancer is bound by a

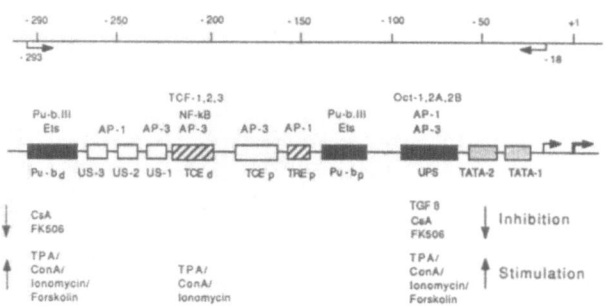

Fig. 1. Scheme of the transcriptional Enhancer of murine Interleukin 2 gene.

The position of the most prominent binding sites of Il-2 enhancer is indicated by boxes. The filled boxes indicate the CsA- and FK 506-sensitive proto-enhancer elements, the distal and proximal Purine boxes, Pu-b$_d$ and Pu-b$_p$, and the upstream promoter sequences, UPS. The dashed boxes indicate the CsA- and FK5 506-insensitive proto-enhancer elements, i.e. the distal T cell element, TCEd, and the proximal TPA responsive element, TREp. The inactive proximal T cell element, TCEp, and the upstream sites, US-1, US-2 and US-3 (the proto-enhancer activity of those has not been tested so far) are indicated by open boxes. The two TATA boxes are indicated by stippled boxes. The activity of Pu-b$_p$ and TREp has been identified with point mutations and deletion mutants, but not in proto-enhancer tests.

variety of ubiquitous and lymphocyte−specific transacting factors, and it is assumed that the cooperative activity of these factors controls the enhancer's activity in T lymphocytes. In order to elucidate the effect of CsA and FK 506 on the activity of single Il−2 enhancer factors, the most prominent factor binding sites

were chemically synthesized, cloned in multiple copies in front of a bacterial CAT indicator gene and tested in transient transfection assays in El4 T lymphoma cells. The inducible activity of the entire Il−2 enhancer and of two enhancer elements, i.e. the distal Purine box, Pu−b$_d$, and the upstream promoter sequence, UPS, was inhibited by low doses of CsA and FK 506. The activity of other enhancer elements, however, remained unaffected by both drugs (5, 6).

The Purine box and UPS motifs show different patterns of DNA binding factors. In nuclear extracts of induced El4 cells we detected one prominent factor binding to both Purine boxes (6). This factor, designated as Pu−box factor III (or NFAT I, see ref. 7), appears to be restricted to lymphoid cells and is rapidly induced upon activation of T cells. Its appearance is specifically blocked by low doses of CsA and FK 506 (5−7). The UPS motif, on the other hand, represents a binding site for Octamer (and AP−1 like) factors. In nuclear extracts of El4 cells, both the ubiquitous Octamer factor Oct−1 and the lymphoid−specific factors Oct−2A and 2B (which are transcribed from the same gene) bind to UPS DNA. In contrast to the Pu−box factor III, the Octamer factors also occur in unstimulated El4 cells, and CsA as well as FK 506 are without any influence on the DNA binding activity of factors. This demonstrates that CsA and FK 506 do not interfer with the occurrence or DNA binding of Octamer factors, but with the establishment of their transacting activity.

CsA and FK506 are bound by cytoplasmic receptor proteins (8, 9). Although the binding proteins of both drugs differ in their chemical structure, they exhibit the same enzymatic activity, i.e. they act as cis−trans peptidyl−prolyl isomerases. Recently, it was found that the FK 506 binding protein corresponds in its sequence to PKC I 2, a cytoplasmic inhibitor of protein kinase C (PKC) (10). This finding suggests that the binding of FK 506 (and CsA) to its cytoplasmic receptor(s) interferes with the activation of T cells via the PKC signal pathway. Candidates for PKC−mediated phosphorylation events are the Octamer factors, in particular Oct−2. For Oct−2 a direct correlation between the state of phosphorylation and its transacting potential has been demonstrated (11), and it is tempting to speculate that FK 506 and CsA impair the phosphorylation of Oct−2. This effect must be T cell−specific, because CsA and FK 506 are without any effect on the activity of Octamer factors in B cells.

References

1. Kahan,B.D. (1989) New England J. Medic. 321, 1725−1738.
2. Macleod,A.M. and Thomson,A.W. (1991) Lancet 337, 25−27.
3. Tocci,M.J., Matkovich,D.A., Collier,K.A., Kwok,P., Dumont, F., Lin,S., Degudicibus,S., Siekierka,J.J., Chin,J. and Hutchinson,N.I. (1989), J. Immunol. 143, 718−726.
4. Serfling,E., Barthelmäs,R., Pfeuffer,I., Schenk,B., Zarius,S., Mercurio,F. and Karin,M. (1989) EMBO J. 8, 465−473.
5. Randak,C., Brabletz,T., Hergenröther,M., Sobotta,I. and Serfling,E. (1990) EMBO J. 9, 2529−2536.
6. Brabletz,T., Pietrowski,I. and Serfling,E. (1991) Nucl. Acids Res. 19, 61−67.

7. Emmel,E.A., Verweij,C.L., Durand,D.B., Higgins,K.M., Lacy,E. and Crabtree,G.R. (1989) Science 226, 1439 – 1441.

8. Siekierka,J.J., Hung,S.H.Y., Poe,M., Lin,C.S. and Sigal,N.H. (1989) Nature 341, 755 – 757.

9. Tropschug,M., Wachter,E., Mayer,S., Schonbrunner,E.R. and Schmid,F.X. (1990) Nature 346, 674 – 677.

10. Goebl,M.G. (1991) Cell 64, 1051 – 52.

11. Tanaka,M. and Herr,W. (1990) Cell 60, 375 – 386.

Institut für Virologie und Immunbiologie der Universität Würzburg, Versbacher Str. 7, D – 8700 Würzburg, F.R.G.

S38

HEMATOPOIETIC GROWTH FACTORS K. Welte

Hematopoiesis is regulated by a complex network of cells and cytokines which maintain an enormous daily production of blood cells. These cytokines belong to a growing familiy of glycoproteins which regulate self-renewal, proliferation and maturation of hematopoietic progenitor cells, and functions of mature blood cells. Based on their in vitro activities to support the growth of colonies of blood cells in semisolid agar cultures they are also known as "Colony-stimulating-factors" (CSFs). Each of the CSFs has both unique and overlapping biological activities (Metcalf, D., Nature 339: 27, 1989). For example, stem cell factor (SCF), Interleukin 3 (IL-3), and Granulocyte-Macrophage-CSF (GM-CSF) stimulate proliferation and differentiation of multipotent progenitor cells, while Granulocyte-CSF (G-CSF), Macrophage-CSF (M-CSF) and Erythropoietin are limited to unipotent precursors of neutrophils, macrophages, and erythrocytes, respectively. Each of these hematopoietic growth factors are currently under investigations in preclinical animal studies and clinical studies (Andreeff, M., Welte, K. Seminars in Oncology 16: 211, 1989). IL-3, GM-CSF and G-CSF can accelerate reconstitution of myelopoiesis following cytotoxic chemotherapy in cancer patients or in patients post bone marrow transplantation. Therefore, they may allow dose escalation of chemotherapeutic agents in the future. Erythropoietin has been shown to correct anemia in chronic kidney failure patients. G-CSF corrects neutropenia and associated clinical symptoms in patients with congenital neutropenia and idiopathic neutropenia. The in vivo activities, toxicities, and clinical uses of CSFs will be considered.

Medizinische Hochschule Hannover, D-3000 Hannover 61, FRG

S37

RECOMBINANT CYTOKINE RECEPTORS: IMMUNOSUPPRESSIVE EFFECTS IN VIVO AND IN VITRO
S. Gillis, Seattle/USA

Abstract not received.

S39

STUDIES ON THE ACTION OF DIOXIN AND RELATED COMPOUNDS ON CELL AND MOLECULAR TARGETS WITHIN THE IMMUNE SYSTEM. W.F. Greenlee*, and T.R. Sutter‡

Background

2,3,7,8-Tetrachlorodibenzo-p-dioxin (TCDD or dioxin) and related compounds can act on specific target cell populations within the immune system to produce a spectrum of age-dependent lesions: thymus atrophy and suppressed cell-mediated immunity in young animals (Vos, 1977); and, suppressed humoral immunity in adult animals (Mantovani et al, 1980; Vecchi et al, 1980). In humans the potential adverse actions produced by dioxin on the immune system appear to be more specific and less severe than in animals. The observed actions of dioxin on immune system target cells are mediated by a specific intracellular receptor protein (designated the TCDD or Ah receptor) (reviewed in Wierda and Greenlee, 1991).

The Receptor Pathway

The major components of the dioxin receptor pathway operating in these and other target cells include recognition (reversible, high affinity binding of dioxin to the Ah receptor); transduction (activation of the dioxin-receptor complex resulting in the binding of the activated complex to specific DNA recognition elements); and response (regulation of specific target genes). It has been proposed that specific target genes under control of the Ah receptor include genes regulating cell growth and differentiation in skin and liver, as well as in organs within the immune system including the thymus and bone marrow (Poland and Knutson, 1982; Greenlee et al, 1987). Functional outcomes of the dioxin-dependent actions on these putative target genes in immune system target cells are postulated to include the alterations in B- and T-lymphocyte maturation characteristic of dioxin immunotoxicity.

Isolation of Novel Dioxin-Responsive Genes

To identify and isolate the postulated growth regulatory genes under control of the Ah receptor, a response-specific cloning strategy was developed in our laboratory (Sutter et al, 1991a). The cell model chosen was a subclone (designated SCC12Fc12c2) of a human squamous cell carcinoma line used to study the mechanisms of dioxin-induced hyperkeratinization and differentiation. Five dioxin-responsive cDNA clones were isolated which include the cDNA for the CYP1A1 gene (Sutter et al, 1991b). Two of the remaining clones were identified as a serine protease inhibitor and a cytokine, respectively. These genes have been shown to be involved in both inflammatory responses and growth regulation. Initial studies on the regulation of their expression indicate that in addition to dioxin, they are co-regulated by serum components, calcium, and protein synthesis inhibitors.

Research in progress on the characterization of the isolated dioxin-responsive clones is focused in three areas: sequencing and chromosome mapping, analysis of the mechanisms of regulation, and elucidation of their biological function and toxicological significance of their regulation by dioxin. Analysis of the actions of dioxin on these genes in immune system target cells may help elucidate the molecular mechanisms for the altered programming of B- and T-lymphocyte maturation produced by dioxin.

References

Greenlee, W.F., R. Osborne, K.M. Dold, L.G. Hudson, M.J. Young, and W.A. Toscano, Jr. (1987). Rev. Biochem. Toxicol. 8: 1.

Mantovani, A., A. Vecchi, W. Luini, M. Sironi, G.P. Canaiani, F., Spreafico, and S. Garattini (1980). Biomedicine 32: 200.

Poland, A. and J.C. Knutson (1982). Annu. Rev. Pharmacol. Toxicol. 22: 517.

Sutter, T.R., M.W. Andersen, J.C. Corton, K. Gaido, K. Guzman, and W.F. Greenlee (1991a). Banbury Report 35 (in press).

Sutter, T.R., K. Guzman, K.M. Dold, and W.F. Greenlee (1991b). Toxicologist 11: 988.

Vecchi, A., A. Mantovani, M. Sironi, W. Cairo, and S. Garattini (1980). Chem. Biol. Interact. 30: 337.

Vos, J.G. (1977). CRC Crit. Rev. Toxicol. 5: 67.

Wierda, D. and W.F. Greenlee (1991). In Principles and Practice of Immunotoxicology, Blackwell Scientific Pub., London (in press).

*Department of Pharmacology and Toxicology, Purdue University, West Lafayette, IN 47907. ‡Department of Environmental Health Sciences, The Johns Hopkins University, Baltimore, MD 21205

S40

AUTOIMMUNITY AND ALLERGY INDUCIBLE BY HEAVY METALS (Au, Hg. Pt): ROLES OF T CELLS, MACROPHAGES, AND CYTOKINES
E. Gleichmann*, M. Kubicka-Muranyi*, C. Stein*, B. Baginski**, H.-C. Schuppe***

Upon administration of relatively low doses of $HgCl_2$, certain mouse strains develop a systemic autoimmune disease. Susceptible strains carry the H-$2A^s$ allele, and $CD4^+$ T cells, presumably of the Th2 subset, are required for the development of disease. T cells of $HgCl_2$-treated mice react to unidentified self-protein(s) altered by Hg^{++}, and such immunogenic Hg-protein complexes are stored in macrophages. Adverse immune reactions similar to those observed in humans can also be induced by weekly i.m. injections into susceptible mice of antirheumatic gold(I) drugs. Both the pathlogical changes and their pathogenesis are very similar to those inducible by $HgCl_2$, an important difference being that gold(I) as such, unlike Hg^{++}, is incapabable of sensitizing T cells. We found, however, that T cells of mice treated with gold(I) responded in an anamnestic fashion to gold(III) respectively macrophages obtained from gold(I)-treated mice. This indiates that gold(I) is oxidized in vivo, presumably in phagocytes, to gold(III) and that the latter elicits adverse immune reactions. Unlike gold(I), gold(III) can irreversibly denature proteins. This property may not only provide the basis for the adverse immune reactions to gold, but also for its unknown pharmacological mechanism.

*Med. Inst. of Environmetal Hygiene, **Inst. of Hygiene, ***Dermatol. Clin., Heinrich Heine University of Düseldorf, Auf'm Hennekamp 50, D-4000 Düsseldorf

1

UNIQUE FLUORESCENT DIHYDROPYRIDINES: IN VIVO STAINING AND IN VITRO LABELING OF L-TYPE Ca^{2+} CHANNELS

T.Moshammer[1], H.-G.Knaus[1], K.Friedrich[1], H.-C.Kang[2], R.Haugland[2] and H.Glossmann[1]

Dihydropyridines (DHP) in radiolabeled form are useful, high affinity probes for L-type Ca^{2+}-channels and are widely employed. We have previously developed ^{125}I-labeled DHP's ([^{125}I]iodipine), ^{35}S-labeled compounds ([^{35}S]sadopine) and the photoaffinity ligand [^3H]azidopine (Glossmann and Striessnig, *Vitam.Horm.* **44**, 155 (1988), *Rev.Physiol.Biochem.Pharmacol.* **114**, 1, 1990). Here we report on the properties of a novel class of fluorescent DHP's (F-DHPs). F-DHPs were characterized with respect to their affinity for the DHP-selective domain of L-type Ca^{2+}-channels, optical properties and their ability to block [$^{45}Ca^{2+}$] influx in GH_3-cells. F-DHPs can be used to purify Ca^{2+} channels from e.g. skeletal muscle transverse tubular membranes using a standard purification protocol (Striessnig and Glossmann, *Meth.Neurosc.* **4**, 210-232, 1991), to study the interaction of competitive resp.allosteric regulators with the Ca^{2+}-channel, to investigate the kinetics as well as the equilibrium binding properties of L-type Ca^{2+}-channel-linked DHP receptors by simply measuring fluoresence. F-DHPs can therefore substitute for the radioactive ligands in almost any aspect. F-DHPs can also be used to visualize L-type Ca^{2+} channels *in vivo* e.g. on GH_3-cells. By employing the technique of enantioselective fluoresence labeling, absolute proof for L-type Ca^{2+}-channel interaction of the F-DHP ligands is provided with a pair of F-DHP's (eudismic ratio $\approx$ 40). The probes may be useful to study lateral mobility of L-type Ca^{2+}-channels by photobleaching recovery microscopy, appearance of L-type Ca^{2+} channels on *Xenopus* oocyte membranes and selection of clones which express L-type Ca^{2+}-channels. Supported by FWF (S45/01-Med and S45/02-Med).

[1] *Institut für Biochemische Pharmakologie, Peter Mayrstr. 1, A-6020 Innsbruck, Austria*
[2] *Molecular Probes, Inc., 4849 Pitchford Ave., Eugene, OR 97402, USA*

2

(±)[^3H]NITRENDIPINE BINDING TO MITOCHONDRIAL DIHYDROPYRIDINE RECEPTORS IN A CYTOSOL-RESEMBLING BUFFER

N.Reider and G.Zernig

Specific binding sites for dihydropyridine- (DHP) Ca^{2+} antagonists located on the inner mitochondrial membrane have been shown to be associated with an inner mitochondrial membrane anion channel; by inhibiting its function, certain Ca^{2+} antagonists might prevent Ca^{2+} overload of ischemically stressed mitochondria (Zernig et al 1990, Mol.Pharmacol. **38**:362). To further determine if binding to the mitochondrial sites might be of relevance for the therapeutic actions of DHP Ca^{2+} antagonists under (patho)physiological conditions, we compared equilibrium binding of the DHP (±)-[^3H]nitrendipine (^3H-NTR) to mitochondrial membranes in a "cytosol-resembling buffer" (Burgess et al 1983, J.Biol.Chem. **258**:15336) to data obtained under optimized conditions. In a buffer containing 500 mM NaCl, 50 mM Tris/HCl (pH 7.4), and 0.1 mM PMSF, ^3H-NTR reversibly bound to mitochondrial membranes of guinea-pig liver with a K_D of 291 ± 42 nM (mean ± SEM, n=4) and a B_{max} of 0.16 ± 0.01 nmol/mg protein (determined according to Bradford 1976, Anal.Biochem. **72**:248), thus essentially confirming previously published results (K_D 586 ± 91 nM (n=11, B_{max} 0.14 ± 0.02 nmol/mg protein [according to Bradford], Zernig and Glossmann 1988, Biochem.J. **253**:49). In the "cytosol-resembling buffer" (20 mM NaCl, 100 mM KCl, 5mM $MgSO_4$, 0.96 mM NaH_2PO_4, 25 mM $NaHCO_3$, 1 mM EGTA, pH maintained at 7.2 by aeration with 5% CO_2 and 95% O_2), ^3H-NTR saturably bound with a K_D of 268 ± 41 nM (n=5) and a B_{max} of 0.010 ± 0.002 nmol/mg. Thus the affinity of ^3H-NTR for the mitochondrial receptors remained essentially unchanged under ionic conditions resembling those of the cytosol, whereas the number of binding sites was considerably decreased.

Supported by FWF grants P7492-MED and K0042-MED and Dr.Legerlotz foundation.

Institut für Biochemische Pharmakologie, P.Mayr-Str.1, A-6020 Innsbruck

3

INTERACTION AMONG CALCIUM-ANTAGONISTS: STUDIES AT THE SINGLE CALCIUM CHANNEL LEVEL AND IN ISOLATED GUINEA-PIG LEFT ATRIA.

S.Braun, N. Frey, and S. Herzig

Calcium-antagonists of different chemical classes are known to display allosteric interactions, when their binding is studied in isolated membranes. However, when the negative inotropic response in myocardial preparations is concerned, a potentiation can be observed, which is much larger (one order of magnitude) than expected.

Measurements of currents through cardiac L-type calcium channels in the presence of nitrendipine and/or bepridil support the idea that the two drugs interact at the same channel molecule, with one of them favouring channel inactivation, and therewith the binding and action of the other.

In isolated guinea pig atria, the interaction is not unique to the combination of bepridil and nitrendipine: bepridil also enhances (by 3- to 10-fold) the negative inotropic potency of nimodipine, nifedipine, (+)-Bay K 8644, and (+)-niguldipine, and (by < 2.5-fold) of (-)-niguldipine, (+)- and (-)-isradipine, and nisoldipine. The ability of bepridil to enhance the potency of nitrendipine is shared by its quaternary derivative CERM 11888 (β-((2-methylpropoxy)methyl)-N-phenyl-N-(phenylmethyl)-1-N-methyl-pyrrolidineethaneamine bromide), and by diltiazem, quinidine and propafenone, but not by nifedipine and gallopamil.

In sum, a combination of dihydropyridines and various non-selective calcium antagonists can lead to a functionally significant interaction.

Abt.Pharmakol.d.Univ., Hospitalstr.4, W-23 Kiel

4

IDENTIFICATION OF CARDIAC Ca^{2+}-CHANNEL SUBUNITS USING SKELETAL MUSCLE ANTIBODIES?

T. Schneider*, S. Freundner-Hagestedt*, W. Nastainczyk*, F. Hofmann**

Voltage activated Ca^{2+}-channels are localized in the plasma membrane of excitable cells and transduce electrical to chemical signals by raising the $[Ca^{2+}]_i$. The L-type Ca^{2+}-channel from T-tubular membranes of the rabbit skeletal muscle consists of four subunits: α_1 - (165 kDa), α_2- (175 kDa), β- (55 kDa) and γ-subunit (32 kDa). The α_1-subunit of the cardiac L-type Ca^{2+}-channel has an apparent M_r of 195 kDa. The cDNA of all mentioned subunits has recently been cloned.
Mono- and polyclonal antibodies were raised in mice against the four skeletal muscle subunits. Peptide-directed antibodies, recognizing a peptide sequence of the Ca^{2+}-channel, were raised in rabbits.
The crossreactivity against the bovine cardiac Ca^{2+}-channel subunits is used to determine the composition of the cardiac Ca^{2+}-channel complex. The different structural composition may reflect the different role in excitation contraction coupling and the specific channel regulation in cardiac and skeletal muscle.

*Medizinische Biochemie, Universität des Saarlandes, D-6650 Homburg/Saar, Germany,
**Institut für Pharmakologie und Toxikologie, TU München, Biedersteiner Straße 29, 8000 München 40, Germany

5

TRH INDUCES OPPOSITE EFFECTS ON CALCIUM CHANNELS IN PITUITARY CELLS BY TWO INDEPENDENT PATHWAYS

Maik Gollasch[*][+], Hermann Haller[#], Günter Schultz[+], and Jürgen Hescheler[+]

Thyrotropin-releasing hormone (TRH) stimulates pituitary secretion by steps involving a rise in the cytosolic Ca^{2+} concentration. Here we addressed to the different pathways by which Ca^{2+} is elevated in pituitary GH3 cells. Using the patch clamp technique in the whole cell configuration and Ba^{2+} as divalent charge carrier through Ca channels, TRH (1 μM) reduced the current by about 55 % in a reversible manner. This hormonal effect was prevented by intracellular infusion of GDPßS but not by pretreatment of the cells with pertussis toxin (PT). Since PT-insensitive G-proteins are known to mediate a hormone-stimulated, IP_3-mediated Ca^{2+} release from intracellular stores, we suppose that the inhibitory effect of TRH on Ba^{2+} currents through Ca channels is caused by the increased intracellular Ca^{2+}. In order to prevent a Ca^{2+} release-dependent inhibiton of Ca channels, we preincubated GH3 cells in a medium free of divalent charge carriers and measured the Na^+ current through Ca channels. When Fura-II was used as indicator for the cytosolic Ca^{2+} concentration, TRH induced a release from intracellular stores only once but had no effect on the intracellular Ca^{2+} concentration during further applications. In line with this observation, TRH reduced the Na^+ current through Ca channels on its first application, but stimulated the current upon the following applications by about 45 %. The stimulation was sensitive to GDPßS and was abolished by pretreatment of cells with PT, suggesting that the stimulatory action of TRH is mediated by a G-protein different from the one that couples the receptor to phosphatidylinositol 4,5-biphosphate hydrolysis.
In conclusion, the present data suggest that TRH increases the intracellular Ca^{2+} concentration by two interacting pathways, that release from intracellular stores causes a secondary blockage of Ca channels and that, especially with empty intracellular Ca^{2+} stores, Ca channels are stimulated *via* a PT-sensitive G-protein.

*Institut für Physiologie, Humboldt-Universität zu Berlin, 1040 Berlin, #Klinikum Steglitz, Abteilung für Innere Medizin, Freie Universität Berlin, 1000 Berlin 45, +Institut für Pharmakologie, Freie Universität Berlin, 1000 Berlin 33

6

TOLBUTAMIDE-SENSITIVITY OF THE ATP-DEPENDENT K^+ CHANNEL IN PANCREATIC B-CELLS: CONTROL BY CYTOSOLIC NUCLEOTIDES.

C.Schwanstecher, C.Dickel, and U.Panten

When applied to the cytosolic face of excised membrane patches of mouse B-cells, physiological concentrations of ADP enhance the K-ATP channel blocking potency of tolbutamide by more than tenfold. The aim of the present study was to gain insight into the mechanism of this ADP-effect. Nucleotides structurally related to ADP were added to the bath solution and the tolbutamide-induced inhibition of the K-ATP currents was measured using the inside-out configuration of the patch-clamp technique. When tested alone, neither nucleotides which increased the opening activity of the K-ATP channel (0.2 mmol/l 2'deoxyadenosine 5'-diphosphate (dADP) or 0.2 -1 mmol/l GDP) nor the channel inhibitor adenylyl-imidodiphosphate (AMP-PNP) (0.05 - 0.2 mmol/l) altered the channel-blocking potency of tolbutamide. However, when the bath solution was supplemented with combinations of channel inhibiting (AMP-PNP 0.05 - 0.2 mmol/l) and channel activating nucleotides (dADP 0.2 mmol/l or GDP 0.2 - 1 mmol/l), the tolbutamide-sensitivity was strongly enhanced. The results suggest that enhancement of tolbutamide-sensitivity requires the simultaneous presence of channel activating and channel inhibiting nucleotides. Most probably ADP regulates tolbutamide-sensitivity by simultaneously occupying an inhibiting (free ADP) and an activating (MgADP) receptor site at the cytosolic face of the B-cell membrane.

Institut für Pharmakologie und Toxikologie, Universität Göttingen, Robert-Koch-Str. 40, D-3400 Göttingen

7

SULFONYLUREA-SENSITIVE POTASSIUM CHANNELS AND THEIR PROBABLE ROLE FOR THE RESTING MEMBRANE POTENTIAL OF MOUSE MOTOR NERVE ENDINGS

Max Deist, Holger Repp & Florian Dreyer

K^+ channels modulated by changes in intracellular ATP-concentration exist in a variety of different cell types including pancreatic β-cells, cardiac myocytes and skeletal and smooth muscle cells. Antidiabetic sulfonylureas like tolbutamide and glibenclamide specifically block these ATP-dependent K^+ channels and have become valuable tools for their identification and characterization. Recently, ATP-dependent K^+ channels have also been identified in the mammalian central nervous system (Ashford et al., Br. J. Pharmacol. 101:531-540, 1990) and in amphibian peripheral nerve fibres (Jonas et al., Pflügers Arch. 418:68-73, 1991). The aim of our work was to collect evidence for the existence of ATP-dependent K^+ channels in mammalian motor nerve endings and for their possible role in modulating transmitter release. Therefore, we studied the influence of tolbutamide and glibenclamide on presynaptic membrane currents in the M. triangularis sterni preparation. Using the subendothelial recording technique (Penner & Dreyer, Pflügers Arch. 406:190-197, 1986), we observed that both sulfonylureas were able to block part of the fast K^+ current in mouse motor nerve terminals. This effect was much more pronounced in glucose-free bath solution. Moreover, with a delay of 5 - 10 min after sulfonylurea-application the frequency of spontaneous quantal transmitter release increased dramatically. Our results strongly suggest that ATP-dependent K^+ channels exist in mammalian motor nerve endings. We hypothesize that the block of these ATP-dependent K^+ channels leads to depolarization of motor nerve terminals thus indicating that this type of K^+ channel is involved in the maintenance of the resting membrane potential.

Rudolf-Buchheim-Institut für Pharmakologie der Justus-Liebig-Universität Gießen, Frankfurter Straße 107, D-6300 Gießen

8

RELAXING EFFECTS OF POTASSIUM CHANNEL OPENERS ON SMOOTH MUSCLE OF KIDNEY PELVIS AND URETER

E. Klaus, H. Englert, M. Hropot, D. Mania, R. Rajagopalan[*], and U. Zwergel[**]

Potassium channel openers (PCOs) relax smooth muscle cells of various organs. In this study, the effects of PCOs on the upper urinary tract were investigated in search of new and selective spasmolytics for an improvement in the treatment of renal colic.
The phasic rhythmic contractions induced by 20-80 mmol/l KCl in isolated rabbit and guinea-pig ureter preparations were diminished by cromakalim and the novel PCO S 0121 ((-)-(3R, 4S, 5'R)-6-Cyano- 3,4 -dihydro- 2,2 -dimethyl- 4 -(2'-oxo-5'-methyl-1'-pyrrolidinyl)-2H-benzo[b]pyran-3-ol). The inhibition of the force and of the frequency of contractions was almost complete at 10^{-5} mol/l. Using microelectrode techniques, cromakalim (5·10^{-7} mol/l) was shown to cause hyperpolarisation in the membrane of ureteral smooth muscle cells (11.3 ± 2.3 mV) as in vascular smooth muscle cells of pulmonary artery (20.6 ± 3.3 mV). S 0121 showed only moderate hyperpolarising activity (3.8 ± 1 mV in ureteral and 13.0 ± 1.3 mV in vascular smooth muscle cells).
Strips of human ureters and renal pelvis obtained after radical nephrectomy (renal cell carcinoma patients) were depolarised with 80 mmol/l KCl. Cromakalim and S 0121 were added cumulatively from 10^{-8} to 10^{-5} mol/l and the resulting tension was recorded. The relaxing effect of S 0121 was shown to be stronger compared to that of cromakalim.
In anaesthetised dogs with one clamped ureter the intraluminal ureteral pressure was decreased after application of PCOs. This relaxant action *in vivo* was more pronounced for S 0121 (100 μg/kg i.v.) than for cromakalim (10 μg/kg i.v.) which are equi-effective doses with respect to blood pressure lowering effects.
In conclusion, these data indicate that PCOs can potently relax smooth muscle of the upper urinary tract.

Hoechst AG, P.O.B. 800320, D-6230 Frankfurt am Main, FRG, [*]Hoechst India Ltd., P.O.B. 7755, Mulund, Bombay 400080, India, and [**]Urol. Universitätsklinik, D-6650 Homburg-Saar, FRG

9

SK&F 96365 (1-{ß-[3-(4-METHOXYPHENYL)PROPOXY]-4-METHOXYPHENETHYL}-1H-IMIDAZOLE HYDROCHLORIDE) INHIBITS A Ca^{2+}-ACTIVATED K CHANNEL IN THE MEMBRANE OF AORTIC ENDOTHELIAL CELLS.
K. Groschner, W. F. Graier and W.R. Kukovetz

SK&F 96365 is known to inhibit receptor-mediated Ca^{2+} entry in a variety of tissues including vascular endothelium. Since Ca^{2+} entry is governed not only by the activity of Ca^{2+} permeable ion channels but also by the membrane potential, we have investigated the effects of SK&F 96365 on K^+ channels of endothelial cells which, for a large part, control the membrane potential.
Inside-out patches were excised from the membrane of cultured pig aortic endothelial cells. In about 50% of the patches, K^+ channels with a slope conductance of 12 pS at 0 mV (K^+ gradient: 5.4/137 mmol/l) were observed. These channels were apparently insensitive to voltage but channel activity was clearly dependent on the Ca^{2+} concentration at the cytoplasmic side. Open probability increased with Ca^{2+} concentrations in the range of 10^{-7} - 10^{-4} mol/l. Addition of SK&F 96365 (3 - 100 μmol/l) to the solution facing the cytoplasmic side of the patches reduced channel activity. At 10^{-5} mol/l Ca^{2+} (0 mV), 30 μmol/l SK&F 96365 reduced open probability of the channels by 53 ± 7 % (N=3) and complete inhibition was obtained with 100 μmol/l SK&F 96365.
The K^+ channel described above, might well contribute to the maintenance of a negative membrane potential and thus a high driving force for Ca^{2+} entry during agonist stimulation of endothelial cells. It is therefore concluded that SK&F 96365 may block Ca^{2+} entry into endothelial cells in part by inhibition of K^+ channels and consequent membrane depolarization.

Department of Pharmacology and Toxicology, University of Graz, Universitätspl. 2, A-8010 Graz, Austria. Supported by the Fonds zur Förderung der wissensch. Forschung (P7290).

10

HEXOPRENALINE AND CALCITONIN GENE RELATED PEPTIDE ACTIVATE CA^{++}-ACTIVATED K^+ CHANNELS IN THE HUMAN MYOMETRIUM
W. Mahnert, W. Schreibmayer, A. Fleischhacker, H.A. Tritthart and N. Adelwöhrer

The role of Ca^{++}-activated K^+ channels in the relaxant mechanism of human myometrium was studied and their regulation by hexoprenaline (a ß-adrenergic agonist of clinical importance in preventing preterm labor) and calcitonin gene related peptide (CGRP) was investigated. Small parts from the fundus and the corpus of vaginally dissected uteri were isolated (age of women 35-50 years). Strips of 1 cm length were cut and contraction isometrically measured. After 60 minutes equilibration at 37 °C and a resting tension of 10 mN spontaneous activity occured and experiments were performed. Single cells were isolated by enzymatic disaggregation with papain and collagenase. Electrophysiological experiments were performed using the patch clamp technique in the cell attached and excised inside out configurations.
Between -20 mV and +20 mV membrane potential we observed K^+-channels with a conductance of 158 pS. The reversal potential of single channel current was measured to be -70 mV ($[K^+]_o$: 5.4 mmol/l; $[K^+]_i$: 140 mmol/l). The channel was sensitive to the free calcium concentration on the cytoplasmic side and open propability (P_0) increased with membrane depolarization. 0.5 mmol/l ATP facing the cytoplasmic side of the patches (at 40 mV depolarization and pCa of 6) did not exert inhibition. Hexoprenaline and CGRP both increased the P_0 of Ca^{++}-activated K^+ channels in the cell attached mode at maintained depolarization. Forskolin failed to activate Ca^{++}-activated K^+ channels. Under isometric conditions the spontaneous acivity of human myometrial strips was suppressed by hexoprenaline (10^{-5} mol/l) and CGRP (10^{-7} mol/l). These effects were antagonized by 2 mmol/l tetraethylammoniumchloride (TEA). Blockade of phasic contractures by forskolin was antagonized by 3 mmol/l glibenclamide but not by TEA. Our results indicate that hexoprenaline and CGRP at the doses tested by us activate Ca^{++}-activated K^+ channels not via activation of adenylate cyclase.

Institute of Medical Physics and Biophysics, University of Graz, Harrachgasse 21/IV, A-8010 Graz, Austria
* Dept. of Gynecology and Obstetrics, University of Graz, Auenbruggerplatz 14, A-8036 Graz, Austria
Supported by the Austrian Science Research Fund (FWF,S4506)

11

ALTERATIONS OF MEMBRANE CURRENTS IN RAT MICROGLIAL CELLS DURING MATURATION
W. Nörenberg, P.J. Gebicke-Haerter and P. Illes

Resident microglial cells are thought to be the source of brain macrophages therefore playing an important role in inflammation and injuries affecting the central nervous system. In the majority of rat microglial cells (60 out of 66) in culture, examined 1 to 7 days after plating, the only voltage-dependent membrane current found under whole-cell clamp conditions was a hyperpolarization-evoked inwardly directed current showing inactivation during large hyperpolarizing voltage steps. The reversal potential was shifted with an increase of extracellular K^+ concentrations as predicted by the Nernst equation for K^+-selective channels. This together with the pronounced inwardly rectifying behaviour and the strong inhibitory effects of extracellularly applied potassium channel blockers (cesium chloride 1 mmol/l, tetraethylammonium chloride 10 mmol/l and barium chloride 0.1 mmol/l) characterize the current as classical potassium inward rectifier. The almost complete lack of other voltage-dependent currents in rat microglia (see also Kettenmann et al., J Neurosci 26:278, 1990), is in contrast to the current pattern found in cells pretreated either with lipopolysaccharide (LPS; 100 ng/ml) an inflammatory constituent of the cell wall of gramnegative bacteria or interferon γ (INF γ, 500 U/ml) a known macrophage activating factor. Similar changes were observed in cells incubated for one week in teflon bags; this measure induces maturation of peripheral monocytes into macrophages. All cells tested under one of these conditions (n=70) displayed in addition to the inward current, a prominent outward current upon membrane depolarization which was abolished by the potassium channel blockers quinine and 4-aminopyridine (1 mmol/l each) and also showed a close relation between reversal potential and K^+-equilibrium potential, thereby resembling the potassium outward currents found in peritoneal macrophages (Randriamampita & Trautmann, J Cell Biol, 105:761, 1987). Since it has been shown that phagocytosis in macrophages is accompanied by activation of in- and outward currents (Ince et al., J Cell Biol, 106:1873, 1988), the described alteration of the membrane current pattern in microglial cells might represent the electrophysiological correlate of the maturation process of microglial precursors to macrophages.

Department of Pharmacology, University of Freiburg, W-7800 Freiburg i. Br., F.R.G.

12

PROPERTIES OF THE $5-HT_3$-RECEPTOR ON N1E-115 NEUROBLASTOMA CELLS STUDIED BY GUANIDINIUM ION INFLUX
M. Barann, J. Graupner, M. Göthert and H. Bönisch

N1E-115 cells, which are known to possess the $5-HT_3$ receptor (Hoyer and Neijt Mol Pharmacol 33:303, 1987), and the ^{14}C-labelled organic cation guanidinium were used to study some properties of the cation channel-linked $5-HT_3$ receptor. Experiments were carried out with cells grown on 24-multiwell culture dishes, and a Ca^{++}- and Na^+-free buffer (Na^+ replaced by choline) was used as a standard condition. After 10-20 min preincubation cells were exposed for 2 min (at 36°C) to ^{14}C-guanidinium (5.5 uM) and thereafter the ^{14}C-content of the cells was determined.
5-HT up to 300 uM caused a concentration-dependent increase of the ^{14}C-guanidinium influx (EC_{50} 30 uM). A similar but less pronounced increase was observed with the $5-HT_3$ receptor agonists 1-(m-chlorophenyl)-biguanide, phenylbiguanide and 2-methyl-5-HT, whereas 5-methoxytryptamine was inactive. The response to 5-HT was antagonized by metoclopramide, by the specific $5-HT_3$ receptor antagonists ICS 205-930 ((3 α -tropanyl)-1H-indole-3-carboxylic acid ester), ondansetron and MDL 72222 (1 α H,3 α (5 α H-tropan-3-yl)3,5-dichlorobenzoate) and by tubocurarine.
In the presence of Ca^{++} (1.8 mM) the 5-HT-mediated guanidinium influx decreased to about 40% and in the presence of Ca^{++} and Na^+ (135 mM) to about 27% of that under the standard conditions. The 5-HT response (% of controls at 36°C) was temperature-dependent: about 300% at 20°C and about 60% at 4°C. Preincubation of the cells with 5-HT (100 uM, 0.5-16 min) caused a time-dependent decrease in the ^{14}C-guanidinium influx which was rapidly reversible; the decrease was fast at 36°C (t/2 = 0.5 min), slower at 20°C (t/2 = 2.5 min) and not detectable at 4°C. The results indicate that the ^{14}C-guanidinium influx is a useful tool to characterize the $5-HT_3$ receptor and that agonists, Ca^{++}, Na^+ and temperature influence the desensitization of the $5-HT_3$-receptor.

Department of Pharmacology, University of Bonn, Reuterstr. 2 b, D-5300 Bonn 1, Germany.

13

STEREOSELECTIVE BLOCK OF CARDIAC SODIUM CHANNELS BY THE ENANTIOMERS OF ASOCAINOL.
J. Gödicke and S. Herzig

The use-dependent block of sodium inward current caused by the (+)-and (-)-enantiomers of the antiarrhythmic agent asocainol was studied using the whole cell patch clamp technique in enzymatically isolated guinea-pig ventricular myocytes. Currents were measured at room temperature in cells (50-100pF) in 20 mM Na^+ containing external solution with pipette resistances ranging from 0.8 to 1 MΩ. Repetitive pulsing from a holding potential of -120 mV to -20 mV with varying test intervals (3s,2s,1s,0.4s,0.22s) in the presence of either (+)- or (-)-asocainol $3 \cdot 10^{-5}$ M led to a use-dependent blockade reaching significantly different levels. With the (+)-enantiomer, steady state block at the intervals tested ranged between 50 and 72%. The (-)-enantiomer was less effective, blockade ranged between 24 and 33%. The time course of onset of block was further analysed. A two-state model used previously by Clarkson (*Circ Res* 65: 1306, 1989) to characterize the stereoselectivity of sodium channel block by RAC 109 (N-diethylaminopropyl-tetralin-1-spirosuccinimide). Based on different rate constants and steady state blocks, constants for binding and unbinding could be calculated for two distinct states (depolarized and rested). Significant differences were obtained for both rate constants describing the depolarized state. Binding of (+)-asocainol [k_{+1} $2.4 \cdot 10^{5}$ $M^{-1}s^{-1}$] is more than 2 times faster than in case of (-)-asocainol [k_{+1} $1.1 \cdot 10^{5}$ $M^{-1}s^{-1}$]. With regard to unbinding, (+)-asocainol [k_{-1} 2.7 s^{-1}] is about 2 times slower than the (-)-form [k_{-1} 6.2 s^{-1}]. No significant differences, however, were found for the rested state. In summary, the differences in potency for inducing use-dependent block are mainly due to variations in affinity during the depolarized state (which in fact comprises binding to both, open and inactivated channels), because of differences in the two rate constants k_{+1} and k_{-1}.

Dept. Pharmacology, University Kiel, Hospitalstr.4, 2300 Kiel, Germany

14

LOCALIZATION OF THE BINDING DOMAIN OF THE INHIBITORY LIGAND FORSKOLIN IN THE GLUCOSE TRANSPORTER GLUT4
B. Hellwig, F.M. Brown, M.F. Shanahan, and H.G. Joost

Insulin-sensitive glucose transport in adipose and muscle tissue is predominantly mediated by a tissue specific transport protein, GLUT4. Ligands of this transporter, namely cytochalasin B, the diterpene forskolin, and several methylxanthines, bind with high affinity to this glucose transporter and reduce its transport activity. These agents label a functionally significant domain of the glucose transporter, since their binding is competitively inhibited by D-glucose. In the present study, we identified a binding region of the inhibitory ligand forskolin with the aid of a photoreactive derivate of forskolin, ^{125}IAPS-forskolin (3-[^{125}I]Iodo-4-azidophenethylamido-7-O-succinyldeacetylforskolin). Plasma membranes obtained from adipocytes by differential centrifugation were irradiated with UV-light in the presence of ^{125}IAPS-forskolin. The covalently labeled GLUT4, a 48 kDa protein, was immunoprecipitated with specific antiserum and was partially digested with trypsin. After separation by denaturing polyacrylamide gel electrophoresis, we identified two labeled fragments of the glucose transporter with apparent molecular weights of 21 and 18 kDa. These fragments contained the intact C-terminus of the GLUT4, since they could also be detected by immunoblotting with antiserum against a peptide corresponding with the C-terminal sequence of the protein. In addition, the tryptic digestion generated a smaller fragment with intact C-terminus (15 kDa) as detected by immunoblotting. This fragment was not labeled by ^{125}IAPS-forskolin. It is concluded that forskolin binds within a region of the GLUT4 corresponding with the membrane spanning domains 7, 8, and 9 (amino acids 285-376).

Institut für Pharmakologie und Toxikologie der RWTH Aachen, Wendlingweg 2, D-5100 Aachen, FRG, and Department of Physiology, University of Southern Illinois Carbondale, Carbondale, USA.

15

EFFECTS OF PHOSPHORYLATION AND DEPHOSPHORYLATION OF THE GLUCOSE TRANSPORTER GLUT4 ON GLUCOSE TRANSPORT ACTIVITY IN ADIPOCYTES
A. Schürmann and H.G. Joost

Glucose transport in insulin-sensitive cells is primarily regulated by the adipose/muscle-type glucose transporter Glut4. It has previously been suggested that the intrinsic activity of the Glut4 is modified by phosphorylation. In the present study, we investigated the effects of protein phosphorylation and dephosphorylation on glucose transport activity reconstituted from adipocyte membrane fractions. In-vitro phosphorylation of plasma membranes and low-density microsomes in the presence of ATP and protein kinase A produced a stimulation of glucose transport activity provided that the cells had been treated with insulin prior to the isolation of the membranes. Conversely, the reconstituted transport activity was reduced after treatment of membranes from insulin-treated cells with alkaline phosphatase; no effect was observed in membranes from basal cells. A potential effect of insulin on the phosphorylation state of GLUT4 was studied in intact adipocytes equilibrated with [^{32}P]phosphate and subsequently incubated with insulin. Glucose transporters were isolated by immunoprecipitation. GLUT4 incorporated significant amounts of [^{32}P]phosphate in the basal state. Insulin failed to alter its phosphorylation state, whereas isoproterenol produced a moderate increase of [^{32}P]phosphate incorporation into Glut4. The present data suggest that the intrinsic activity of the Glut4 is modified by protein phosphorylation. This effect is indirectly controlled by insulin through an unidentified factor. However, the phosphorylation of the Glut4 does not appear to mediate the insulin-induced translocation of glucose transporters.

Institut für Pharmakologie und Toxikologie der RWTH Aachen, Wendlingweg 2, D-5100 Aachen, FRG.

16

NONHYDROLYZABLE GTP ANALOGS SUPPRESS 2-DEOXYGLUCOSE UPTAKE OF GLUT1 GLUCOSE TRANSPORTER-EXPRESSING OOCYTES
M. Wellner and K. Keller

Molecular cloning has led to the identification of five different glucose transporters of the facilitative diffusion type which according to the time of their publication are referred to as Glut1 through Glut5. Xenopus oocytes have been shown to faithfully translate, process and insert a number of proteins after the injection of heterologous mRNA. Using this expression system all different glucose transporter cDNA clones encode a functional glucose transport protein. Xenopus oocytes also proved to be extremely helpful in addressing the question to transport kinetics of an individual glucose transporter isoform. In addition, the cytoplasm of the oocyte can be altered by microinjetion of substrates/proteins and the regulatory response to such perturbation can then be studied. Here we studied the effect of coinjected non-hydrolyzable GTP analogs (i.e., GTPγS and GppNHp) on the glucose transporter activity that has been expressed from Glut1 cDNA under the control of the bacteriophage SP6 promoter of the pXOV vector. 2-Deoxyglucose uptake measurements on individual oocytes and Western blot analysis led to the following results:
1. Non-hydrolyzable GTP analogs cause an effective suppression of 2-deoxyglucose uptake.
2. The extent of inhibition is dependent on the intracellular concentration of the analog which can be determined rather precisely.
3. The inhibition is specific for GTP since ATP and GDP analogs are not effective.
4. The effect is on the uptake system and not on the translocation of glucose transporter from an intracellular pool.

Supported by the DFG
Institut für Pharmakologie, Freie Universität Berlin, Thielallee 69-73, 1000 Berlin 33

17

DUAL EFFECT OF SPERMINE ON MITOCHONDRIAL CALCIUM TRANSPORT

I. Rustenbeck, W. Münster, and S. Lenzen

The polyamine spermine in physiological concentrations lowers the external Ca^{2+} concentrations to which mitochondria respond to levels close to those present in the cytoplasm of resting cells. This effect has been attributed to an allosteric activation of the mitochondrial Ca^{2+} uniporter uptake system. Using a Ca^{2+}-sensitive minielectrode with a microincubation chamber in combination with a computerized data acquisition and evaluation system we could show that spermine exerts a dual effect on mitochondrial Ca^{2+} uptake of rat liver, heart, and brain. When the steady state of extramitochondrial free Ca^{2+} was lowered by 200 µM spermine from 0.44 µM to 0.26 µM, the initial velocity of Ca^{2+} uptake was not increased, but rather reduced to 66%. The half maximally effective concentrations of 50 µM for the former and 180 µM for the latter effect demonstrate that these are two distinct phenomena, one representing an enhanced accumulation capacity of the mitochondria, the other an inhibition of the transmembrane transport velocity. This second property puts spermine in line with other polycationic inhibitors of mitochondrial Ca^{2+} uptake. The presence of 0.5 mM Mg^{2+} further reduced the uptake velocity, while it did not influence the Ca^{2+} accumulation capacity. An antagonism between Mg^{2+} and spermine on the Ca^{2+} accumulation became apparent at higher concentrations of Mg^{2+}. Thus polyamine metabolism and Mg^{2+} provide a means of flexible coupling between cytoplasmic Ca^{2+} concentrations and mitochondrial Ca^{2+} transport.

Institut für Pharmakologie und Toxikologie, Universität Göttingen, D-3400 Göttingen

18

PHOSPHOLAMBAN PHOSPHORYLATION AND CALCIUM UPTAKE IN MICROSOMAL FRACTIONS FROM RABBIT AORTA

P. Karczewski and R. Vetter.

In vascular smooth muscle (VSM) sarcoplasmic reticulum (SR) calcium uptake is thought to contribute to vasodilation. Phospholamban (PLB) was shown to be present in the SR of various VSM types. It has been proposed that phosphorylation (PHOS) of PLB may control the SR calcium uptake in VSM. Crude microsomal fractions (CM) were prepared from rabbit aorta. In CM protein PHOS by exogenous cyclic AMP-dependent protein kinase (cAMP-PrK) and oxalate-supported calcium uptake was studied. Low molecular substrates of about 6, 19 and 21 kDa were phosphorylated by cAMP-PrK. The 6 kDa protein was identified as PLB by its molecular weight shift. There was no detectable endogenous PHOS of PLB. The mean value of CM calcium uptake was 1.4 nmole/min/mg of protein. Pretreatment of CM with 0.03 % digitonin decreased the calcium uptake by 35 %. Under phosphorylating conditions (in the presence of cAMP-PrK) calcium accumulation increased to maximally 124 % of controls. Under these conditions PHOS of PLB was found to be significantly elevated as detected by back-phosphorylation. The data are consistent with a role of PLB PHOS in the modulation of SR calcium uptake in VSM.

Institute of Cardiovascular Research, Robert-Rössle-Straße 10, O-1115 Berlin, Germany

19

ENHANCED SENSITIVITY OF BLOOD PLATELET CALCIUM-METABOLISM TO HALOTHANE IN MALIGNANT HYPERTHERMIA

H.S.Fink*, S.Maak, H.Hentschel & U.Till

Malignant Hyperthermia (MH) is a pharmacogenetic disorder which occurs in predisposed individuals exposed to volatile anaesthetics such as halothane. Recently, the susceptibility to MH was linked to the Ca release channel of the muscle sarcoplasmic reticulum (ryanodine receptor). We have shown that abnormalities in the regulation of cytosolic free Ca can also be detected in Quin2-loaded blood platelets from patients and pigs.

In human platelets suspended in a "Ca free" medium the resting level of cytosolic Ca was about 90 nM. Halothane (Hal) induces a dose-dependent, rapid Ca release from intracellular stores both in normal and in MH derived cells, but the resulting increase in cytosolic Ca is significantly higher in the latter (2 mM Hal: 117 ±12 nM vs. 218 ±117 nM; 4 mM Hal: 225 ±35 nM vs. 417 ±201 nM; $p < 0,001$). In order to determine the extracellular Ca influx the rise in cytosolic Ca caused by elevation of external Ca up to 1 mM was measured. Whereas the basal level only slightly increased in MH-platelets ($\Delta[Ca^{++}]_i = $ 41 ±10 nM vs. 48 ±23 nM) the Ca influx was significant higher in presence of halothane (2 mM Hal: $\Delta[Ca^{++}]_i = $ 69 ±12 nM vs. 135 ±63 nM; 4 mM Hal: 127 ±33 nM vs. 258 ±111 nM; $p < 0,001$).

To get a distinct value that combines several aspects of the platelet Ca homeostasis as well as the results obtained at different halothane concentrations the parameter SHCa (Sensitivity to Halothane of platelet Ca homeostasis) was introduced. This parameter allowed a good discrimination between MH-susceptible patients and controls. The use of genetically well-defined pigs rendered it possible to test the presented method. The rate of false positive and false negative results were about 4% and 3%, respectively. Moreover, a susceptibility to MH can also be detected in about two third of heterozygous animals.

* Present address: Institute of Pathological Biochemistry, Medical Academy of Erfurt, Nordhäuser Str. 74, O-5010 Erfurt, Germany

20

THROMBIN STIMULATION RAISES CYTOSOLIC FREE Na^+ IN HUMAN PLATELETS - STUDIES USING THE NOVEL FLUORESCENT DYE SBFI. W.Siffert, M.Borin.

Human platelets were loaded with the fluorescent Na^+ dye sodium-binding benzofuran isophtalate (SBFI) by incubation with its acetoxymethyl ester. Calibration of fluorescence in terms of $[Na^+]_i$ was done by measuring the 345/385 nm excitation ratio (em: 500 nm) at various $[Na^+]_0$ in the presence of gramicidin D. Basal $[Na^+]_i$ was 26 mM. Ouabain (0.5 mM) raised $[Na^+]_i$ to 56 mM within 1h. Activation of Na^+/H^+ exchange by exposing platelets to propionic acid also raised $[Na^+]_i$, an effect that could be mimicked by the Na^+ ionophore monensin. Transient acidification of platelets by storage in acidic (pH 6.7) buffer evoked a brief $[Na^+]_i$ transient upon resuspension of platelets into pH 7.4 medium. Stimulation of platelets with thrombin (0.5 U/ml) increased $[Na^+]_i$ by 16 mM in the presence of Ca^{2+}_0. In contrast to the transient rise in $[Na^+]_i$ following pH_i recovery from acidification, this latter $[Na^+]_i$ rise was sustained and $[Na^+]_i$ did not return to its resting value within 1 h after thrombin addition. This suggests a thrombin-mediated inhibition of the Na^+,K^+ ATPase. In the absence of Ca^{2+}_0, an additional thrombin-induced influx of Na^+ was noticed. This additional Na^+ influx could be prevented by Mn^{2+} and La^{3+}, i.e. ions which diminish receptor-mediated Ca^{2+} entry. This indicates that Na^+ can enter stimulated platelets via a Ca^{2+} influx pathway.

Max-Planck-Institut f. Biophysik, Kennedyallee 70, D-6000 Frankfurt/M. 70

21

THE AFFINITY OF DIFFERENT LOCAL ANESTHETIC DRUGS AND CATECHOLAMINES
TO THE CONTRALUMINAL TRANSPORT SYSTEM FOR ORGANIC CATIONS IN
PROXIMAL TUBULES OF RAT KIDNEYS
E. Brändle, G. Fritsch*, J. Greven, K.J. Ullrich*

The transport system for organic cations at the renal proximal tubules is an
important site for xenobiotic elimination. However, only a few
informations are available on the molecular requirement of a substance
which is transported by this system. To study the cellular uptake of ^{3}H-
TEA (tetraethylammonium) and its inhibition by different local anesthetic
drugs and catecholamines the capillary stopped flow microperfusion
method described by Ullrich et al (Pflügers Arch 400: 250-256, 1984) was
used. ^{3}H-TEA concentration in the peritubular capillaries decreased in a
time and concentration dependent manner. This cellular uptake of ^{3}H-TEA
could be described by a facilitated diffusion model [J_{max}=0.57±0.08
pmol*sec^{-1}*cm^{-1}, K_m=0.28±0.01 mmol/l]. Between the pK_a values of the
local anesthetic drugs [range: 2.8 and 8.9] and their app. K_i values a
significant correlation was found [r=-0.949, N=13]. Hydrophobic
substitution in form of an alkyl chain in alpha position or at the nitrogen
increased the inhibitory potency of the catecholamines, while hydroxyl
substitution in beta position decreased the affinity. In contrast, however,
the app. K_i values of catecholamines with complex substitutions at the
benzene ring (-CH_2OH,-$NHCONH_2$, -$OOCN[CH_3]_2$, -Cl,-NH_2] were not
directly correlated to the hydrophobicity. **Conclusions:** The hydrophobicity
and the pK_a value are two important physicochemical parameters, which
influence the affinity of a molecule to the transport system for organic
cations at the contraluminal side of renal proximal tubules. However the
different inhibitory potency of catecholamines with complex substitutions
at the benzene ring could not be explained by these parameters.

Address: Department of Pharmacology, Wendlingweg 2, 5100 Aachen,
* MPI für Biophysik, Kennedyallee 70, 6000 Frankfurt 70, Germany

22

INJURY OF BLOOD BRAIN BARRIER AFTER FREEZE LESION IN MICE:
TIME COURSE AND PHARMACOLOGICAL TREATMENT.
K.F. FUNK and M. BLASCHKE

A slight freeze lesion by application of a liquid nitrogen
cooled rod of 2 mm diameter on the scull for 15 sec causes
injury of the blood brain barrier (BBB) - measured by
penetration of injected dyes - , and induces local brain
edema - measured by increase of water content.
Both processes proceed with different time course showing
a very soon appearing maximum in dye penetration followed
by a later maximum in water increase. Dye penetration
seems to be independent from the molecular weight of the
dyes used as to be seen from the similar curves of the
protein bound EVANSBLUE and the free moving FLUORESCEIN.
The BBB-injury was nearly resistant to treatment with
cerebroprotective drugs. The same is to be stated about
the local brain edema by previous results.

Department of Pharmacology,
Medical Academy "Carl Gustav Carus" Dresden,
Karl-Marx-Str. 3   8080 DRESDEN

23

PROSTANOID BIOSYNTHESIS IN THE TISSUE OF DIFFERENT
ORGANS OR TUMORS AND THE INFLUENCE OF DRUGS
P. MENTZ, CH. GIESSLER, A. TAMPE, A. GÜNTHER, H.-
A. GITT", T. WALTHER", K. FRANK"

Prostanoids are substances occuring in many
tissues where they could be formed in different
amounts. Out of these mediators prostacyclin
(PGI_2) and thromboxane A_2 (TXA_2) are of
outstanding importance. The experiments dealt with
a comparison of tissue capacity for PG-
biosynthesis under special conditions. After a
short period (3 min) the incubation medium of
small tissue slices showed the following amounts
of prostanoids (pg/mg wet weight): PGI_2: 2-106, 6-
oxo-PGF_1alpha: 24-746, TXB_2: 16-284. The
analysis was performed by a specific and sensitive
enzyme immunoassay. Out of the investigated organs
stomach, lung and renal medulla showed a
relatively high PG-formation, while myocard, aorta
and skin had a low capacity of biosynthesis.
Sensibilization of the animals with ovalbumin and
addition of the antigen to the incubation medium
induced a 2-10 fold rise of the released PGs.
Malignant tumor growth of the skin is linked with
an enhanced PG-biosynthesis. Besides these
pathophysiological conditions drugs also may exert
an significant influence on PG formation.
Actovegin or insulin/glucose induced an increase
of the substances, while indomethacin , verapamil
and propranolol reduced the PG formation by the
organs. The results show, that the PG-biosynthesis
of different tissues may be influenced by
pathophysiological conditions and drugs with some
relevance for diagnosis and therapy.

Department of Pharmacology and Toxicology, Martin-
Luther-University, O-4020 Halle, Leninalle 4, FRG,
"Clinic of Dermatology, University Leipzig, O-
7010, Liebigstraße 21, FRG

24

MYOCARDIAL   BIOSYNTHESIS   OF   PROSTACYCLIN   AND
THRMBOXANE B_2 AND THE INFLUENCE OF CARDIAC LOADING
BY HYPOXIA AND DRUGS
P. MENTZ, K.E. PAWELSKI, CH. GIESSLER

Investigations in cardiac tissue of rats, guinea
pigs and rabbits indicate a close connection of
the heart action and the biosynthesis of
prostanoids. Auricles show a higher prostanoid
formation than ventricles. Arachidonic acid and
the endoperoxide PGH_2 stimulate the myocardial
formation of PGI_2 and TXB_2. Cardiac loading by
aortic stenosis, coronary ligation or pacing
induced a decrease of contractility and marked
changes in the stimulated and non stimulated PGI_2
biosynthesis of the tissue from auricles and
ventricles. Cardiac and antianginous drugs
increase the PGI_2 and TXB_2 formation under in
vitro conditions. On the other hand some
antianginous substances as well as indomethacin
and PGE_1 or iloprost inhibit the myocardial PG
formation and exert a protective effect against
cardiac damage. The changes in the prostanoid
biosynthesis may be due to an increased
availability of substrate, an alteration of enzyme
activity or the functional state of the heart. The
results show that the biosynthesis of the
investigated prostanoids in the myocardium may
play an important role in the regulation of the
functional state of the heart.

Department of Pharmacology and Toxicology, Martin-
Luther-University, Leninallee 4, O-4020 Halle/S.
FRG

25

EFFECT OF THE PGE_2 DERIVATIVE NOCLOPROST ON HUMAN PLATELET FUNCTION

E. Glusa, K. Jacobsen* and I. Amon*

Nocloprost, the 9ß-chloro,16,16-dimethyl-prostaglandin E_2, may be useful in the therapy of gastric ulceration. Derivatives of PGE_2 methylated at position 15 or 16 may display proaggregatory activity in contrast to PGI_2 and PGE_1. Therefore, the influence of nocloprost on human platelets was investigated. The aggregation was measured turbidimetrically. Thromboxane B_2 was determined by radioimmuno assay. In platelet-rich citrated plasma, nocloprost alone (≥ 0.1 µmol/l) caused an aggregation with a biphasic course at higher concentrations. Aggregation induced by nocloprost (1 µmol/l) corresponded to that induced by ADP (5 µmol/l). The thromboxane formation in platelets by nocloprost was not significantly different from that induced by ADP. Nocloprost-induced aggregation occurred also in hirudinized plasma. Comparable aggregation of washed platelets was induced by nocloprost (1 µmol/l) and thrombin (0.1 IU/ml). The nocloprost-induced aggregation was completely inhibited by iloprost (10 nmol/l), while indomethacin and daltroban (50 µmol/l, each) diminished the aggregation by 70-80%. At lower concentrations (<0.1 µmol/l) nocloprost did not influence the aggregation induced by ADP or other aggregating agents. PGE_2 did not induce platelet aggregation; at 10 µmol/l, it diminished the ADP-induced aggregation by about 20%. However, preincubation of the platelets with PGE_2 (0.1 and 1 µmol/l) significantly inhibited the nocloprost-induced aggregation. The concentrations of nocloprost required for its therapeutic use as anti-ulcer agent are lower by three orders of magnitude than those which induce platelet aggregation.

Institute of Pharmacology and Toxicology, Medical Academy Erfurt, O-5010 Erfurt and * Asche AG, D-2000 Hamburg, FRG.

26

ARTERIAL VASORELAXATION INDUCED BY ILOPROST IS PREVENTED BY BLOCKERS OF ATP-DEPENDENT K^+ CHANNELS

Hella Gollasch[+*], Jürgen Hescheler[#] and Mark T. Nelson[*]

Recent findings suggest that vasorelaxation induced by the stable prostacyclin analog iloprost is caused by a membrane hyperpolarizing K^+ conductance of smooth muscle cells. To determine the K^+ conductance activated by iloprost, the effects of the ATP-dependent K^+ channel blockers glibenclamide and tetrapentylammonium (TPeA) on iloprost-induced vasorelaxation of rabbit mesenteric arteries were examined.
Iloprost relaxed $5*10^{-6}$ M noradrenaline-preconstricted arteries with an $ED_{50} = 2*10^{-8}$ M. The maximal effect was observed at $3*10^{-7}$ M with a relaxation to 12 ± 4 % of preconstricted values (n = 19, mean $\pm$ S.E.M). Glibenclamide ($3*10^{-6}$ M) and TPeA (10^{-5} M) reversed the $3*10^{-7}$ M iloprost-induced vasorelaxation to 80 ± 16 % (n = 12) and to 76 ± 12 % (n = 7) of preconstricted values, respectively. Both K^+ channel blockers had no effect on tension before and during noradrenaline-induced constriction. Pretreatment of the arteries with glibenclamide or TPeA inhibited the relaxing effect of iloprost. Vasorelaxation induced by the ATP-dependent K^+ channel opener lemakalim (10^{-8} M) was completely reversed by glibenclamide ($3*10^{-6}$ M). The data suggest that iloprost induces vasorelaxation primarily by opening of ATP-dependent K^+ channels in arterial smooth muscle cells.

[+]Institut für Physiologie, Humboldt-Universität zu Berlin, D-1040 Berlin, [*]Department of Pharmacology, University of Vermont, Burlington, VT 05405, [#]Institut für Pharmakologie, Freie Universität Berlin, D-1000 Berlin 33

27

A SPECIFIC ENZYME LINKED IMMUNOSORBENT ASSAY FOR 11DH-THROMBOXANE B_2 USING A MONOCLONAL ANTIBODY

M. Reinke*

A monoclonal antibody against 11DH-thromboxane B_2 ($MAB-1E-DHTBR_1$), which may be used in a specific enzyme linked immunosorbent assay (ELISA) is described. The MAB recognizes the acyclic form of 11DH-thromboxane B_2 as found in basic range of pH with a detection limit of 4.6 pg/sample and a binding affinity of 6.1×10^9 l/mol (Scatchard Plot). Only negligible crossreactivity could be found for thromboxane B_2 (0.05%), 2,3-dinor-thromboxane B_2 (0.06%) and prostaglandin D_2 (0.08%). The suitability of the assay was checked by measurement of standard dilutions of $11DH-TXB_2$, supplemented with 10% of human serum, which yielded unchanged sensitivity. Recovery experiments showed an accuracy of r=0.982. Validity was confirmed by a good correlation between radioimmunoassay and ELISA (r=0.975). Measurements of 11DH-thromboxane B_2 in human serum and urine demonstrated the practical applicability of the MAB in ELISA. Using different clotting times the serum level of 11DH-thromboxane B_2 ranged from 0.8 (1.3) ng/ml (30 min) to 54.7 (24.6) ng/ml (4 h). After administration of aspirin the 11DH-thromboxane B_2 level of human urine dropped from 3.9-5.4 ng/ml to 0.4-1.6 ng/ml after 6 h.

* Dept. of Medicine IV, Univ. of Erlangen-Nürnberg, Kontumazgarten 14-18, D- 8500 Nürnberg, Germany.

28

THE RELATIONSHIPS BETWEEN THE ARACHIDONIC ACID-METABOLITES AND THE CONTENT OF CATECHOLAMINES IN WHOLE RAT BRAINS AFTER ETHANOL ADMINISTRATION

K. R. Lutnicki, E. Trebas-Pietras, J. Wróbel

The influence of the AA-metabolites on the content of catecholamines in rat brain after ethanol ingestion was assessed. The experiments were carried out on 50 male albino rats. The animals were pretreated with compounds: 2(12-hydroxydodeka-5,10-diynyl) 3,5,6-trimethyl-1,4-benzoquinone (AA 861) as a 5 lipoxygenase inhibitor (100 mg/kg b.w. i.p.), BW 755 C as a 5 lipoxygenase cycloxygenase dual inhibitor (100 mg/kg b.w. i.p.) and CGS 13080 - TXA_2 as a synthetase inhibitor (1 mg/kg s.c.) 30 minutes before ethanol administration. As a control rats administered with only ethanol (positive control group) and saline (negative control group) were used. Each group consists of 10 animals. Two hours after ethanol administration the rats were sacrified and the levels of catecholamines according to Laverty and Taylor method were assessed.
Ethanol decreased the content of noradrenaline (NA) and dopamine (DA) in rat brain in comparison with saline treated group. The compound AA 861 enhanced the NA- and DA-brain contents, decreased as well the level of NA in comparison with the ethanol treated group. The BW 755 C slightly decreased the level of NA in brains and significantly enhanced the content of DA in comparison with control group administered with ethanol alone. In the group of the animals pretreated with CGS 13080 increased levels of NA and DA in brains were assessed.

Department of Pathophysiology, Medical Academy, Jaczewskiego 8, 20084 Lublin, Poland

29

CONTACT ACTIVATION OF THE INTRINSIC COAGULATION CASCADE TRIGGERS STIMULATION OF THE 5-LIPOXYGENASE PATHWAY IN HUMAN PERIPHERAL MONOCYTES

I. Weide and Th. Simmet

We have previously demonstrated that clotting of whole human blood in vitro results not only in the generation of cyclooxygenase-derived thromboxane $(TX)B_2$ but also in the production of vasoconstrictory and edema-promoting cysteinyl-leukotrienes (CYS-LT). We have now investigated whether the contact-mediated coagulation process might be able to stimulate the 5-lipoxygenase (lox) pathway in human peripheral monocytes (PM). When 5×10^6 or 15×10^6 human mononuclear cells (MNC) containing $11.4 \pm 0.6\%$ monocytes and $88.6 \pm 0.6\%$ lymphocytes were added to autologous whole human blood allowed to clot in vitro at 37°C for 60 min a cell number-dependent increase in CYS-LT serum levels to $165.7 \pm 6.5\%$ and $333.2 \pm 48.5\%$, respectively, was observed. Similarly supplementation of autologous whole human blood with PM 0.5×10^6 or 1.5×10^6 purified from MNC by differential centrifugation (90.4 ± 0.8% purity) led to increased CYS-LT serum levels (174 ± 10.5% and 244.2 ± 18.2%, repectively). Furthermore, incubation of PM 0.5×10^6 in autologous platelet-rich plasma resulted in a time-dependent production of CYS-LT reaching 452.6 ± 68.8 pg/ml at 60 min. PM incubated in parallel in Hank's balanced salt solution did not produce any detectable CYS-LT. The CYS-LT were determined radioimmunologically and were further characterized by reverse phase HPLC. Since in whole human blood the CYS-LT production in contrast to the TXB_2 formation is not affected by exogenous human α-thrombin nor by the thrombin inhibitors hirudin (1.4 μM) or D-Phe-Pro-Arg-CH_2Cl (100 μM) the stimulation appears to be independent from endogenous thrombin formation. The stimulus triggering 5-lox activity is under further investigation.
Ruhr-University, Department of Pharmacology, Universitätsstr. 150, W-4630 Bochum 1, F.R.G.

30

LEUKOTRIENE INACTIVATION IS A POTENTIAL TARGET FOR LEUKOTRIENE RECEPTOR ANTAGONISTS. M. Grimberg, C. Haberl, W. Wilmanns, and C. Denzlinger
Leukotrienes are potent mediators of allergy and inflammation. Their inactivation in vivo proceeds via hepatobiliary and renal elimination and by metabolic degradation. We studied whether these mechanisms are affected by the cysteinyl leukotriene receptor antagonists FPL 55712 (sodium 7-[3-(4-acetyl-3-hydroxy-2-propylphenoxy)-2-hydroxypropoxy]-4-oxo-8-propyl-4H-1-benzopyran-2-carboxylate), LY 163443 (1-[2-hydroxy-3-propyl-4-((4-(1H-tetrazol-5-ylmethyl)phenoxy)methyl)phenyl]ethanone), or MK-571 ([3-(3-[2-(7-chloro-2-quino-linyl)ethenyl]phenyl)([3-(dimethylamino-3-oxo propyl)thio] methyl)thio]propanoic acid), respectively. Anesthetized rats and homogenates of rat liver were used as experimental models. In the anesthetized rat, FPL 55712 (5 or 20 μmol kg^{-1} h^{-1} administered intravenously) was a strong inhibitor of the hepatobiliary elimination both of [^{3}H]leukotrienes and of leukotrienes elicited in vivo. LY 163443 (25 μmol kg^{-1} h^{-1}) reduced only the biliary secretion of [^{3}H]leukotriene D$_4$ significantly. Inhibition of [^{3}H]leukotriene elimination by MK-571 (15 μmol kg^{-1} h^{-1}) was compensated for by a drug-induced increase in bile flow. The urinary leukotriene elimination, quantitatively less important in the rat, was not significantly reduced by the leukotriene receptor antagonists. FPL 55712, LY 163443, or MK-571 enhanced the metabolic stability of [^{3}H]leukotriene C$_4$ or [^{3}H]leukotriene D$_4$, respectively, in suspensions of rat liver homogenate. This corresponded to a reduced binding of [^{3}H]leukotrienes to the homogenates.
From our data we conclude that both pathways of leukotriene inactivation, i.e. elimination from blood and metabolic degradation, may be impaired by leukotriene receptor antagonists. This could be due to similarities of binding sites of leukotriene receptors and of binding sites involved in leukotriene inactivation. Inhibition of leukotriene inactivation by the leukotriene receptor antagonists may counteract the leukotriene antagonistic properties of these drugs.
Medizinische Klinik III, Klinikum Grosshadern, Ludwig-Maximilians Univerität, D-8000 München 70

31

TISSUE AND PLASMA KINETICS OF NAPROXEN AND PHENYLBUTAZONE IN DOGS
Rikea Zech, R. Scherkl, A. Hashem and H.-H. Frey

In nonsteroidal antiinflammatory drugs (NSAIDs) with short elimination half-lives in plasma, a discrepancy appears between elimination half-life and clinical effect. We have therefore studied the tissue kinetics of one drug having a long (naproxen) and one having a short elimination half life (phenylbutazone) in dogs. Tissue fluid was obtained from so called tissue cages implanted on both sides over the shoulder. On one side an inflammatory response was induced by injecting 1 ml of 2 % carrageenan into the chamber. The concentrations of both drugs were determined throughout the experiments in plasma and tissue fluid from both sides. Experiments with single doses and with treatment for one week were performed.
Naproxen, having an elimination half-life of about 72 h in dogs, accumulated more readily in the inflamed site but attained finally on both sides the plasma concentration and remained in equilibrium with it. In the case of phenylbutazone, concentrations in the tissue fluid fell with a definitely longer half-life than plasma concentrations and exceeded the latter ones after some hours. This allows a lower dosage than calculated on the basis of plasma concentrations in the case of phenylbutazone, and possibly also other NSAIDs having a short plasma half-life.

Department of Pharmacology and Toxicology, School of Veterinary Medicine, Freie Universität Berlin, Koserstr. 20, W-1000 Berlin 33

32

CHARACTERIZATION OF THE OUTFLOW OF ENDOGENOUS SEROTONIN FROM THE ISOLATED RABBIT SMALL INTESTINE.
A. Reimann, B. Hering, H. Schwörer and K. Racké.
Serotonin (5-HT) is present in high concentrations in the enterochromaffin cells (ECs) of the intestinal mucosa from where it is secreted into the lumen as well as into the portal circulation. In the present experiments a possible differential release of 5-HT from the mucosal and serosal side of the small intestine was studied by the use of a modified Ussing technique.
Segments of the rabbit small intestine were cut along the mesenteric border. Using modified Ussing chambers, made of Plexiglas, the mucosal and serosal sides of the intestine were incubated separately in Krebs-HEPES solution. The outflow of 5-HT and its metabolite 5-hydroxyindoleacetic acid (5-HIAA) was determined by HPLC with electrochemical detection.
In the absence of test drugs, the spontaneous outflow after 1 h of incubation in vitro amounted to 2.6 ± 0.57 pmol/cm^2/10 min 5-HT and 25 ± 6.4 pmol/cm^2/10 min 5-HIAA at the serosal side (n=14) and to 12 ± 3.0 pmol/cm^2/10 min 5-HT and 57 ± 12,8 pmol/cm^2/10 min 5-HIAA at the mucosal side (n=7). The outflow of 5-HT at the serosal side was only marginally increased, when the muscarine receptor agonist oxotremorine (up to 10 μmol/l) was added to the incubation medium either at the mucosal or serosal side or at both sides. However, in the presence of tetrodotoxin (TTX, 1 μmol/l) oxotremorine, either added to the serosal side or to both sides, increased the outflow of 5-HT at the serosal side about 5fold. On the other hand, oxotremorine had no marked effect on the outflow of 5-HT at the mucosal side, neither in the absence nor presence of TTX. Nicotine (up to 100 μmol/l) enhanced the outflow of 5-HT at the serosal side by about 70 % and this effect was partially attenuated in the presence of TTX.
The present experiments indicate that the release of 5-HT from basal side of the ECs of the rabbit small intestine can be increased by activation of muscarine receptors located directly at the ECs. However, in the absence of 72 TTX this direct stimulation of 5-HT release is markedly attenuated by the simultaneous release of a supposed inhibitory neurotransmitter.
Supported by the Deutsche Forschungsgemeinschaft (Ra 400/3-1)
Pharmakologisches Institut der Universität Mainz, Obere Zahlbacher Str. 67, D-6500 Mainz, FRG.

33

INFLUENCE OF DIFFERENT SOLVENTS ON THE FUNCTIONALITY AND VIABILITY OF THE ISOLATED PERFUSED GUT
H. Wentges, S. Klee, F.R. Ungemach and A. Pospischil*

In the isolated perfused jejunum of the rat the influence of different solvents [ethanol, glycerol formal (GF) and poly-ethyleneglycol 400 (PEG)] and of hypoxia (N_2) on different parameters of intestinal function and viability (absorption of water, Na^+ and glucose, release of K^+ and LDH) and on the morphology of the gut segment were investigated in order to test the sensitivity of these criteria and the suitability of this perfusion model.
The perfused gut segment remained morphologically and functionally intact over at least 2h. The solvents used exerted no negative effects at a concentration of 1%. They rather tended to increase water absorption. Ethanol and GF induced a beginning impairment of function, viability and morphological integrity at 3% whereas 10% and hypoxic conditions lead to a remarkable damage. PEG showed no relevant deleterious effects but only an osmotic-induced reduction of water flow.

	Control	Ethanol	Gly.Form.	PEG 400	N_2
water (ml/cm)	0.25	0.08	0.09	0.03	0.03
glucose (S/M)	4.47	1.10	1.01	6.10	0.89
K^+ (S/M)	0.81	1.63	2.15	1.04	1.80
LDH (U/cm)	0.31	0.98	1.20	0.56	1.03

water absorption; S/M:serosal/mucosal conc.; LDH in the perfusate. Solvent conc.: 10%. Perfusion for 2h

CONCLUSIONS:
(1) The perfused jejunum remains intact for at least 2h. (2) Absorption of water, Na^+, K^+ and glucose are only parameters of intestinal function but not of viability. (3) As suitable viability parameters glucose-S/M, K^+-S/M as well as LDH can be regarded. (4) The viability parameters are sensitive so much to indicate a beginning morphological damage. (5) Ethanol and GF induce a manifest organ damage at concentrations >3% whereas the impermeable PEG exerts no damage but leads to a strong reduction of absorption processes even at lower hyperosmolarity.

Institute of Pharmacology and Toxicology, FB Vet.Med., Freie Univeristät Berlin, Koserstr. 20, D-1000 Berlin 33
*Institute of Veterinary Pathology, University of Zürich

34

STUDIES ON BENZOQUINONE ADDUCTS DURING METABOLISM OF BENZENE
E. Krewet, W. Popp, B. Gansewendt*, K. Norpoth

Chromatographic separation techniques for the analysis of compounds formed during in vitro reactions of p-benzoquinone with deoxyguanosine or guanine were used to examine urine and tissue samples of male Wistar rats exposed to ^{14}C-benzene (3,3 mCi, 80 ppm) by inhalation. Radioactivity was measured by liquid scintillation counting in 24-hour urine samples collected 6 days after the end of exposure, in tissues (blood, liver, bone marrow, spleen, thymus) and isolated DNA, RNA, protein. The ^{14}C-label showed a marked decrease in urine samples 48 hours after the end of exposure but remained unchanged from the 4. to the 6. day. After separation of known benzene metabolites from urine samples eight unknown ^{14}C-labeled compounds, excreted within the first 4 days, could be detected. Three of them may be p-benzoquinone adducts when comparing their chromatographic properties with those of compounds formed during incubation experiments. Radioactivity was also detected in tissues 6 days after the end of exposure and corresponding results from DNA analysis will be presented.

Address: Institute of Hygiene and Occupational Medicine, University Medical Center, Hufelandstr. 55, D-4300 Essen 1, FRG
*Institute of Occupational Health, Ardeystr. 67, D-4600 Dortmund, FRG

35

GLUTATHIONE S-TRANSFERASE CLASS MU ACTIVITY AND LUNG CANCER RISK
J. Brockmöller, D. Gross, R. Kerb, N. Drakoulis, J. Siegle, R. Loddenkemper*, and I. Roots

Environmental carcinogens, especially those of the tobacco smoke, are of predominant impact in the etiology of lung cancer in humans. Glutathione S-transferases (GST's) are capable of detoxifying several toxic compounds and their activated metabolites. Genetic deficiency of GST class Mu isoenzymes has been suggested to be a lung cancer risk factor (Seidegard et al., Carcinogenesis 11: 33). However, the conjugation activity towards the specific substrate trans-stilbene oxide ex vivo in cancer patients may be confounded by secondary phenomena. Thus, the recent availability of genetic probes for detection of the GST Mu deficiency (using the PCR technique) which has been shown to be in almost complete correlation with enzyme activities (J. Brockmöller et al., Biochem. Pharmacol., in press) is of special value in epidemiological studies.
104 patients (smokers) with lung cancer and 92 reference patients (smokers) have been tested by ex vivo phenotyping for GST Mu activity and by genotyping using the PCR technique.

	Low activity < 10	High activity > 20 pmol/min/10^6 lymphocytes
Lung cancer:	n=58 (PCR- : n=58)	n=46 (PCR+ : n=46)
	Mean activity: 2.7	Mean activity: 74.9
Controls:	n=50 (PCR- : n=50)	n=42 (PCR+ : n=42)
	Mean activity: 1.5	Mean activity: 81.0

PCR- denotes the absence of an amplifyable GST Mu genomic fragment, indicating a deletion of part (or in total) of the GST Mu gene.

Conclusion: An unambiguous diagnosis of GST class Mu deficiency was obtained by PCR. The proposed overrepresentation of persons with hereditably low GST class Mu activity could not be detected by enzymatic and molecular genetic methods among lung cancer patients studied in Berlin.
Institut für Klinische Pharmakologie, Klinikum Steglitz, Freie Universität Berlin, Hindenburgdamm 30, D-1000 Berlin 45, and *Krankenhaus Heckeshorn, Berlin 39, FRG

36

INDUCTION OF ETHOXYRESORUFIN O-DEETHYLASE ACTIVITY IN EXTRAHEPATIC TISSUE OF MOUSE EMBRYOS BY BENZO[A]PYRENE.
Diether Neubert and Ulrich Räuchle

The basal activity of P450-dependent monooxygenases in extrahepatic fetal or embryonic tissue of rodents has been reported to be not measurable, and almost no information is available on the inducibility of such monooxygenase activities. We have therefore tested whether such enzyme activity, as revealed e.g. by ethoxyresorufin O-deethylase (EROD) may be inducible by benzo[a]pyrene (B[a]P).

NMRI mice received B[a]P by gavage on days 10, 11 and 12 of pregnancy, and the EROD activity was measured in the embryos without the liver ("rest-embryo") or in limb buds pooled from several litters on day 13 of gestation.

	EROD activity*
"rest-embryo"	
controls	< 0.2
3 x 150 mg B[a]P/kg body wt	2.2 ± 0.4
limb buds	
controls	< 0.2
3 x 150 mg B[a]P/kg body wt	2.3 ± 0.6
maternal liver	
controls	31 ± 5
3 x 150 mg B[a]P/kg body wt	208 ± 26

* (pmoles x mg protein (homogenate)$^{-1}$ x min^{-1})

Without induction, EROD activity was not measurable in the "rest-embryos" or limb buds. Following three doses of 50 mg B[a]P/kg body wt the activity was just detectable, and at higher doses clearly measurable. However, the increase was very small when compared with non-induced maternal liver (< 1/14). The rate of induction achieved in the extrahepatic tissue was only about 1/17 of that observable in fetal liver under similar experimental conditions (cf. Räuchle and Neubert, this meeting).

Institut für Toxikologie und Embryopharmakologie, Freie Universität Berlin, Garystrasse 5, D-1000 Berlin 33, Germany

37

INDUCTION OF THE ACTIVITY OF ETHOXYRESORUFIN O-DEETHYLASE IN HEPATIC TISSUE OF LATE-STAGE MOUSE EMBRYOS BY BENZO[a]PYRENE
Ulrich Räuchle and Diether Neubert

It is generally believed that the activity of monooxygenases in rodent liver at the late embryonic stage is low or even absent, and almost no information is available on its possible inducibility. We have studied the inducibility of ethoxyresorufin O-deethylase (EROD) in early fetal liver (day 13 of gestation) by benzo[a]pyrene (B[a]P) in the mouse. After pretreatment for 3 days with B[a]P, livers from 13-day-old mouse embryos were dissected, and the tissue from one litter was pooled, homogenized, and the enzymatic activity measured fluorometrically.

Liver (day 13)	n =	EROD activity*	P=
Controls	24	0.5 ± 0.2	
B[a]P pretreatment:			
3 x 1 mg/kg body wt	15	0.9 ± 0.2	<0.01
3 x 25 mg/kg body wt	17	6.9 ± 3.1	<0.01
3 x150 mg/kg body wt	11	38.2 ±7.9	<0.01

* (pmoles x mg homogenate protein^{-1} x min^{-1})

Data shown in the table indicate that the basal activity on day 13 of gestation is about 2% of that in maternal liver. The monooxygenase activity depending on the P450IA-type is inducible in fetal liver with doses as low as 1 mg B[a]P/kg body wt, which is much lower than the doses necessary for induction of B[a]P-hydroxylases. Subsequent to 150 mg B[a]P/kg the EROD activity reaches values of the non-induced maternal liver.

Institut für Toxikologie und Embryopharmakologie, Freie Universität Berlin, Garystrasse 5, D 1000 Berlin 33, Germany

38

POSTNATAL DEVELOPMENT OF RATS AFTER PRENATAL TREATMENT WITH DIHYDROERGOTAMINE.
Jutta Hartmann, Ibrahim Chahoud, Gerd Bochert, Uta Lübbe, Diether Neubert

Dihydroergotamine (DHE) has also been suggested for therapy of hypotonia during pregnancy. In the present study the effect of prenatal treatment with DHE on postnatal development in rat pups was investigated. Dams were dosed with 20, 60 or 100 mg DHE/kg body wt, respectively. 50 rats per group were treated daily s.c. from day 15 of pregnancy till birth (fetal period). Variables of postnatal development of offspring (day 1 - day 21) were recorded. Since litter size influence these variables only the data of litter size 10 were presented.

Body weight is presented as mean ± S.D.; mortality, eye opening and incisor eruption is presented as a relative, cumulative frequency.

Variable	Control	DHE (mg/kg) 20	60	100
body weight				
day 1	5.5 ± 0.5	5.4 ± 0.2	5.3 ± 0.4	5.1 ± 0.4
day 21	24.4 ± 3.3	25.6 ± 1.9	25.8 ± 1.8	18.4 ± 3.2
mortality (%)				
day 2-7	3.1	0.9	2.4	4.0
day 8-14	5.1	0.9	3.3	11.1
day 15-21	5.5	0.9	6.0	12.4
eye opening (%)				
day 16	79	54	100	37
incisor eruption (%)				
day 9	56	60	80	17

Under the chosen experimental conditions the dose of 20 mg DHE/kg body wt can be considered as NOEL. The dose of 100 mg/kg obviously had a toxic effect on the offspring exposed during the fetal period.

Institut für Toxikologie und Embryopharmakologie, Freie Universität Berlin, Garystr. 5, 1000 Berlin 33

39

POSTNATAL DEVELOPMENT AND BEHAVIOUR OF RAT OFFSPRING AFTER EXPOSURE TO 2,3,7,8-TETRACHLORODIBENZO-p-DIOXIN DURING THE LATE FETAL AND POSTNATAL PERIOD.
Renate Thiel, Maria Korte, Ibrahim Chahoud, and Diether Neubert

Little direct evidence has been obtained, up till now, on effects of 2,3,7,8-tetrachlorodibenzo-p-dioxin (TCDD) on the CNS. We therefore studied the influence of this compound on the pysiological development and on behaviour during the postnatal period in rats, because a lack of blood-brain barrier functions may facilitate revealing possible effects on the CNS. Pregnant Wistar rats were treated on day 19 of gestation with an initial s.c.-injection of 300 or 1000 ng TCDD/kg body wt, the controls received the vehicle (toluene/DMSO) only. The treatment of the dams during lactation and of the offspring after weaning was continued weekly with a maintenance-dose (120 or 400 ng TCDD/kg body wt). Landmarks of postnatal development such as body weight gain, eye opening, fur development, incisor eruption and some reflexes were monitored. To avoid a possible influence of the litter size, only data of litters with 9 to 11 pups were selected. The body weight in both TCDD-exposed groups was reduced, significantly only in the high dose group on day 14 and 21 postnatally. The weight gain from day 1 to day 21 was: i) control: 4.5-fold, ii) 300/120: 4.4-fold, iii) 1000/400: 3.9-fold. The following results were obtained:

Parameter	Day	Control (N = 40)	TCDD ng/kg body wt s.c. 300/120 (N = 60)	1000/400 (N = 72)
physiological development				
fur development	7	85%	67%* (100%)	67%* (100%)
incisor eruption	10	80%	83%	76%
eye-opening	15	62%	45% (69%)	28%* (100%)
		(N = 40)	(N = 39)	(N = 41)
developmental reflexes				
righting	6	48%	74%*	66%
cliff-drop-aversion	8	45%	49%	59%
forelimb-grasp	8	53%	49%	61%
rota rod	24	83%	32%* (79%)	20%* (85%)

% = rats with positive response; * = p < 0.05 (Chi-Square)

The reduced rates of the responding animals correlated with a reduced body weight. No effect was observable (percentage in parenthesis) when offspring with the same body weight were compared. Obviously TCDD did not lead to permanent changes of the variables tested.

Institut für Toxikologie und Embryopharmakologie, Freie Universität Berlin, Garystr. 5, D-1000 Berlin 33. Supported by the grant no. 0765002 from the Bundesministerium für Forschung und Technologie (BMFT).

40

CONCENTRATION OF 2,3,7,8-TCDD IN LIVER AND ADIPOSE TISSUE OF RAT OFFSPRING AFTER CONTINUOUS EXPOSURE
Elisabeth Koch, Maria Korte, Renate Thiel, Martin Mayer, Ibrahim Chahoud, and Diether Neubert

Female Wistar rats were treated with a single loading-dose of 50, 120 or 250 ng ^{14}C-TCDD/kg body wt 4 weeks prior to mating. Up to mating, during pregnancy and the lactation period weekly maintenance-doses of 20% of the loading-dose were injected. After weaning (at 3 weeks of age) the F1-generation was treated with the same dose regime (loading-/maintenance-doses). During the phase of rapid growth (4th to 8th week) this dosing schedule was insufficient to keep the tissue concentrations of TCDD constant. Therefore, we treated the adult animals with a second loading-dose. The concentrations of 2,3,7,8-TCDD were measured in the offspring (F2-generation). Results obtained in the highest dose group (250/50 ng TCDD/kg body wt) are compiled in the table (pg TCDD/g wet weight).

Tissue	Number of samples	Day postnatally 3	7	14	21
Liver	5	721±41	946±135	1845±274	1671±112
br. ad. tissue *	3	420±18	456±17	416±24	288±25
wh. ad. tissue *	3	---	693±105	700±122	413±35

* = pooled material from one litter

The concentration of TCDD in the liver tissue doubled between day 3 and 14 postnatally and stayed about constant thereafter. In both adipose tissues the concentrations of TCDD remained constant up to day 14 postnatally and declined during the following week. The concentration ratio: liver/white adipose tissue declined from day 7 (ratio: 1.4) to day 21 (ratio: 4.1)) apparently due to redistribution and growth phenomena.

Institut für Toxikologie und Embryopharmakologie, Freie Universität Berlin, Garystr. 5, D-1000 Berlin 33, Germany

41

TISSUE CONCENTRATIONS IN LACTATING WISTAR RATS AFTER SINGLE OR REPEATED TREATMENT WITH 2,3,7,8-TETRACHLORO-DIBENZO-P-DIOXIN (TCDD).

Maria Korte, Renate Thiel, Elisabeth Koch, Ralf Stahlmann, Diether Neubert

Polychlorinated dioxins as highly lipophilic substances are excreted effectively via mother's milk. We studied the time-related changes of TCDD concentrations in liver tissue and adipose tissue during the lactation period after single exposure or continuous exposure. Pregnant Wistar rats were pretreated on day 19 of gestation with a subcutaneous injection of 300 ng TCDD/kg body wt. Subsequently, half of the animals received no further treatment (group 1) whereas the rest was treated with a weekly maintenance-dose of 120 ng TCDD/kg body wt (40% of the loading-dose; group 2). On days 3, 7, 14 and 21 postnatally TCDD concentrations were determined in maternal tissues by liquid scintillation counting. The following results were obtained:

	Dose (ng/kg b.wt)	Concentration (ng TCDD/g)			
		Day postnatally			
		3	7	14	21
Liver	300	2.53	1.39	0.14	0.03
	300/120	1.89	1.88	0.99	0.81
Abdominal fat	300	0.89	0.63	0.39	0.10
	300/120	0.43	0.79	0.83	0.53

After single treatment TCDD concentrations declined rapidly in the tissues. After multiple injections the concentrations in liver tissue declined by about 50% within the second week. However, the concentrations stayed rather constant in the abdominal fat, indicating that the dosing regime used guaranteed almost constant tissue levels of TCDD.

These studies were supported by grant No. 0765002 from the Bundesministerium für Forschung und Technologie.

Institut für Toxikologie und Embryopharmakologie, Freie Universität Berlin, Garystr. 5, 1000 Berlin 33, Germany

42

ELUCIDATION OF THE SENSITIVE PERIOD FOR INDUCING CLEFT PALATES BY TCDD IN MICE.

Stephan Klug, Elisabeth Wildi, Keisuke Yamashita, and Diether Neubert.

The teratogenic potential of 2,3,7,8-tetrachlorodibenzo-*p*-dioxin (TCDD) is largely confined to the induction of cleft palates (CP) in mice (besides causing dilatations of the renal pelvis). Such an effect may also be induced by other polychlorinated or polybrominated dibenzo-*p*-dioxins or dibenzofurans.
Using a combined *in vivo* / *in vitro* approach we have attempted to elucidate the period of palatal development which is susceptible to the action of TCDD. The former data on the sensitive stages (Neubert and Dillmann, Naunyn-Schmiedebergs's Arch Pharmacol 272:243-264,1972) were reevaluated using another route of administration. In our NMRI strain gestational day 11 represents the most susceptible period for induction of CP by TCDD.
Furthermore, organ cultures of palate anlagen were initiated from 13-day-old mouse embryos (method cf: Shiota et al. Acta Anat 137: 59-64,1990) in order to see whether TCDD induces a corresponding effect *in vitro*. In contrast to dexamethason, addition of TCDD to the culture medium did not (in contrast to *in vivo*) dose-dependently and reproducibly interfere with palate closure:

	ng/ml	n=	Palates completely fused
Controls	0	40	90%
Dexamethason	200,000	17	13%
TCDD	1.5	26	77%

From our data it is unlikely that the interference of TCDD with palate development is mainly mediated through processes occurring at the very late stages of palate closure.

These studies were supported by grant # 07VDX019 from the Bundesministerium für Forschung und Technologie.
Institut für Toxikologie und Embryopharmakologie, Freie Universität Berlin, Garystr. 5, D-1000 Berlin 33, Germany

43

MOLECULAR MODELLING OF THE TERATOGENIC ACTIVITY OF CHIRAL α-BRANCHED ALIPHATIC ACIDS RELATED TO VALPROIC ACID

R. Kühne*, R.-S. Hauck and H. Nau

The antiepileptic drug valproic acid (VPA) acts as an effective teratogen in the human and in several experimental animals. To better understand the structural requirements of teratogenic effects, measured as rates of exencephaly in mice, a series of analogs of valproic acid was studied by means of the molecular modelling software package SYBYL. We demonstrated that all aliphatic acids used for analysis including VPA, 2-n-propyl-4-pentenoic acid (4-en), 2-n-propyl-4-pentynoic acid (4-yn) and 2-ethylhexanoic acid (2-EHXA), exhibit a high conformational flexibility. However, employing the SYBYL-Multifit procedure, we found that teratogenically active and inactive compounds occupy different spacial regions in relation to the carboxylic group. A comparison of molecular volumes both of teratogens and nonteratogens reveals zones of excluded ("forbidden") volumes of teratogenically active compounds. The stereoisomers with high teratogenic potency (S-4-en, S-4-yn and R-EHXA) occupied spacial volumes which were distinctly different from those occupied by their respective antipodes (R-4-en, R-4-yn and S-EHXA). Based on the conformations calculated with the Multifit procedure, the shapes of molecular electrostatic potentials were also calculated. We found that the potential shapes of teratogenic and nonteratogenic acids were quite different. These findings indicate a possible mechanism of action involving a conformationally specific binding site which could be useful in helping to formulate a computer assisted risk assessment of potentially teratogenic compounds.

* Institute of Drug Research, Alfred-Kowalke-Str. 4, 0-1136 Berlin.
Institute of Toxicology and Embryopharmacology, Free University Berlin, Garystrasse 5, D-1000 Berlin 33, Germany.

44

VALPROIC ACID-INDUCED SPINA BIFIDA: A MOUSE MODEL

K. Ehlers, H. Stürje, H.-J. Merker, and H. Nau

Prenatal exposure to the antiepileptic drug valproic acid (VPA) has been associated with the formation of spina bifida aperta in the human. Until now, a direct relationship between VPA application and spina bifida has not been experimentally demonstrated. VPA was known only to induce exencephaly in mice, a defect of the anterior neural tube. Maximal sensitivity toward production of this defect was on day 8 of gestation (plug day = day 0). The closure of the posterior neuropore occurs later in the development of mice than the closure of the anterior neuropore. To investigate whether there is a direct relationship between VPA application during pregnancy and induction of spina bifida in mice, we administered various doses of the drug on day 9 of gestation, at three time intervals (at 0 h, 6 h, 12 h). This administration of VPA produced spina bifida aperta and spina bifida occulta in mice. High doses of VPA (3x450 mg/kg; 3x500 mg/kg) induced a low rate of spina bifida aperta in the lumbosacral region. High incidences of spina bifida occulta, a less serious form of spina bifida, were induced with lower doses. This malformation was demonstrated in double-stained fetal skeletons by measurements of the distance between the cartilaginous ends of each vertebral arch. The occurence of this defect and its localization was dose-dependent. The lumbar region was affected by all doses investigated (3x300 mg/kg; 3x350 mg/kg; 3x400 mg/kg; 3x450 mg/kg; 3x500 mg/kg). The sacral/coccygeal region was affected additionally, but with higher doses (3x400 mg/kg; 3x450 mg/kg; 3x500 mg/kg). A comparison of the results obtained with day 16 and 17 control fetuses showed that the pattern of gaps present in the lumbar and sacral region of the spinal cord in treated groups was drug-specific and not related to a developmental delay. Our results indicate that multiple administrations of VPA on day 9 of gestation in mice result in a low incidence of spina bifida aperta and a high incidence of spina bifida occulta, and provides a relevant model for the study of human spina bifida defects.

Institute of Toxicology and Embryopharmacology, Free University Berlin, Garystrasse 5, D-1000 Berlin 33, Germany.

45

DISSOCIATION OF THE TERATOGENIC, ANTICONVULSANT AND NEUROTOXIC ACTIVITY OF VALPROIC ACID AND RELATED COMPOUNDS BASED ON STEREOCHEMICAL CONSIDERATIONS

R.-S. Hauck, M.M.A. Elmazar[*], and H. Nau

The widely used anticonvulsant drug valproic acid (2-n-propylpentanoic acid, VPA) is teratogenic and neurotoxic in the human and experimental animals. We synthesized the enantiomers of several chiral VPA related carboxylic acids. The teratogenic, anticonvulsant and neurotoxic activities were investigated in NMRI mice. Exencephaly was used as teratological endpoint. The anticonvulsant activities were determined using the pentylenetetrazol seizure threshold test; the Rotarod test was used for investigating the neurotoxicity (sedation). The teratogenic activity of e.g. 2-n-propyl-4-pentenoic acid (4-en-VPA) and 2-n-propyl-4-pentynoic acid (4-yn-VPA) enantiomers was found to be enantioselective. In contrast, no significant differences between the activities of the enantiomers were found regarding the anticonvulsant as well as the neurotoxic activity. a) The *teratogenic activity* drastically decreased in the sequence: S-4-yn-VPA > S-4-en-VPA > VPA > R-4-en-VPA > R-4-yn-VPA. b) The *anticonvulsant activity* decreased as follows: VPA = R-4-en-VPA ≈ S-4-en-VPA > R-4-yn-VPA = S-4-yn-VPA. c) The *neurotoxic activity* decreased in the sequence: VPA > R-4-en-VPA > S-4-en-VPA > R-4-yn-VPA = S-4-yn-VPA. Pharmacokinetic studies indicated that the stereoselective teratogenicity is due to intrinsic activities of the enantiomers and not to pharmacokinetic differences. The dissociation of the enantioselective teratogenicity from the - not enantioselective - anticonvulsant and neurotoxic activity of these compounds opens a new and promising field of research toward the rational and scientific development of novel antiepileptic drugs.

* Alexander von Humboldt grant. Department of Pharmacology and Toxicology, Faculty of Pharmacy, Mansoura University, Mansoura, Egypt. Institute of Toxicology and Embryopharmacology, Free University Berlin, Garystrasse 5, D-1000 Berlin 33, Germany.

46

EMBRYOTOXIC EFFECTS OF VALPROIC ACID (VPA), 4-enVPA, AND 2-enVPA: COMPARATIVE STUDIES WITH SPECIES OF VARIOUS LEVELS OF ORGANISATION

Frank Kirschbaum and Axel Oberemm

Testing for embryofeto-toxicity as part of a savety evaluation is exclusively performed, up to now, on mammalian species. We are studying non-mammalian systems in order to assess their possibility for revealing the potency of chemicals to interfere with normal development. Species used comprized lower vertebrates, a chordate (tunicate), and a coelenterate. We analysed embryotoxic effects and tried to define the NOEL-values (hatching of normal shaped animals). As model substances we used VPA and 4-enVPA which are teratogenic in mice and induce abnormal development in culture of mammalian embryos and 2-enVPA which is inactive in these systems.

Species	NOEL-values, concentration in mM		
	VPA	4-enVPA	2-enVPA
Coelenterate: Hydractinia	1.0	1.0	10.0
Chordate: Ciona	1.0	1.0	10.0
Teleosts: Brachydanio	0.025	0.01	0.08
Melanotaenia	0.01	0.01	
Amphibians: Ambystoma	0.3	0.3	3.0
Hyperolius	0.01	0.03	0.3
Xenopus	0.03	0.3	0.3

In six of the seven systems studied the two derivatives teratogenic in mammalian systems (VPA and 4-enVPA) are also similarly active in the non-mammals, while the derivative inactive in mammals (2-enVPA) shows an order of magnitude lower activity to induce abnormal development in the lower animal species. However, in Xenopus laevis it was not possible to distinguish between 2-enVPA and 4-enVPA which exhibit opposite diverse activities in mammals.
Additional studies are necessary in order to validate the usefulness of these developmental models as alternative systems for screening the potency of chemicals to induce abnormal development.

Institut für Toxikologie und Embryopharmakologie, Freie Universität Berlin, Garystr. 5, D-1000 Berlin-33

47

VALPROIC ACID INDUCED ABNORMAL DEVELOPMENT OF THE CENTRAL NERVOUS SYSTEM (CNS) OF THE AXOLOTL: STAGE-DEPENDENT EFFECTS.

Axel Oberemm and Frank Kirschbaum

Neural tube defects are common human birth defects, their causes, however, are still unknown (Gordon 1985, J. Embryol. exp. Morph. 89, Suppl., 229-255). Experimental data with mammals (mouse, hamster, rat) have shown that the antiepileptic drug valproic acid (VPA) can induce malformations of the CNS. We have initiated studies to assess the possibility of using lower vertebrates (which present several advantages compared to mammals) for revealing the potency of chemicals to induce abnormal development. In three species of amphibians we indeed were able to induce abnormal development of the CNS by application of VPA (Oberemm and Kirschbaum 1991, Naunyn Schmiedeberg's Arch. Pharmacol. Suppl. Vol. 343, R117 468): The most obvious and uniform effects occurred in Ambystoma mexicanum (axolotl) following a pulse exposure to 5 and 10 mM VPA during gastrulation (from stage 9 up to 12 of controls). This type of exposure, however, does not indicate which developmental stages are sensitive to VPA treatment. We therefore successively advanced the pulse exposure (up to stages of early cleavage, stages 7-10 of controls), delayed it (treating stages of late gastrulation and neurulation, stages 11-13 and 14-18 of controls) and applied VPA continuously (from stage 9 to hatching of controls). The strongest effects on neurulation and on closure of the neural tube occurred if the period of treatment combined stages of blastula and early gastrula (complete failure of neural tube closure; death at days 6-8 after exposure). Pulse application during later stages of gastrulation also altered the process of neurulation, but less seriously, and yielded minor malformations (successive closure of the neural tube at late stages of controls, similar to exencephaly in mammals). Application during neurulation itself did not influence normogenesis of neurulation and caused no malformations of the CNS. Surprisingly, continuous exposure had a relatively minor effect: Delayed closure of the neural tube and malformations very much resembling exencephaly in mammals.

Institut für Toxikologie und Embryopharmakologie, Freie Universität Berlin, Garystr. 5, 1000 Berlin 33, Germany

48

CHROMOSOME PREPARATION FROM THE ZEBRAFISH EMBRYO - ANOTHER TOOL FOR TESTING CHEMICALS IN THIS ORGANISM

K. Schreeb, G. Groth, W. Sachsse*, and K.J. Freundt

The embryo of the zebrafish (Brachydanio rerio) serves already for examining teratogenic effects. Test criteria are morphological changes inside the developing fish egg. Following xenobiotics like dimethylformamide and its metabolites, or alkylamines, p-benzoquinone, chloroacetaldehyde and cyclohexanol frequently malformations of the heart and of the skeleton or death of the embryo can be observed (Arch Pharmacol Suppl 341, No 82 (1990); dto. Suppl 343, No 121 (1991). Cahiers de notes documentaires No 140, 712 - 715 (1990)). For going more into the details we prepared - to our knowledge for the first time - the chromosomes of the zebrafish from their embryos as another tool for the investigation of chemically induced disturbances.

Fertilized eggs of the zebrafish were singly kept in small glass vessels containing fish cell buffer. After 24 hours of development a high concentration of colchicine (3 mg/ml) was added. Four hours later chorion and yolk sac were removed and a hypotonic treatment of 20 minutes aqua bidest. was applied. In order to minimize loss of cells, fixation of the embryo was performed on the slide itself - a modification of the method of Tarkowski (Cytogenetics 5: 394 - 400 (1966)).
This technique is easy to handle and the results are reproducible. The chromosome number of the zebrafish prooved to be (2n =) 48.

The examination of the chromosomes from the zebrafish embryo can be recommended for testing and this will, in addition to teratogenesis, reveal structural aberrations in the genome and thus at least open the approach to mutagenesis.

*Institut für Genetik der Johannes Gutenberg-Universität, Saarstraße 21, D-6500 Mainz

Institut für Pharmakologie und Toxikologie, Fakultät für Klinische Medizin Mannheim, Universität Heidelberg, Maybachstraße 14-16, D-6800 Mannheim 1

49

DIFFERENTIATION AND MATURATION OF VARIOUS TISSUES IN ORGANOID CULTURE AS A TOOL IN TOXICOLOGY AND PHARMACOLOGY

B. Zimmermann

Behaviour of cells in culture depends on cell density. In low-density cultures (e.g. monolayers), cells proliferate, but loose many specific differentiation markers. At high density, cells are able to maintain a specific microenvironment, which is neccessary for cell-specific differentiation and maturation. Furthermore, the different cellular subtypes of an organ sort out at high density and form histotypic structures - organoids. Therefore, this type of culture is called "organoid culture". In general, all types of cells and tissues can differentiate into histotypic structures and maintain the differentiated status in such high density cultures. Methodology: A suspension of single cells is obtained by enzymatic treatment of collected fetal organs and sedimented by centrifugation. Five to ten ul of the sediment is placed on a membrane filter at the medium/air interface and grown under standard conditions. Pore-size of the filter influences the micromilieu and thus quality and quantity of histotypic organization. Examples: Fetal lung cells form vesicles and acini (alveolar-like structures) comprising mainly type II-pneumocytes, which produce large amounts of surfactant. Limb bud mesenchymal cells undergo chondrogenesis with all stages of cartilage differentiation, maturation and, finally, degeneration. Endochondral mineralization can be induced. Also in organoid cultures from calvarial osteoblasts, mineralization occurs as in vivo. Fetal liver cells form histotypic aggregates with bile capillaries; blood precursor cells, that are also present, differentiate according to their lineages. Nervous tissue shows neuronal differentiation and forms myelinated axons, synapses and ventricle-like spaces; very often, a medium/nervous tissue barrier is formed, which is probably a prerequisite of proper neuronal differentiation in vitro. Due to the tissue-like reorganization and differentiation of the cells at high density, this type of culture may prove useful for studies in organ toxicology and pharmacology.

Institute of Anatomy, Free University of Berlin, Königin-Luise-Str. 15, D-1000 Berlin 33, FRG

50

REACTIVATION OF HUMAN ACETYLCHOLINESTERASE INHIBITED BY MONOCROTOPHOS OR PARAOXON

W. Biederbick, M. Wentz, H. Thiermann, L. Szinicz

Treatment of organophosphorus insecticide poisoning is based on muscarinic blockade with atropine and acetylcholinesterase (AChE) reactivation with oximes, in Germany mostly obidoxime. The use of a new oxime, pyridinium-1-(((4-(aminocarbonyl)-pyridinio)-methoxy)methyl)-2-((hydroxyimino)-methyl)-dicholride (HI 6) for treatment of organophosphorus compound poisoning was reported by Kusic et. al. (Hum.Exp.Toxicol. 10:113, 1991).
In order to compare the reactivating potency of the oximes lyophilized type XIII AChE (Sigma, St. Louis) from human erythrocytes was inhibited by monocrotophos or paraoxon for 5 minutes at pH 7,4 and 37,0° C and then reactivated by obidoxime or HI 6 (both 10 μmol/l) for 20 minutes (monocrotophos) and 30 minutes (paraoxon). AChE activity was measured titrimetrically.
After incubation with monocrotophos and reactivation with obidoxime there was an increase in AChE activity from 16.5 % ± 6.6 % (with monocrotophos alone) to 30.2 % ± 10.8 % (n = 20). Addition of HI 6 to monocrotophos inhibited AChE resulted in a significantly higher activity compared to the former oxime, i. e. an increase from 16.5 % to 46.2 % ± 7.4 % (n = 20). With paraoxon (6.1 % ± 2.0 %) inhibited AChE obidoxime (76.4 % ± 9.2 %; n = 16) was more effective then HI 6 (25.8 % ± 6.1 %; n = 16). These results and the lower toxicity of HI 6 compared to obidoxime warrant further experiments in order to improve the treatment of organophosphorus compound poisoning.

Institut für Pharmakologie und Toxikologie, Akademie des Sanitäts- und Gesundheitswesens der Bundeswehr, BSW, Ingolstädter Landstr. 100, D-8046 Garching, FRG.

51

EFFECTS OF ATROPINE AND [2-(HYDROXYIMINO-METHYL]-3-(O-DIMETHYLCARBAMOYL)-PYRIDINIUM-(1)]-METHYLIODIDE (HGA 1) UPON MOTOR PERFORMANCE AND NEUROBEHAVIOUR OF SOMAN POISONED MICE

I. Steidl, M. Wentz, and L. Szinicz

The conventional therapy of organophosphorus compound poisonings with atropine (AT) and presently used oximes is insufficient after soman (SO), mainly because of lacking oxime efficacy.
Searching for an alternative the efficacy of the new oxime HGa 1 was testet in soman poisened mice.
White male NMRI mice, 10/group, received SO, 0,1 mg/kg (50% LD$_{50}$) s.c., SO and immediately thereafter AT, 10 mg/kg i.p. or SO and HGa 1 1.2 mikromol/kg i.p.(= ED$_5$, parameter running time), or SO and AT + HGa 1. After the injection(s) the animals were allowed to run for 60 min on a rotating (14 rpm) mash wire drum (20 cm diam.). The neurobehavioural status (Irwin, Psychopharmacologia 13, 222-257 (1968)) was checked in each animal before the injection and after the running period.
SO reduced significantly the running time, AT and AT + HGa 1 improved the running time in SO poisoned mice, whereas HGa 1 alone showed no significant improvement in comparison neither to the SO poisoned group nor to the group with AT therapy. SO caused a change of several neurobehavioural parameters, AT and AT + HGa 1 improved in part the changes caused by soman. HGa 1 alone showed no improvement on pathologic neurobehavioural status.
The data indicate that the new oxime HGa 1 does not further improve the therapeutic efficacy of atropine on soman poisoning.

Institut für Pharmakologie und Toxikologie,
Akademie des Sanitäts- und Gesundheitswesens der Bundeswehr, BSW, Ingolstädter Landstr. 100, D(W)-8046 Garching (FRG)

52

EFFECT OF PYRIDINIUM,1-{[(4-CARBAMOYL-PYRIDINIO) METHOXY] METHYL}-2-(HYDROXYIMINO-METHYL) DICHLORIDE MONOHYDRATE (HI6) IN SOMAN POISONING

S. de la Motte, L. Szinicz

HI6 is effective in certain organophosphate-poisonings, where obidoxime is ineffective (Rousseaux, Can J Physiol Pharmacol, 67:1183, 1989). But little is known about the effects of the drug on vital functions.
Circulatory and respiratory parameters were investigated in guinea pigs anesthetized with urethane (1.7 g/kg). 2 min after poisoning with 192 ug/kg Soman (12xLD50) iv, animals were treated iv with either NaCl 0.9%, or 15 umol/kg Atropine (A), or 100 umol/kg HI6 (H), or with A plus H. Survival rates were 0/4, 0/4, 0/4 or 4/4 in the respective groups. All animals in all groups suffered respiratory arrest 2.5-3.5 min after S. No effect of H alone was found. With A treatment respiratory rate (RR) recovered to 20% of pretreatment values for several minutes. A+H improved RR slowly within 20 min to a "steady state" of 70%. Heart rate (HR) was decreased to 20% by S. Improvement of HR occured immediately after H to 40%, with A to 70%, and with A+H to 100%.
Although Atropine seems essential for immediate survival, HI6 treatment also contributes markedly to the recovery of the animals. With respect to the low lipid solubility of the oxime, and the time of occurance of the effect, it may be assumed that the recovery of circulation is mediated by peripheral mechanisms, whereas the recovery of respiration may also be of central origin.

Akademie des Sanitäts- und Gesundheitswesens der Bundeswehr, Institut für Pharmakologie und Toxikologie, Ingolstädter Landstr. 98, W-8046 Garching-Hochbrück, FRG.

53

CARDIOVASCULAR AND RESPIRATORY EFFECTS OF N-HYDROXY-AMINOCARBONYL-N',N',N',-TRIMETHYLAMMONIUM BROMIDE (HW2) AND ATROPINE IN SOMAN POISONED GUINEA PIGS
F. Worek, W. Biederbick, M.L. Wentz, L. Szinicz

The therapy of soman (SO) poisoning is insufficient until now, mainly because of ineffective restoration of nicotinic signs of poisoning. Searching for more effective oximes, HW2 was tested in SO poisoning. Female Pirbright-White guinea pigs were anesthetized with urethane (1.8 g/kg). The trachea, a. carotis and v. jugularis were canulated and circulatory and respiratory parameters were measured. After stabilization of the parameters SO (0.032 mg/kg = 2*LD50) or saline (2 ml/kg) were injected i.v. and 2 min later atropine (A, 10 mg/kg) or HW2 (100 umol/kg) or A+HW2 or saline were given (n=6 in each group). The observation period was 60 min. After SO and SO+HW2 rapid respiratory depression and respiratory arrest within 4 min and circulatory failure within 10 min was observed in all animals. The therapy with A restored the respiratory parameters to 80% of base line values throughout the observation period. Heart rate and mean arterial pressure increased to 120% and remained above base line for 60 min. The combined therapy with A+HW2 did not further improve circulatory and respiratory parameters. All animals in the SO+A and SO+A+HW2 groups survived the 60 min period. An interesting effect of HW2 was an immediate and complete relaxation of SO induced muscular spasm. No reactivation of erythrocyte acetylcholinesterase was observed in HW2 treated animals.
The results suggest that the efficacy of SO poisoning therapy in guinea pigs with A cannot be further improved by HW2.

Institut für Pharmakologie und Toxikologie, Akademie des Sanitäts- und Gesundheitswesens der BW, BSW, Ingolstädter Landstr. 100, D-8046 Garching

54

INVESTIGATIONS ON THE INFLUENCE OF ACETYLCHOLINE-ESTERASE - Na^+, K^+-ATPASE INTERACTIONS BY ORGANO-PHOSPHATES IN VITRO
H. Bleyer and M. Rohde

In a working hypothesis on the complex mode of action of highly toxic organophosphate compounds, it was postulated that the organophosphate intoxication is represented as a sum of disturbances in the intercellular mechanisms of regulation and not only explained by inhibition of acetylcholine-esterase.
In acceptance of former findings by other authors to the inhibition of kidney mitochondrial Na^+, K^+-ATPase with DFP, a possible cooperation of membrane enzymes of synaptical structures of rat ZNS and the influence by organophosphate compounds exemplified by acetylcholine-esterase and Na^+, K^+-ATPase of a synaptical fraction was studied.
The highly toxic organophosphates Soman, Sarin, VX and Paraoxon inhibit dose-dependently the basal as well as the NaCl + KCl activated acetylcholine-esterase in vitro.
The differences in the inhibition values in both experimental groups were not significantly ascertained. Concerning an influence on the Na^+, K^+ activated, Mg^{2+} dependent, as well as Mg^{2+} activated ATPase activity it was found out that only the Na^+, K^+ activated ATPase is inhibited by Sarin (10^{-3} - 10^{-6} mol/l).
To sum up the discussion, the organophosphate intoxication appears to be an accumulation of acetylcholine following to disturbances of functional interactions of membrane enzymes, and not by a direct effect of organophosphates.
Dept. of Toxicology, MMS, E.-M.-Arndt-University of Greifswald, R.-Petershagen-Allee 38, O-220 Greifswald, FRG

55

THE THERAPEUTIC VALUE OF NEW DIMERCAPTOSUCCINIC ACID ESTERS IN ACUTE ARSENIC TRIOXIDE POISONING IN MICE.
*U.Paepcke, H.Kreppel, H.Thiermann, M.M.Jones, and P.K.Singh

The effect of various esters (DMDMS, DEDMS, DnDMS, DiPDMS ##) of dimercaptosuccinic acid (DMSA) on survival in acute arsenic poisoning and on arsenic elimination from the body was investigated. Mice were injected s.c. with either 65 µmol/kg arsenic trioxide (survival study) or 42.5 µmol/kg arsenic trioxide containing a tracer dose of 73-arsenite (elimination study). 30 min later equimolar amounts (0.7 mmol/kg) of the newly synthetized compounds, saline (controls) or DMSA were given i.p. or via gastric tube (i.g.). In the survival study lethality was recorded over 30 d in mice injected with 65 µmol/kg arsenic trioxide (n = 7/group). In the elimination study the arsenic content of various organs (blood, liver, kidneys, lungs, spleen, small intestine, large intestine, brain, testes, muscle and skin) was measured at 30 min, 2 h, 4 h, 6 h and 8 h after the arsenic injection using a gamma counter (n = 6/group).
All control animals died within 4 d. Treatment with DMDMS, i.p. or i.g., and DEDMS, DnPDMS and DiPDMS, i.p., did not reduce lethality either. Given i.p., DnPDMS, DEDMS and DiPDMS reduced lethality to 2/7, 1/7 and 1/7, respectively. In DMSA treated mice lethality was 3/14 (i.g.) and 0/14 (i.p.). Observed lethality was well correlated to the organ arsenic mobilization. It is concluded that DnPDMS, DEDMS and DiPDMS, i.p., are effective arsenic antidotes, but are not superior to DMSA. Different substitution of the DMSA molecule resulted in altered therapeutic efficacy. The dependence of the antidotal efficacy on the route of administration indicates differences in resorption or metabolization of the analogues.

##Dimethyl-, diethyl-, di-n-propyl-, diisopropyl-meso-2,3-dimercaptosuccinate.
*Institut für Pharmakologie und Toxikologie der Akademie des Sanitäts- und Gesundheitswesen der Bundeswehr, BSW, Ingolstädter Landstr. 100, 8046 Garching, FRG

56

EFFECT OF DI(ACETYLTHIO)- AND DI(BENZOYLTHIO)SUCCINIC ACID (DATSA, DBTSA) AS ARSENIC ANTIDOTES. *H.Kreppel, U.Paepcke, F.X.Reichl, P.K. Singh, and M.M. Jones

Dimercaptosuccinic acid (DMSA) is reported to be more effective than dimercaptopropanol (BAL) in reducing lethality and body arsenic content in acute arsenic poisoning. In the present study the therapeutic effect of DATSA and DBTSA, newly synthetized analogues of DMSA with shielded thiolgroups ("prodrugs"), was investigated in experimental arsenic poisoning.
The efficacy of 0.7 mmol/kg DATSA and DBTSA, i.p. or via gastric tube (i.g.), was compared to DMSA and saline (controls). Antidotes were given 30 min after 65 µmol/kg arsenic trioxide (survival study) or 42.5 µmol/kg arsenic trioxide containing a tracer dose of 73-As (elimination study). Lethality was recorded over 30 d in mice injected with 65 µmol/kg arsenic trioxide (n = 7 or 14/group). In the elimination study, the arsenic content of various organs (blood, liver, kidneys, lungs, spleen, small intestine, large intestine, brain, testes, muscle and skin) at 30 min, 2 h, 4 h, 6 h and 8 h after the arsenic injection was measured using a gamma counter (n = 6/group).
14/14 control animals died within 4 d. Given i.g., DATSA and DBTSA increased the survival rate to 2/7 and 3/7, and given i.p. to 6/7. Following therapy with DMSA, however, animals recovered more rapidly, and 11/14 (i.g.) and 14/14 (i.p.), respectively, animals survived. In all organs investigated, DATSA and DBTSA markedly reduced the arsenic content, however the time-course was dependent on the route of application: Following therapy i.g., a similar extend of organ arsenic elimination was observed within 3.5 - 5.5 h as was found already 1.5 h after treatment i.p. The efficacy of DATSA and DBTSA in reducing the organ arsenic content was close but not superior to the effect of DMSA.

*Institut für Pharmakologie und Toxikologie der Akademie des Sanitäts- und Gesundheitswesen der Bundeswehr, BSW, Ingolstädter Landstr. 100, 8046 Garching, FRG

57

PYRUVATE METABOLISM IN LIVERS OF GUINEA PIGS PERFUSED WITH ANTIDOTES AFTER ACUTE EXPERIMENTAL POISONING WITH As_2O_3

F.X. Reichl, H. Kreppel, and W. Forth

An increased pyruvate content in livers of guinea pigs was observed after acute experimental poisoning with As_2O_3 (Reichl et al. 1988, Arch. Tox. 62: 473-475).
The relative effectiveness of British Anti-Lewisite (BAL), dimercaptopropanesulfonic acid (DMPS) and dimercaptosuccinic acid (DMSA) was compared by determining their effect on pyruvate metabolism in perfused livers of guinea pigs after acute experimental poisoning with As_2O_3.
Guinea pigs received As_2O_3, 10 mg/kg s.c., as a single injection. One hour after the injection the livers were perfused (35 ml/min) with Krebs-Henseleit buffer and glucose (10 mmol/l) for 80 minutes. After 40 minutes of perfusion either 0.1 or 0.7 mmol/l BAL, DMPS, or DMSA were added to the perfusate for 40 min. Samples of the effluent were collected every 10 min; lactate and pyruvate were determined enzymatically.
As compared to controls, a significant increase in the pyruvate efflux was observed in perfused livers of guinea pigs treated with As_2O_3. After influx of DMSA and DMPS (0.1 and 0.7 mmol/l), respectively, the pyruvate efflux decreased and reached control values without arsenic treatment. On the other hand the pyruvate efflux was further decreased after influx of BAL (0.1 and 0.7 mmol/l).

Walther Straub-Institut für Pharmakologie und Toxikologie der LMU München, Nußbaumstr. 26, 8000 München 2

58

DOES ALUMINIUM INFLUENCE CASOMORPHIN-MEDIATED BEHAVIOUR IN RATS ?

H. Stark, C. Schmidt, R.Schmidt, G. Poeggel and H-G. Bernstein

Aluminium is a well-known neurotoxin in animals and man. A hypothesis was formulated by Banks and Kastin (Banks W.A., Kastin A.J.: Neurosci. & Biobehav. Rev. 13, 47-53, 1989) to explain the effects of the metal on multiple neurobiological phenomena. According to these authors aluminium is capable of altering the transport of certain neuropeptides through the blood-brain barrier, thereby changing CNS processes. We used long-term administration of aluminium (subcutaneous injection of $AlCl_3$) to rats to prove this idea in behavioural experiments. The first results are showing that casomorphin-evoked analgesia (as tested by electric tail root stimulation) was enhanced in aluminium-treated animals. Though other explanations of this effects cannot be excluded, it seems to us that the results are in favour of an increase transport of the peptide into the brain thereby providing a greater amount of casomorphin to analgesia-mediating receptors. Additionally, we observed a decrease of memory formation in rats after chronical aluminium administration.

Institute of Neurobiology and Brain Research, Brenneckestr. 6, O-3090 Magdeburg, FRG

This research was supported by a grant of BMFT of FRG.

59

INTERACTION OF DIETHYLDITHIOCARBAMATE (DEDTC) AND PYRROLIDINEDITHIOCARBAMATE (PDTC) WITH ZINC IN VIVO

V.Eybl, M.Koutenská, J.Koutenský, J.Sýkora, V.Smolíková, M.M.Jones[+]

DEDTC has been used as immunomodulating drug. Chemical evidence suggests that PDTC might prove to be quite superior for this purpose. Several metals may be chelated by DEDTC in vitro. In this paper the influence of both dithiocarbamates (DTCs) on the zinc kinetics has been compared. The experiments were performed in male mice (ICR, Velaz). The influence of DEDTC and PDTC on the whole body burden (w.b.b.) and the organ distribution of Zn was studied. The mice were given always a single dose of $^{65}ZnCl_2$ (with carrier) corresponding to 0.14 mg Zn^{2+}/kg. DTCs applied ip immediately after the iv Zn injection at drug:Zn molar ratio of 200:1 increased significantly the w.b.b. of Zn at 48th h. The content of Zn in the liver was not increased. The content of Zn in the kidneys was increased due to PDTC. Both DTCs decreased the w.b.b. of Zn when administered on the 2nd, 4th and 7th day after the i.v. Zn injection. DTCs were injected i.p. always at drug:Zn molar ratio of 200:1. The experiment was finished on the 9th day. However, only little changes in the Zn content of the organs were found. DTCs applied p.o. simultaneously with $ZnCl_2$ (10:1) remarkably enhanced the Zn absorption during 24h. The w.b.b. was increased. The Zn-content of the liver was increased due to DTCs. The Zn content of the kidneys was increased only by DEDTC administration but decreased by PDTC application. The results show that the Zn-DTCs complexes may be formed in vivo.

Dept.of Pharmacology and CRL, Charles Univ. Medical Faculty, 301 66 Pilsen, ČSFR; [+]Dept. of Chemistry, Vanderbilt Univ., Nashville, TN, 37 235 U.S.A.

60

EFFECT OF DIETHYLDITHIOCARBAMATE AND ITS DERIVATIVE N-(4-METHOXYBENZYL)-N-DITHIOCARBOXY-D-GLUCAMINE ON TRACE METAL LEVEL IN MICE

D.Kotyzová, J.Koutenský, M.M.Jones[+], V.Eybl

Diethyldithiocarbamate (DEDTC) and its derivative N-(4-methoxybenzyl)-N-dithiocarboxy-D-glucamine (MeOBDCG) have been proposed as agents for treatment of metal intoxications. These metal chelators could have also serious influence on the body levels of essential metals. In the experiments performed in male ICR mice the effect of DEDTC and MeOBDCG on the tissue distribution of some essential metals was studied. The chelators were administered in a sigle dose or repeatedly. The level of Ca,Mg,Fe,Cu and Zn were measured in the liver, kidneys and in the brain. Elements were estimated using atomic absorption spectrometry and the dry-ashing procedure for tissue solubilization. Particular attention was paid to the tissue levels of Zn and Cu. The influence of the chelators on the tissue level of these elements was studied also in the acute experiments without/with additive administration of $CuCl_2/ZnCl_2$. The most significant changes were seen in the cooper and zinc distribution after DEDTC application. In the experiments with $CuCl_2/ZnCl_2$ treated mice both antidotes increased the amount of Cu in the brain. DEDTC also increased the content of Cu and Zn in the liver. In the experiments in which Cu/Zn were not injected the influence of dithiocarbamtes were less expressive.

Department of Pharmacology, Charles University Faculty of Medicine, CS-301 66 Pilsen, ČSFR

[+]Department of Chemistry, Vanderbilt University, Nashville, TN 37 235 U.S.A.

61

EFFECTS OF LONG TERM LEAD EXPOSURE ON THE CHOLINERGIC AND ADRENERGIC RECEPTOR SYSTEMS IN MICE
S. Schulte, K. Mengel, W.E. Müller, K.D. Friedberg

The precise mechanism of the neurotoxic effects of lead is still controversial. Neurotoxicity of long term low level exposure to lead in adult and juvenile mouse brain and its influence on the central cholinergic and adrenergic membrane receptors have been studied.

Lead was administered for periods of 10, 30 and 90 days to adult mice. Exposure of juvenile animals was initiated on the day of conception in their mothers and continued after birth and during weaning until 30 days postpartum. Both groups, adult mice and pups or their mothers, were given a solution of 1, 10, 100 and 1000 ppm lead nitrate in their drinking water, which was available ad libitum.

Radioligand binding studies were performed in vitro to determine apparent receptor densities (B_{max} values) and affinities (K_D values) in brain membranes of the lead exposed mice. Saturation studies of ligands for α_1- and α_2-adrenoceptors, β-adrenoceptors and muscarinic receptors were carried out. In addition, the binding of a selective muscarinic agonist and an antagonist to putative subtypes in mouse cerebral cortex was investigated. Inhibition curves of ^{3}H-QNB labelled membranes were determined with the m_1-antagonist pirenzepine and the m_2-agonist carbachol to distinguish between high and low affinity agonist and antagonist states in the cortex.

No gross changes in density or affinity of the membrane receptors investigated were seen in animals treated with lead. Similarly the properties of high and low affinity muscarinic receptor binding were unchanged in all the groups exposed to lead.

In conclusion, our results show up to now that lead does not affect any of the investigated neurotransmitter receptor systems in mouse brain under the experimental conditions used.

Institut für Pharmakologie und Toxikologie der Fakultät für klinische Medizin Mannheim der Universität Heidelberg, Maybachstr. 14-16, D-6800 Mannheim 1, FRG

62

COMPARATIVE STUDIES ON THE INDUCTION OF DEALKYLATION OF METHACETIN, PHENACETIN AND CAFFEINE BY 2,3,7,8-TCDD OR 2,3,4,7,8-PCDF IN LIVERS OF A NON-HUMAN PRIMATE.
Birgit Jödicke*, Ursula Kastner, Hans Helge* and Diether Neubert.

A breath-test using [3-^{14}CH$_3$]-caffeine as a sensitive tool in monitoring a monooxygenase induction by 2,3,7,8-tetrachlorodibenzo-p-dioxin (TCDD) in vivo (Krüger et al. Chemosphere 20, 1173, 1990) schowed the rate of ^{14}CO$_2$ exhalation from methacetin or phenacetin not to be increased. Therefore, we studied the inducibility of dealkylation of methacetin or phenacetin in liver homogenates of *Callithrix jacchus* one week after treatment with TCDD or 2,3,4,7,8-pentachlorodibenzofuran (PCDF).

| µM | Methacetin | | Phenacetin | | Caffeine(C3) |
	(19)	(197)	(21)	(204)	(991)
Controls	1.2 ± 0.4 =100%	4.8 ± 1.1 =100%	0.2 ± 0.1 =100%	1.0 ± 0.4 =100%	0.2 ± 0.1 =100%
TCDD 1 µg/kg body wt	467% 368% 328%	350% 261% 297%	380% 185% 250%	214% 179% 142%	285% 225% 246%
PCDF 1 µg/kg body wt	355% 335% 375%	286% 257% 211%	245% 210% 155%	159% 132% 203%	265% 210% 205%

The rates at similar substrate concentrations in marmosets without induction were: methacetin > phenacetin > caffeine. The single doses of TCDD or PCDF used in this study induced a clear-cut and comparable increase in the dealkylation rate of methacetin, phenacetin and caffeine. The finding that methacetin or phenacetin (in contrast to caffeine), after subcutaneous injection, cannot serve as substrates in monitoring the inducing effect of TCDD with a breath-test must have pharmacokinetic reasons, and cannot be explained by a lack of response of the monooxygenases involved.

Supported by grant # 0765002 from the Federal Ministry for Research and Technology (BMFT). Institut für Toxikologie and Embryopharmakologie, Garystr. 5, 1000 Berlin 33 and *Kinderklinik, Heubnerweg 6, 1000 Berlin 19, Freie Universität Berlin, Germany

63

TCDD-INDUCED INCREASE IN THE DEALKYLATION OF METHACETIN, PHENACETIN AND CAFFEINE IN MOUSE LIVER HOMOGENATES.
Birgit Neubert*, Ursula Kastner, Hans Helge* and Diether Neubert.

The hepatic O- or N-dealkylations of methacetin (metha), phenacetin (phena) and caffeine (caff) are apparently all catalysed by P450IA-type monooxygenases, although it has not yet been proven that the same P450-isozyme (e.g P450IA2) is involved. We investigated whether differences are detectable in the inducibility of these 3 substrates subsequent to a single s.c. dose (100 ng/kg body wt) of 2,3,7,8-tetrachlorodibenzo-p-dioxin (TCDD). The dose was chosen to be just sufficient to initiate such an inducing effect in the liver. Full enzyme kinetics were established for all the substrates, but only the results for one substrate concentration are presented here.

	substrates	(µM)	pmoles aldehyde formed x mg wet weight^{-1} x minute^{-1} (M ± SD)		factor	Mann-Whitney-test (p =)
controls	metha	46	11.55 ±	1.94		
TCDD	metha	46	17.15 ±	1.81	1.5	0.002
controls	phena	80	2.43 ±	0.60		
TCDD	phena	80	4.21 ±	0.89	1.7	0.006
controls	3-caff	200	0.50 ±	0.12		
TCDD	3-caff	200	0.89 ±	0.18	1.8	0.002
controls	7-caff	200	0.34 ±	0.09		
TCDD	7-caff	200	0.30 ±	0.03	0.9	0.273

controls: n = 8.   TCDD: n = 6

The mouse does not seem to be very sensitive to the inducing effect of TCDD, but the results indicate that the activity of all 3 substrates is found induced in the mouse 4 days after exposure to this rather small dose of TCDD, and no pronounced difference in the susceptibility for induction between these substrates was obvious. From these results no preference in choosing one of the substrates for analysing biological actions of polychlorinated dibenzo-p-dioxins and dibenzofurans would be justified. However, only the N3-demethylation of caffeine was found to be inducible by TCDD, while demethylation of the 7-CH$_3$ group of caffeine does not readily respond to this type of induction, as has been shown before in breath-tests in vivo with other species (Krüger et al. Chemosphere 20, 1173, 1990).
Supported by the Federal Ministry for Research and Technology (BMFT), grant # 0765002. Institut für Toxikologie and Embryopharmakologie, and *Kinderklinik (Kaiserin Auguste Victoria Haus), Freie Universität Berlin, Garystr. 5, 1000 Berlin 33, Germany

64

INDUCTION BY BENZO[a]PYRENE OF THE DEALKYLATION OF CAFFEINE, PHENACETIN AND METHACETIN BY HEPATIC MONOOXYGENASES IN MICE AND MARMOSETS
Diether Neubert, Ursula Kastner, Birgit Jödicke

The capacity of mouse liver homogenates to dealkylate the substrates caffeine, phenacetin and methacetin 24 hrs after an oral pretreatment with 50 mg benzo[a]pyrene/kg body wt for 3 days was compared. The goal was to test whether the substances are suitable as substrates for the detection of B[a]P-type inductions, and also applicable for a breath-test (to be used experimentally, and possibly also with ^{13}C in man).

| | Phenacetin | | Methacetin | Caffeine | |
	(14 µM)	(76 µM)	(41 µM)	C3- (218 µM)	C7- (204 µM)
Control	100%*	100%	100%	100%	100%
B(a)P	32% 58% 44%	336% 625% 994%	234% 202% 318%	278% 360% 418%	128% 125% 178%

* controls: SD = ± 35%; each row: values of 3 pooled livers

It was found (Table) that the rate of dealkylation of all three substrates responded to the inducing effect of B[a]P. However, the induction of phenacetin O-deethylation occurred only at high substrate concentrations, indicating that only one of two metabolic reactions (to be distinguished by kinetic data) responded. There was evidence for only one enzyme reaction in the case of methacetin demethylation. Caffeine 3-demethylation was much more susceptible to the action of B[a]P than 7-demethylation. Similar results were obtained in marmosets, but there was only evidence for one phenacetin deethylating reaction.

Institut für Toxikologie und Embryopharmakologie, Freie Universität Berlin, Garystrasse 5, D-1000 Berlin 33, Germany

65

THE TOXICOLOGICAL RELEVANCE OF PARACETAMOL-INDUCED
INHIBITION OF HEPATIC RESPIRATION AND ATP-DEPLETION.
O. Strubelt, M. Younes*, A. Röbke, and C. Magnussen

In order to elucidate the role of mitochondrial dysfunction for paracetamol-induced hepatotoxicity, the effects of paracetamol on the
oxygen consumption and the ATP-content of the isolated perfused
rat liver were correlated with parameters of hepatic viability and
hepatotoxicity. 5 g/l paracetamol reduced the oxygen consumption
of the livers by about 80% and hepatic ATP-content by 96%.
Hepatotoxicity was evident by a nearly complete interruption of
bile secretion, a marked release of enzymes (GPT, LDH) in the perfusate, by a depletion of hepatic glutathione and by an accumulation of calcium in the liver. Paracetamol-induced hepatotoxicity
could be completely prevented by using livers from non-fasted rats
as well as by addition of fructose to the perfusate of livers from
fasted animals. Both treatments resulted in an increased energy
supply from anaerobic glycolysis as evidenced by a large release
of lactate and pyruvate into the perfusate, but did not inhibit paracetamol-induced decline of oxygen consumption. The decrease in
hepatic oxygen consumption depended on the dose of
paracetamol and first occurred at a concentration of 0.2 g/l
(-10%). LDH and GPT release, on the other hand, were elevated at
2 and 5 g/l and calcium accumulation occured at 5 g/l paracetamol
only. The oral administration of the high dose of 5 g/kg
paracetamol in vivo to rats exerted strong hepatotoxicity but
produced maximal serum levels of 800 mg/l paracetamol only and
did not decrease hepatic oxygen consumption as measured in
vitro.
Conclusions: In the isolated-perfused rat liver in vitro, high
concentrations of paracetamol can produce "chemical hypoxia" by
attacking mitochondria resulting in hepatic injury. Such high
concentrations of paracetamol, however, are not attained in vivo.
"Chemical hypoxia" thus seems not to be relevant to the well-
known hepatotoxic action of paracetamol.
Institut für Toxikologie der Medizinischen Universität zu Lübeck,
Ratzeburger Allee 160, D-2400 Lübeck, and
*Max von Pettenkofer-Institut für Toxikologie, BGA, Postfach
330013, D-1000 Berlin 33.

66

STUDIES ON COVALENT BINDING OF A POTENT ß-BLOCKING DRUG IN
TISSUE PROTEINS AND COLLAGEN OF RATS
A. Baumann, and K.-U. Möritz

Toxic effects of drugs and their metabolites may be caused
by covalent binding to cellular macromolecules. The potent
ß-blocking drug B 24/76 (dl-1-(2,4-dichlorphenoxy)-3- 2-(3,4-
dimethoxyphenyl) ethylamino -propan-2-ol is a highly lipophilic compound with an extensive binding to plasma proteins.
Since interstitial and intracellular volumes are about 13
times larger than plasma volumes and 98 % of all proteins
are located extravascularily we directed our attention to the
covalent binding of the substance to tissue proteins and its
possible toxicological consequences.
³H-B 24/76 was given orally to male Wistar rats in a dosage
of 10 mg/kg. After 24 h the animals were sacrificed and lung,
liver, heart, kidney, muscle were taken. We extracted the
tissue homogenates exhaustivily with methanol and considered
the covalent protein binding by means of liquid scintillation
counting.
The highest binding was found in the liver with 11 % of the
radioactivity distributed in this organ while muscle, lung,
kidney and heart showed almost no activities. We couldn' t
see any differences of the binding strenght in the individual fractions of particles in the cell and the cytosol
of this tissue. In respect to the binding to collagens we
found that 7 % of the radioactivity distributed to the lung
were covalently bound to this protein. Since these structure
proteins have a great half-life such an irreversible binding
can cause damage.
Our results are discussed in connection with other biochemical and histological investigations as to their relevance
for toxic effects by the ß-blocker.

Institute of Pharmacology and Toxicology, University of
Greifswald, Friedrich-Loeffler-Straße 23d,
O-2200 Greifswald, FRG

67

DELETERIOUS ACTIONS OF DICHLOROMETHANE ON
REVERSIBLE HEMORRHAGIC SHOCK IN RATS

J.R.Kullik, M.Weise, M.Klapperstück, P.Hoffmann.

The effects of dichloromethane (DCM) exposure on
hemodynamic, electrocardiographic and paraclini-
cal parameters in hemorrhagic shocked rats were
investigated. Acute DCM exposure (12.4 mmol/kg,
po) increased the blood volume necessary to be
withdrawn in order to induce the shock (30 mm
Hg, 20 min). DCM exposed animals showed a delayed restitution of arterial blood pressure, a
prolonged depression of central venous pressure,
a reduction of the cardiac performance as well
as an increased incidence of cardiac arrhythmias
(atrioventricular blocks). Furthermore, a pronounced metabolic acidosis, a reduced oxygen saturation of the blood and a hyperkaliemia in the
posthemorrhagic period as well as a pronounced
leukocytosis, thrombocytopenia and signs of a
hypocoagulability with simultaneous activation
of the fibrinolytic system (disseminated intravascular coagulation) were observed in DCM exposed rats.
The results demonstrate that an acute DCM exposure impaired recovery from reversible hemorrhagic shock.

(Supported by the BMFT Grant No. 01HK011R)

Institute of Industrial Toxicology,
Faculty of Medicine
Martin-Luther-University Halle-Wittenberg
Franzosenweg 1a, Halle/S., O-4020 , Germany

68

GLIATOXICITY IN IN-VITRO CELL CULTURES INDUCED BY
2.5-HEXANEDIONE
W. Grüning*, F. Boegner#, H. Altenkirch*, G. Stol-
tenburg+, P. Marx#, M. Wagner°

2.5-hexanedione (2.5 HD) is the most neurotoxic
metabolite of n-hexane. In animal studies an axono-
pathic mechanism consisting of the accumulation of
10 nm neurofilaments could be demonstrated. So far
only few studies have considered a possible effect
of 2.5 HD on Schwann cells, glia cells or both.
Our cell culture model offers the possibility of
qualitative differentiation and quantification of
toxic effects for neurons and glia cells selectively. We prepared pure neuronal, pure glial and
mixed cultures from dorsal root ganglia (DRG) of 6
to 14 day old chick embryos (E6 - E14). DRG were
chosen because they project to the central as well
as to the peripheral nervous system. Cells were
cultivated in serum containing F12-medium with
nerve growth factor (NGF) and the neurotrophic
matrix factor (NTF B 82). Methods of investigation
included phase contrast microscopy and scanning
electron microscopy.
In mixed cultures we observed severe toxic alteration of glial cells at a concentration of 0.25%
2.5 HD, whereas neurons and neurites remained almost unaffected. We could demonstrate similar glia-
toxic effects on mixed cultures of sympathetic
ganglia, myelon and brain.

*Department of Neurology, Spandau Hospital, Free
University Berlin, F.R.G.
#Department of Neurology, Klinikum Steglitz, Free
University Berlin, F.R.G.
+Institute of Neuropathology, Klinikum Steglitz,
Free University Berlin, F.R.G.
°Bundesgesundheitsamt, Berlin, F.R.G.

69

DNA ADDUCTS FORMED BY URINARY EXTRACTS FORM SMOKERS, PASSIVE SMOKERS AND NON-SMOKERS
G. Scherer, A. Krätschmer and F. Adlkofer

It has been assumed that the elevated mutagenic activity in smokers' urine is predominantly caused by aromatic amines. Pyrolysis products of proteins such as 3-amino-1,4-dimethyl-5H-pyrido[4,3-b]indole (Trp-P1), 3-amino-1-methyl-5H-pyrido[4,3-b]indole (Trp-P2), 2-amino-1-methyl-6-phenylimidazo[4,5-b]pyridine (PhIP), 2-amino-6-methyldipyrido[1,2-a:3',2'-d]imidozole (Glu-P1), 2-aminodipyrido[1,2-a:3',2'-d]imidazole (Glu-P2) and 2-amino-3-methyl-9H-pyrido[2,3-b]indole (MeAαC) are possible candidates for this activity. An in vitro assay for detecting DNA-binding capacity of complex mixtures has been established according to published methods. The assay includes incubation of the test substance with calf thymus DNA in the presence of rat liver S9, cofactors and 3'-phosphoadenosine5'-phosphosulfate (PAPS), subsequent isolation of the DNA and ^{32}P-postlabelling analysis (P1 version) for DNA adducts. This method has been applied to benzo(a)pyrene (BaP), some aromatic amines (4-aminobiphenyl, MeAαC, Trp-P1, Trp-P2, Glu-P2) and condensates of cigarette smoke (CSCs, both from mainstream smoke and from environmental tobacco smoke). The major DNA adducts of BaP and most of the aromatic amines seem to be visuably similar to those reported in the literature. The autoradiographs obtained with CSCs show the characteristic diagonale radioactive zone (DRZ) observed with DNA isolated from smokers or from mice treated with CSC. The adducts obtained with urine extracts so far do not match with those of any of the aromatic amines tested.

Analytisch-biologisches Forschungslabor Prof. F. Adlkofer, Goethestr. 20, 8000 München 2, Germany

70

ON TWO INTOXICATIONS WITH DISINFECTANTS
F. Riemer[1] and J. Resler[2]

In a state of an acute psychosis, caused by abuse of alcohol, a 23-year-old man ingested according to his own statement 20 tablets of the disinfectant chloramin[R] (19.6 g of tosylchloramide sodium) with suicidal intent. About one hour later the patient was hospitalized. No symptoms of poisoning were observed. A gastric lavage was carried out and after this charcoal and magnesium sulfate were instilled into the stomach. The drug could be detected in the stomach contents and also in the urine by means of TLC and the UV-spectrum after separation by TLC.

A 53-year-old man drank an unknown amount of a brown liquid in the morning. At the time of hospitalization the patient showed severe symptoms of poisoning: deep coma, respiratory global-insufficiency, anuria. In spite of intensive care therapy the man died on the same day. By means of TLC and the UV-spectrum the liquid could be identified as the disinfectant stallosept[R]. The main ingredients detected after reaction with fast red salt AL were 1,2,4-xylenol, 1,3,5-xylenol, and m-cresol.

[1]Institute of Pharmacology and Toxicology, [2]Clinic of Internal Medicine, University of Greifswald, F.-Loeffler-Straße 23, O-2200 Greifswald, FRG

71

FUNCTIONAL IMPORTANCE OF TYROSINE RESIDUES IN CYTOCHROME P-450 ENZYMES
G.-R. Jänig, J. Blanck, W. Schwarze, H. Schrauber, and K. Ruckpaul

The function of tyrosine residues in cytochrome P-450 has been analysed by means of chemical modification aimed to get deeper insight into the structural basis of the different substrate specificity of P-450 enzymes and mechanisms of electron transfer between P-450 and NADPH-cytochrome P-450 reductase. P-450 LM2 (IIB4) and P-450 LM4 (IA2) as representative enzymes of different gene families were chemically modified with tetranitromethane. Nitration of two tyrosine residues of each enzyme inhibits the activity of P-450 LM2 as well as of P-450 LM4 by about 80%. HPLC tryptic peptide mapping reveals for P-450 LM2 that Tyr-235 and Tyr-380 are nearly fully nitrated, while Tyr-348, Tyr-484 and Tyr-111 are partially labeled. Analyses of P-450 LM4 show that mainly Tyr-243 and Tyr-271 are labeled, whereas Tyr-71, Tyr-188 and Tyr-365 are modified to a lower extent. Binding of metyrapone to P-450 LM2 prior to treatment with tetranitromethane reveals protection of Tyr-380 from nitration and a lower extent of inactivation suggesting its location at the active center. Based on this assignment a computer-graphic model of the substrate binding site of this P-450 was developed (Schwarze et al. (1988) Biochem. Biophys. Res. Comm. 150, 996-1005). Analyses of the phase distribution of the P-450 LM2 and P-450 LM4 reduction in dependence of the molar ratio of reductase to P-450 suggests that a 1:1 complex of P-450 and reductase represents the reactive species of an effective electron transfer. The impaired electron transfer capability of P-450 enzymes on nitration is attributed to a disturbed complex formation with NADPH-cytochrome P-450 reductase.

Department of Biocatalysis, Central Institute of Molecular Biology, O-1115 Berlin-Buch, Germany

72

CROSS-REACTIVITIES WITHIN THE CYTOCHROME P-450 SUPERFAMILY: THEORY AND EXPERIMENTS
W. Schwarze, M. Henning, E. Grau, and K. Ruckpaul

Cytochrome P-450 enzymes are important in the oxidative metabolism of numerous endogeneous compounds such as steroids, bile acids, fatty acids, prostaglandins, leukotrienes and biogenic amines. Many of these enzymes also metabolize a wide range of compounds including drugs, environmental pollutants, carcinogens, natural plants products, and alcohols. Cytochromes P-450 represent a gene superfamily comprehending at present about 154 members which have been assigned to 27 families (Nebert et al. (1991) DNA and Cell Biol. 10,2). The members differ in gene structure, sequence, membrane binding, substrate specificity and immunochemical reactivity. This contribution represents a systematic study of cross-reactivity within this superfamily: 1) Statistical examination of published experimental results: Monoclonal antibodies (MAbs) and polyclonal antibodies (= PAbs) do not cross-react with members of foreign families. All of PAbs but only a few of MAbs cross-react with all members of the same subfamily independently of affiliation to species, gene or tissue localization. 2) ELISA: PAbs against cytochrome P-450 XI B1 do not cross-react with any member of the tested eight foreign families. 3) Prediction of cross-reacting epitopes: Epitopes were predicted on the basis of hydrophobicity and flexibility profils according to (Hopp and Woods (1981) Proc. Nat. Acad. Sci. 78, 3824, and Karplus and Schulz (1985) Naturwissenschaften, 72, 212). If such epitopes are parts of conserved amino acid regions, then cross-reactivity of such epitopes is concluded. The results obtained by the three topics are in agreement with each other.

Central Institute of Molecular Biology, Robert-Rössle-Str. 10, O-1115 Berlin-Buch

73

COMPUTER MODELLING OF CYTOCHROME P-450 II B4 SUB-
STRATE BINDING SITE, W. Schwarze, J. Jäger, G.-R.
Jänig, and K. Ruckpaul

The unique capability of cytochrome P-450 II B4 to
convert a great variety of drugs and other xenobiotics is not understood until now, and the three
dimensional structure of the membrane bound enzyme
is not available. To get deeper insight into struc-
ture-activity relationships of P-450 II B4, a series of tertiary amines as substrates was investigated with respect to (1) selected physicochemical
parameters as substrate enzyme interaction (binding,
spin shift, reduction rate, turnover), (2) the substrate structures by quantum-chemical methods, and
(3) the substrate binding amino acid(s) by the method of chemical modification. From these data a
three dimensional conception of substrate-enzyme
interaction area was developed and its reliability
proved by quantum-chemical methods (minimization of
the interaction energy). The results show, that (1)
substrates with a butterfly-like conformation, that
means with about parallel benzene rings, are pre-
fered for binding (2), the tetrapeptide Phe-377
until Tyr-380 in a ß-like strand conformation should
provide the major contributions to the substrate-
enzyme interaction (Schwarze et al. (1988) Biochem.
Biophys. Res. Commun. 150 (3), 996). Numerous computer graphics of substrate conformations and sub-
strate-tetrapeptide arrangements are shown and discussed in relation to binding and spin shift. The
influence of water and peptide environment on the
substrate structure, and vice versa the influence
of the substrate on the tetrapeptide structure (induced fit) was quantum-chemically investigated
(Jäger et al. (1988) J. Mol. Structure 170, 181).

Central Institute of Molecular Biology, Robert-
Rössle-Str. 10, O-1115 Berlin-Buch

74

ENZYMATIC CHARACTERIZATION OF THE P450IA1 AND IA2
GENE PRODUCTS FROM GENETICALLY ENGINEERED V79
HAMSTER CELLS.
Barbara Heinrich-Hirsch, Thomas Schulz-Schalge, Dorothea Hofmann,
Catherine Wölfel*, Johannes Doehmer*, and Diether Neubert.

Two V79 derived cell lines, XEM2, expressing rat P450IA1 and
XEMdMZ, expressing rat P450IA2, were investigated for their capacity
for O-dealkylation of different phenoxazone ethers.
The activities of ethoxy-, methoxy-, benzoxy- and pentoxyresorufin O-
dealkylases (**EROD, MROD, BROD, PROD**) were determined in a
fraction free of cytosol. In the cytosol a NADPH-dependent reduction
of resorufin could be demonstrated, which could be inhibited by
addition of 30 μM dicoumarol, suggesting the presence of a NAD(P)H-
oxidoreductase. The addition of dicoumarol to the homogenates showed
no influence to the EROD activity. The following results were obtained:

	EROD	MROD	BROD	PROD
IA1	17.6 ± 1.1	1.5 ± 0.3	1.6 ± 0.2	< 0.2
IA2	10.7 ± 1.5	30.7 ± 2.8	1.4 ± 0.1	2.0 ± 0.3
V79	<0.2	<0.2	-	-

Values given as pmoles resorufin x mg protein^{-1} x min^{-1}

Appreciable EROD activities were detectable in both cell lines, yet
more pronounced in the IA1 expressing cell line. MROD activity was
predominantly observed in the P450IA2 expressing cell line. Distinct,
but only marginal activities were determined for BROD and for PROD
only in IA2 expressing cells.
Our data confirm findings from *Namkung et al. (Molec. Pharmacol. 34,
628-637, 1988)* that methoxyresorufin is a specific substrate for rat
P450IA2, and that this substrate may help to differentiate the induction
of the P450IA subforms. The significance of these findings for the
human P450IA2 form has still to be elucidated.

Institut für Toxikologie und Embryopharmakologie, FU Berlin, W-1000 Berlin 33;
*Institut für Toxikologie, Johannes-Gutenberg Universität, W-6500 Mainz

75

THE PROTON PUMP INHIBITOR PANTOPRAZOLE IS A WEAK SUBSTRATE
FOR CYTOCHROME P450 DEPENDENT ENZYMES
W.A.SIMON

The gastric acid antisecretory compound omeprazole (5-
methoxy-2-((4-methoxy-3,5-dimethyl-2-pyridinylmethyl)-sul-
phinyl)-1H-benzimidazole, OME), a member of the new class
of H^+,K^+-ATPase inhibitors, is known to interact with the
metabolism of other drugs in vitro and in vivo. In this
study, two other substituted benzimidazoles, pantoprazole
(5-difluoromethoxy-2-((3,4-dimethoxy-2-pyridinylmethyl)-
sulphinyl)-1H-benzimidazole, PANTO) and lansoprazole (2-
((3-methyl-4-(2,2,2,-trifluoroethoxy)-2-pyridinylmethyl)-
sulphinyl)-1H-benzimidazole, LANSO) are compared for their
ability to inhibit cytochrome P450 dependent biotransformation in vitro with regard to three representative reactions: O-dealkylation of 7-ethoxycoumarin (EC), N-demethy-
lation of ethylmorphine (EM) and hydroxylation of lonazolac
(LONA). These reactions can be followed in microsomes from
phenobarbital pretreated rats representing the cytochrome
P450IIB1 subfamily. As shown in presence of known inhibitors of cytochrome P450, e.g. SK&F 525A, metyrapone, chlor-
promazine and nitrendipine, different enzymes seem to be
responsible for these three indicator reactions of the
cytochrome P450IIB1 complex. These reactions are inhibited
to a different extent by the three H^+,K^+-ATPase inhibitors. PANTO shows the lowest inhibitory activity versus the
three reactions (K_i, μmol/l): EC, 138; EM, 104; LONA, 128.
A greater effect is observed with OME: EC, 38; EM, 68;
LONA, 20. LANSO exceeds OME in inhibiting the three enzymes: EC, 17; EM, 34; LONA, 8. The biotransformation rate of
the substituted benzimidazoles themselves is increased in
microsomes from B: phenobarbital induced rats (P450IIB1)
versus A: control rats (P450IIA), determined as % remaining
parent compound after 30 min of incubation in microsomes:
PANTO A:100, B:53, OME A:37, B:22 and LANSO A:72, B:28.

Abteilung Biochemie I, Byk Gulden Pharmazeutika,
7750 Konstanz, Germany.

76

INHIBITION OF COUMARIN - 7 - HYDROXYLASE IN
VIVO IN MICE
H. Sigusch[*#], J. Mäenpää[#], A. Rautio[#], H.
Kraul[*#], and O. Pelkonen[#]

5 substances (8-methoxypsoralen, 5,8-
dimethoxypsoralen, metyrapone, miconazole and
clotrimazole) found to be strong inhibitors of
mouse cytochrome 2a-4 in vitro (IC50 1.9 - 42
μM) were tested to inhibit coumarin
hydroxylation in vivo. DBA/2 mice (male, age 10
- 12 weeks) received 3 μmol coumarin i.p.
without and with pretreatment of the inhibitors
(10 mg/kg bw). Excretion of 7-OH-coumarin (7HC)
was determined in urine fluorometrically after
ß-glucuronidase and sulfatase hydrolysis and
chlorform extraction.

| | 7HC excretion (% of dose) ||
	control	pretreatment
8-methoxypsoralen	6.17 (0.57)	0.57 (0.11)
metyrapone	6.40 (2.64)	1.28 (0.51)
5,8-dimethoxy-psoralen	6.94 (2.87)	2.29 (1.09)
miconazole	5.30 (3.16)	4.00 (0.80)
clotrimazole	5.61 (2.37)	5.76 (1.31)

n=4., $\bar{x}$ (SD)

The in vivo elimination of 7HC corresponds well
with the IC50 found in vitro. 8-methoxypsoralen
and metyrapone (IC50 values 1.9 and 10.0 μM,
respectively) the strongest in vitro inhibitors
were also found to be the potentest inhibitors
of coumarin hydroxylation in vivo.

* Present address: Department of Clinical
Pharmacology, University of Jena, Bachstraße
18, O-6900 Jena, FRG
Department of Pharmacology and Toxicology,
University of Oulu, SF-90220 Oulu, Finnland

77

UROPROTECTIVE ACTIVITY OF SODIUM MERCAPTOETHANESULFONATE (MESNA) IN MAN AND pH-DEPENDENT VELOCITIES OF 2-CHLOROACETALDEHYDE INACTIVATION BY THIOL GROUPS.
A. Küpfer, J.R. Idle, T. Cerny

The oxidative metabolism of ifosfamide produces important quantities of cytotoxic aldehydes, particularly 2-chloro-acetaldehyde (Cl-AA) which can be inactivated by thiol-containing compounds. For the prevention of hemorrhagic cystitis in ifosfamide treated patients, sodium mercapto-ethanesulfonate (mesna, Uromitexan) is co-administered for maximal uroprotection. The chloroalkyl group of Cl-AA is able to react irrevesibly with the mesna thiol group and the velocity of this reaction might be critical for optimal uroprotection. To study the kinetics of this reaction, we have incubated Cl-AA solutions (0.3 mM) with mesna (5 mM final concentration) in sodium phosphate buffer 0.2 M at pH 4.5, pH 6.5 and pH 8.5. At timed intervals, the reaction was stopped with formaldehyde (0.1 M final concentration). Cl-AA concentrations were determined by GLC with ECD detection (Tenax packed column at 100°C using dichloromethane as the internal standard). At pH 4.5 and pH 6.5, Cl-AA disappeared with a half-life of approx. 10 min. By contrast, at pH 8.5 the Cl-AA half-life was 0.5 min which represents a 20-fold increase of Cl-AA inactivation. Dimercaptopropanol (British Anti-Lewisite, BAL) and sodium dimercaptopropanesulfonate (Dimaval) exhibited the same pronounced pH-dependence of Cl-AA inactivation. From these data we conclude that Cl-AA consumption by mesna and other thiol containing compounds is strongly influenced by surrounding pH conditions. Thus, high urinary pH should be maintained for optimal uroprotective action of mesna whereas to low urinary pH might increase the risk of Cl-AA uro-toxicity and possibly also of Cl-AA neurotoxicity in ifosfamide treated cancer patients.

Dept. of Clinical Pharmacology, University of Berne, Murtenstrasse 35, CH-3010 Berne, Switzerland

78

INFLUENCE OF BILE ACIDS ON STIMULATED LIPID PEROXIDATION AND HYDROGEN PEROXIDE PRODUCTION IN RAT LIVER MICROSOMES

A. Barth, and M. Bernst

In living organism antioxidant mechanisms include enzymes and small molecules such as glutathione, vitamins C and E, which react directly with free radicals. Bile acids were found to be effective antioxidants by scavenging peroxyl radicals via direct oxidation to ketoderivatives (De Lange R.J. and A.N. Glazer Archs. Biochem. Biophys. 276: 19, 1990). We investigated the in vitro influence of different bile acids on the NADPH-Fe^{2+}-stimulated lipid peroxidation (LPO) and hydrogen peroxide production (H_2O_2) in rat liver microsomes. LPO was determined as production of thiobarbituric acid reactants (TBAR), H_2O_2 was estimated colorimetrically. Different tri- di- and monohydroxylated bile acids were given to the incubation mixture in concentrations ranging from 10^{-5} to 10^{-3} M. Sodium salts of cholic, tauroglycocholic and deoxycholic acids as well as chenodeoxycholic, ursodeoxycholic, lithocholic acids and cholesterol did not alter the microsomal production of TBAR. H_2O_2 formation was significantly decreased by sodium deoxycholate whereas cholesterol increased H_2O_2 production up to 4 times.
These results show that bile acids were not able to protect microsomal membrane lipids against peroxidative damage. Cholesterol mediated H_2O_2 formation as source of hydroxyl radicals had no toxic effect in our incubation mixture, TBAR were not enhanced significantly.

Present address: Instistute of Pharmacology and Toxicology, Friedrich Schiller University Jena, Löbderstraße 1, 0-6900 Jena

79

THE EFFECT OF OXYGEN RADICALS ON THE CONTRACTILITY OF SKINNED MUSCLE FIBRES FROM THE PIG MYOCARDIUM.
H. Löwe, I. Baeger, I. E. Blasig

Oxygen radicals have been implicated as mediators of cellular injury in myocardial ischemia-reperfusion. As could be shown by Kaneko (Am. J. Physiol. 256, H368, 1989) sarcolemmal membranes are alterated by oxygen free radicals resulting in depression in calcium pump activities. We studied the effect of oxygen radicals on the contractility of skinned muscle fibres from pig hearts prepared by the method of Herzig: Muscle fibres were skinned in glycerol with 1% triton X100. The contraction of the fibres was tested in medium containing in mM:10 ATP, 12 MgCl₂,5 EGTA, 20 imidazole, 5 NaN₃, 5 phosphoenolpyruvate and pyruvatkinase (ca. 20 U/ml); pH 6.7;20° C. Defined calcium concentrations were prepared by the method of Fabiato (J. Physiol. /Paris/ 75, 463, 1979). After control contractions (I) the preparations were incubated for 10 min. in a solution containing a radical generating system: 140 mM KCL, 20 mM imidazole, 20 mM xanthine, 0.05 U/ml xanthinoxidase. To compare the fiber contraction before and after the radical injury, we tested the fiber again after the incubation (II). A third group was incubated for 10 min. in a solution without radical generating system (III). To identify the generated radicals, using esr-technique, we added to the solution 100 mM DMPO, a spin trapping substance. Results: The generation of superoxide anions in the incubation solution could be detected directly by esr-technique. The radicals caused a reduction of the fiber contractility (Ca^{++}-concentration: $4.79*10^{-5}$ M) from 100.4 +/- 1.26% (I), 85.4 +/- 1.6% (III) to 52.0 +/- 15.5% (II) (p<0.01) and a right shift of the hill-plot (contractility over Ca^{++}-concentration). The following EC50 values were determined:2.82 +/- $0.66 * 10^{-6}$ M Ca^{++} (I), 5.47 +/- $2.06 * 10^{-6}$ M Ca^{++} (II) (p<0.05), 3.79 +/- $0.72 * 10^{-6}$ M Ca^{++} (III) (n.s.). The hill coefficients of the groups were not different. In additional experiments we could show, that the calcium induced contraction of the radical defected fibres could be sensitized by application of $5*10^{-4}$ M APP 201-533 (3-Amino-6-methyl-5-phenyl-1,2-dihydro-pyrid-2-on) in the same manner as in the controls.

Present adress: Institute of Drug Research, Alfred-Kowalke-Str. 4, O - 1136 Berlin, Germany

80

CALCIUM SENSITIZING EFFECTS OF PYRIDINE DERIVATIVES ON SKINNED MUSCLE FIBRES FROM THE PIG MYOCARDIUM.
H. Löwe, I. Baeger, V. Hagen

Some pyridine derivatives show positive inotropic activities. Two bipyridines, amrinone (3-amino-2-oxy-5-/pyrid-4-yl7-1,2-dihydropyridine) and milrinone (1,6-dihydro-2-methyl-6-oxo-/3,4-bipyridine/-5-carbonitril) are in clinical trials as cardiotonics. We synthetized two other pyridine derivatives with cardiotonic activities: 3-cyano-2-morpholino-5-/pyrid-4-yl7-pyridine (122-14) and 3-cyano-2-/3-diethylamino-propylamino-5-/pyrid-4-yl7-pyridine (122-60). The knowledge about the pharmacodynamic mechanisms of cardiotonic pyridines is insufficient. Some of them partially inhibit the phosphodiesterase III followed by an increase of the cellular cAMP levels. We tested the calcium sensitizing effects of amrinone, milrinone, 122-14 and 122-60 in medium concentrations of 0.5-1.0 mM on the contractility of skinned muscle fibres from pig hearts using the method of Herzig et al.: Muscle fibres from the right ventricle were skinned in glycerol with 1% triton X100. The contractions of the skinned fibres were tested in a medium containing in mM:10 ATP, 12 MgCl₂,5 EGTA, 20 imidazole, 5 NaN₃,5 phosphoenolpyruvate and pyruvatkinase (ca. 20 U/ml); pH 6.7; 20 °C; Different calcium concentrations were prepared by the method of Fabiato (J. Physiol. /Paris/ 75, 463, 1979). The sensitizing effect was tested in of Ca^{++}-concentrations of $6.17*10^{-7}$ M and $1.45*10^{-6}$ M. Results: Amrinone, milrinone and 122-14 did`nt show Ca^{++}-sensitizing effects. But 122-60 induced dose-dependently an increase of the contractility (p<0.01) in doses between 10^{-6} to 10^{-5} M. Tests of the dependence of the contraction from the calcium concentration showed in control groups an EC50 of 1.01 +/- $0.13*10^{-6}$ M Ca^{++}, and in 122-60 groups an EC50 of 0.72 +/- $0.1*10^{-6}$ M (p<0.01). The Hill-plot (contractility over the calcium concentration in the medium) did`nt show different Hill-coefficients in presence and in absence of 122-60 (1.99 +/- 0.73, n=6). 122-60 is a new, calcium-sensitizing substance for skinned fiber contraction of pig hearts.

Present adress: Institute of Drug Research, Alfred-Kowalke-Str. 4, O-1136 Berlin, Germany

R 54

81

EFFECT OF ANTICOAGULANT AND ANTITHROMBOTIC AGENTS ON EXTRINSIC AND INTRINSIC ACTIVATION OF COAGULATION
J. Hauptmann and B. Kaiser

Naturally occurring and synthetic inhibitors of the coagulation enzyme thrombin exert anticoagulant effects in vitro (ex vivo) and antithrombotic effects in vivo. To characterise the anticoagulant effect common clinical tests are used: Thrombin time (TT), prothrombin time (PT) and activated partial thromboplastin time (PTT). TT is a measure of the antithrombin activity of a given substance, PT and PTT reveal inhibitory effects on the extrinsic and intrinsic pathways of the coagulation system as well. The anticoagulant effects of various blood coagulation inhibitors and established anticoagulant/antithrombotic agents were compared: Hirudin, heparin, heparin-like agents (LMW-heparin, pentosan polysulfate, sulfated lactobionic acid amides), and a number of synthetic inhibitors of serine proteinases, that had been shown to inhibit thrombin with varying potency, were added to blood plasma in vitro and coagulation was triggered by addition of exogenous thrombin (TT) or extrinsic (PT) and intrinsic (PTT) activation. The concentrations necessary for doubling the respective clotting times were estimated; reciprokes of the concentrations (on μmolar basis) were taken as "potencies" in the three assays. Hirudin showed the highest potency in all assays, similarly potent was heparin. Pentosan polysulfate and sulfated lactobionic acid amides showed higher potencies in inhibiting intrinsic than extrinsic system activation and were least active in inhibiting thrombin. The synthetic thrombin inhibitors ranked in the three assays according to their inhibition constants.

Institute of Pharmacology and Toxicology, Medical Academy Erfurt, Nordhäuser Str. 74, Erfurt, O-5010

82

GENERATION OF THROMBIN IN CITRATED, R-HIRUDINIZED AND HEPARINIZED WHOLE BLOOD
B. Kaiser, J. Fareed [*], J.M. Walenga [*], D. Hoppensteadt [*]

The generation of thrombin was studied in vitro in whole blood of healthy volunteers anticoagulated either by citrate, r-hirudin or heparin (final concentrations 10, 25, 50 μg/ml). Blood was activated either by glass or dextrane sulfate (contact activation; CA) as well as by thromboplastin/calcium chloride (extrinsic activation; EA) and by ellagic acid/cephaloplastin/calcium chloride (IA) and incubated 10 (CA, EA, IA) or 30 (CA) min at 37°C. Thereafter, generation of thrombin was quantitated by measuring the plasma levels of prothrombin fragment 1+2 (F1+2) and thrombin-antithrombin III-complex (TAT) utilizing ELISA methodology. After EA or IA no blood clotting occurred in all r-hirudinized samples and in heparinized blood at the highest concentration used. Despite inhibition of clotting F1+2 levels were increased both in r-hirudinized and in heparinized blood. However, in blood anticoagulated with heparin F1+2 levels after EA, IA and especially after CA were markedly lower than in r-hirudinized blood. Furthermore, in r-hirudinized blood an increase of TAT levels was found. The enhancement of F1+2 and TAT levels by r-hirudin was concentration-dependent and was lower in the higher r-hirudin concentration. The results indicate that in r-hirudinized whole blood significant amounts of thrombin can be generated which may elicit thrombin-mediated feedback mechanisms.

Institute of Pharmacology and Toxicology, Medical Academy, Nordhäuser Str. 74, Erfurt, O-5010
[*]Department of Pathology, Loyola University Medical Center, Maywood, IL 60153

83

STUDIES ON PROFIBRINOLYTIC AND ANTICOAGULANT PROPERTIES OF CALCIUM PENTOSAN POLYSULPHATE
H.-P. Klöcking, M. Richter, and J. Hauptmann

Calcium pentosan polysulphate (BEGO 0391, Bene Arzneimittel GmbH Munich) is a new derivative of the sulphated polysaccharide, pentosan polysulphate, which was prepared to improve the enteral absorption of pentosan polysulphate. The pro-fibrinolytic and anticoagulant properties of BEGO 0391 were compared to those of sodium pentosan polysulphate (SP54, FibrezymR) in vitro and in vivo.
Both substances showed in vitro in citrated human and rat plasma anticoagulant effects. The concentrations in plasma doubling clotting times were between 38-85 μg/ml plasma. BEGO 0391 reduced at doses of 1 to 5 mg per kg experimental macrothrombosis and disseminated intravascular coagulation in rats. The acute tissue-type plasminogen activator (t-PA) release was studied in the isolated perfused pig ear. At a concentration of 10 μg/ml perfusion solution, both BEGO 0391 and SP54 were able to increase the t-PA release by about 100 %. The t-PA releasing effect in vivo was studied in rats after i.v. administration of 5 mg/kg. Compared to the control (saline) BEGO 0391 caused a statistically significant increase in t-PA release. Determination of the partial thromboplastin time (PTT) served to establish the anticoagulant effect after intravenous and oral administration of 5 mg/kg. The PTT values were significantly prolonged up to 4 h after administration. The elimination half life of BEGO 0391 was about 1 h. Oral administration of BEGO 0391 resulted in an absorption of 10-20 % whereas the absorption of SP54 amounted to about 1 % only.

Institute of Pharmacology and Toxicology, Medical Academy Erfurt, Nordhäuser Straße 74, O-5010 Erfurt

84

EFFECT OF HEPARIN, LOW MOLECULAR WEIGHT HEPARINS AND SULFATED LACTOBIONIC ACID AMIDE ON HUMAN PLATELET AGGREGATION IN TYRODE'S SOLUTION, CITRATED AND HIRUDINIZED PLASMA
E. Glusa and C. Asche

Heparin is known to promote platelet aggregation possibly by a direct effect due to its polyanionic structure. In the course of heparin treatment side effects occur such as haemorrhagic complications and thrombocytopenia. To reduce the deleterious effects low molecular weight (LMW-)heparins habe been developed. The present paper deals with the influence of heparin, LMW-heparins and sulfated lactobionic acid amide (LW 10082) on human platelet aggregation. Aggregation was measured turbidimetrically. Heparin and its derivatives inhibited the thrombin-induced aggregation of washed platelets in the absence of antithrombin III; heparin being the most potent inhibitor. In citrated plasma heparin at anticoagulantly effective concentrations increased minimum ADP-induced aggregation to 80% of the maximum. Heparin was more potent than the LMW-heparins. This effect was inhibited by aspirin and daltroban. The lactobionic acid amide neither inhibited nor potentiated the aggregation in plasma. However, in hirudinized plasma at physiological calcium ion concentrations heparin and related compounds at concentrations higher than those required for anticoagulation did not enhance the aggregation induced by ADP or collagen. In contrast to hirudinized plasma, in citrated plasma with low calcium ion level (<40μmol/l) ADP was found to cause formation of thromboxane A_2 in platelets. These results suggest that the aggregation-promoting effect of heparin and LMW-heparins is due to the generation of thromboxane A_2 in citrated platelet rich plasma.

Institute of Pharmacology and Toxicology, Medical Academy Erfurt, O-5010 Erfurt, FRG

85

ANTITHROMBOTIC ACTIVITIES OF APROSULATE SODIUM (LW 10082)
A SYNTHETIC BIS-LACTOBIONIC ACID AMIDE
W. RAAKE

Aprosulate sodium (LW 10082), a synthetic bis-lactobionic acid amide and the most potent substance of a homologous series of related compounds, was evaluated for its anti-coagulatory and antithrombotic activities. It has a molecular weight of 2388 dalton and exhibits a low anticoagulatory activity compared to heparin and low molecular weight heparins. In a concentration of 2.5 - 50 µg/ml in vitro no effect was seen on Protrombin time and only a slight effect was observed on the Heptest clotting time. Activated partial thromboplastin time (APTT) was the only coagulation parameter which shows a dose-dependent increase, but compared to heparin it demonstrates only 25 % of the APTT prolongation. Depleting plasma of antithrombin III (AT III) did not change the results of the assays; this means that AT III is not required for the anticoagulant activity. At concentrations up to 0.1 mg/ml in platelet-rich plasma, no agent-induced effect (ADP, collagen, arachidonic acid, ristocetin, epinephrine) on platelet aggregation was observed. In different animal models (Wessler-test, Harbauer-model, laser induced coagulation, and the rat jugular vein clamping model) in rabbits and rats, the compound demonstrated interesting antithrombotic activities. In contrast to its low anticoagulatory activity, the antithrombotic activity of LW 10082 proved to be as potent as that of a low molecular weight heparin when a dose range of 0.5 - 5.0 mg/kg b.w. was used. The anticoagulant as well as the antithrombotic activity of Aprosulate sodium were neutralized by protamine. In equigravimetric doses protamine neutralized 70 % of the Heptest clotting time and the thrombin time. When the protamine dose was increased to 2.0 times the dosage of Aprosulate, a complete antagonism to the anticoagulant and antithrombotic effects took place.
The mode of action of Aprosulate is not finally enlightened, but by preliminary results it is supposed that it acts on the intrinsic pathway.

Luitpold-Werk, Chemisch-pharmazeutische Fabrik, Zielstattstraße 9, W-8000 München 70, FRG

86

EFFECT OF THROMBIN ON THE MIGRATION AND PROTEIN KINASE C IN ENDOTHELIAL CELLS

K.-U. Möritz[1], S. Wolff[2], R. Fermum[1] and E. Teuscher[2]

Thrombin plays a role in the angiogenesis. Protein kinase C (PKC) is a key regulatory enzyme involved in both signal transduction and cellular proliferation. As a step towards understanding the thrombin signal transduction in endothelial cells, we have examined the chemotaxis effects and subcellular distribution and activation state of PKC after exposure for 2 h of thrombin on aortic and capillary endothelial cells. At concentration range from 1-10 IU/ml, thrombin increased the migration and PKC activity in both cytosolic and particulate-fraction. Thrombin elicited a marked redistribution of the PKC from cytosol to membrane.
The present investigation suggests that PKC translocation is part of the signal transduction system in capillary cells for stimuli such as thrombin and that its effects on migration are mediated in part through activation of PKC.

[1]Department of Pharmacology and Toxicology and

[2]Department of Pharmacy, University of Greifswald, O-2200 Greifswald, FRG

87

The A_2 Adenosine Receptor: Guanine Nucleotide Modulation of Agonist Binding Is Enhanced by Proteolysis
Ch. Nanoff, K.A. Jacobson, and G.L. Stiles

Agonist binding to the A_2 adenosine receptor (A_2AR) and its regulation by guanine nucleotides was studied using the newly developed radioligand ^{125}I-2-[4-(2-{2-[(4 aminophenyl)methylcarbonylamino]ethylaminocarbonyl}-ethyl)phenyl]ethylamino-5'-N-ethylcarboxamidoadenosine (^{125}I-PAPA-APEC) and its photoaffinity analog ^{125}I-azido-PAPA-APEC. A single protein of M_r 45,000, displaying the appropriate A_2AR pharmacology, is labeled in membranes from bovine striatum, PC 12 cells and frog erythrocytes. Incorporation of ^{125}I-azido-PAPA-APEC into membranes from rabbit striatum, however, reveals two specifically labeled peptides (M_r 47,000 and 38,000), both of which display A_2AR pharmacology. Inhibition of protease activity leads to a decrease in the amount of the M_r 38,000 protein, with only the 45,000 protein remaining. This suggests that the M_r 38,000 protein is a proteolytic product of the M_r 47,000 A_2AR protein. In membranes containing the intact undigested A_2AR protein, guanine nucleotides induce a small to insignificant decrease in agonist binding, which is atypical of stimulatory G_s-coupled receptors. This minimal effect is observed in rabbit striatal membranes prepared in the presence of protease inhibitors, as well as in the other tissued studied. Binding to rabbit striatal membranes that possess the partially digested receptor protein, however, reveals a 50% reduction in maximal specific agonist binding upon addition of guanine nucleotides. Inhibition of proteolysis in rabbit striatum , on the other hand, results in a diminished ability of guanine nucleotides to regulate agonist binding. Thus, the enhanced effecitveness of guanine nucleotides in rabbit striatal membranes is associated with the generation of the M_r 38,000 peptide fragment.

Departments of Medicine and Biochemistry, Duke University Medical Center, Durham, N.C. 27710 (C.N., G.L.S.), and Laboratories of Chemistry, National Inst. of Diabetes, NIH, Bethesda, MD. 20892, USA.

88

SENSITIZATION AND DESENSITIZATION OF THE ACETYLCHOLINE CONTRACTION OF GUINEA PIG ILEUM - POSSIBLE ROLE OF THE "SILENT" MUSCARINIC M2 RECEPTORS

Jutta Bergmann

Muscarinic agonists need intracellular and extracellular sources of Ca^{++} to induce the phasic and tonic part of contraction, and they are their own inhibitors, too (desensitization).
To investigate this complex mechanism of action and to find out a functional role for the high number of the silent M2 receptor subtype, we compared four concentration-response curves:
1. contraction in a normal solution (M3 subreceptor activation),
2. so-called Ca^{++} influx contraction in a Ca^{++} free solution,
3. inhibition of a submaximal acetylcholine-induced normal contraction,
4. inhibition of a submaximal acetylcholine-induced Ca^{++} influx contraction.
These curves varied strongly for different agonists, and we found a new dose-dependent effect - sensitization of the submaximal acetylcholine-induced contractions by low agonist concentrations whereas the inhibition needs higher concentrations. The parallel shift to the right of the sensitization/desensitization curve of oxotremorine by the M2 selective Antagonist AF-DX 384 (11-(2-(dipropylaminomethyl)-1-piperidinyl)-ethylaminocarbonyl)-5,11-dihydro-6-H-pyrido(2,3-b)(1,4)-benzodiazepine-6-one) in a concentration which has no effect on the contraction suggests a functional role of this receptor subtype.

Central Institute of Molecular Biology
Robert-Rössle-Str.10
O-1115 Berlin

89

HUMAN MYOCARDIAL ADENYLATE CYCLASE ACTIVITY UPON
STIMULATION OF DIFFERENT RECEPTOR SYSTEMS
O.-E.Brodde, A.Broede, S.Bals, and H.-R.Zerkowski[1]

In the human heart β-adrenoceptors play an important role in regulation of cardiac function by mediating positive inotropic and chronotropic effects.
Additional (submaximal) positive inotropic effects
can be induced, however, by endogenous substances
such as serotonin (5-HT), angiotensin II and hista-
mine.In this study we compared the effects of these
substances on adenylate cyclase activity in human
right atrial membranes with those of isoprenaline
and two other well known adenylate cyclase activators, prostaglandin E_1 (PGE_1) and glucagon. 5-HT,
histamine,glucagon and PGE_1 (1-100 µmol/l) caused
concentration-dependent activation of adenylate
cyclase; at 100 µmol/l maximal activation amounted
to (activation of adenylate cyclase by 100 µmol/l
isoprenaline = 100 %): 27 ± 6 % histamine (n=5);
28 ± 5.5 % PGE_1 (n=4);20 ± 3 % glucagon (10 µmol/l,
n=4); 57 ± 15 % 5-HT (n=5). Angiotensin II (0.01 -
10 µmol/l) did not affect adenylate cyclase activity. These results indicate that in the human right
atrium submaximal (compared to the isoprenaline-
effects) positive inotropic effects caused by 5-HT
and histamine are associated with submaximal activation of adenylate cyclase. Angiotensin II appears
to evoke its positive inotropic effect by a cyclic
AMP independent mechanism.

Biochem. Forschungslabor, Med. Klinik & Poliklinik,
Abtlg. Nieren- & Hochdruckkrankheiten, and [1]Abtlg.
Thorax- & Kardiovaskuläre Chirurgie, Universitäts-
klinikum Essen, Hufelandstr. 55, D-4300 Essen, Fed.
Rep. of Germany

90

STIMULATION OF CHICKEN CARDIOMYOCYTE β-ADRENOCEPTORS
UP-REGULATES MUSCARINIC RECEPTORS AND G_i-PROTEIN
ALPHA-SUBUNITS BY A DIFFERENT MECHANISM[1]

C.Reithmann and K.Werdan

Long-term β-adrenoceptor (β-AR) agonist exposure leads
to a desensitization of adenylyl cyclase stimulation
mainly due to a down-regulation of β-AR by the agonist
exposure. Additionally, persistent adenylyl cyclase
stimulation has recently been reported to induce
alterations of the adenylyl cyclase inhibitory pathway
such as of inhibitory receptors and of the inhibitory
G-protein (G_i). The aim of the present study was to
investigate the mechanisms by which the β-AR agonist-
induced alterations of adenylyl cyclase inhibitory
components are mediated.
Exposure of chicken cardiomyocytes for 3 days in the
presence of 10 uM isoproterenol leads - in addition to
a down-regulation of β-AR by 60 % - to an increase in
the level of muscarinic acetylcholine receptors (mAChR)
by about 30 % and of the alpha-subunits of the inhibitory
G-proteins (G_{ia}) by about 100 %. An increase in the level
of mAChR can also be induced by cardiomyocyte treatment
in the presence of the weak β-AR agonists, celiprolol
(10 uM) and xamoterol (10 uM), but not in the presence of
the β-AR-independent adenylyl cyclase stimulators, prostaglandin E_1 (10 uM) and forskolin (10 uM). In contrast,
exposure of the cells to prostaglandin E_1 and forskolin
up-regulates the level of G_{ia} to a similar degree as the
β-AR agonist exposure, whereas treatment with celiprolol
and xamoterol does not alter the level of G_{ia}.
The data presented indicate that the β-AR agonist-induced
up-regulation of mAChR and G_{ia} in chicken cardiomyocytes
is mediated by a different mechanism. The increase in
the level of G_{ia} seems to be a cyclic AMP-mediated
process whereas the up-regulation of mAChR is apparently
due to a β-AR-specific, at present unknown mechanism.

Medizinische Klinik I, Universität München
Marchioninistr. 15, D-8000 München 70

91

IN VIVO TREATMENT WITH POSITIVE AND NEGATIVE
INOTROPIC AGENTS DIFFERENTIALLY AFFECTS MYO-
CARDIAL β-ADRENOCEPTORS, G-PROTEIN EXPRESSION
AND FORCE OF CONTRACTION IN RATS
T. Eschenhagen, B. Geertz, B. Hertle, U. Mende, C. Memmesheimer,
A. Pohl, W. Schmitz, H. Scholz, and M. Steinfath

Chronic β-adrenergic stimulation induces downregulation of β-adrenoceptors (β-AR) and upregulation of the inhibitory G-protein (Gi)
accompanied by an increased potency for the negative inotropic effect
(NIE) of carbachol (Carb) in rat hearts (Mende et al., Naunyn-
Schmiedeberg's Arch Pharmacol 342: R24, 1990). To further characterize the underlying mechanism we investigated the influence of different positive and negative inotropic agents on myocardial β-AR density, Giα-protein and Gα-mRNAs. In addition, we studied the positive
inotropic effect (PIE) of forskolin (F) as well as the NIE of Carb in the
presence of F or isoprenaline (Iso) in electrically driven papillary
muscles. Rats were treated by a 4-day subcutaneous infusion (mg/kg
d) of Iso (2.4), Carb (9.6), Ouabain (Ouab; 6.5) or 0.9 % NaCl (Ctr,
n=9-12 each). Compared to Ctr, Iso decreased β-AR density (62±4 vs
35±2 fmol/mg protein), increased Giα2- and Giα3-mRNA by 42 and
53 %, resp. and Giα-protein by 25 %. This was accompanied by a decreased potency for the PIE of F (pD2 6.4±0.1 vs 5.9±0.1) and increased potency for the NIE of Carb in the presence of Iso (pD2
6.9±0.1 vs 7.5±0.1) as well as in the presence of F (pD2 6.3±0.1 vs
7.1±0.1). Conversely, treatment with Carb decreased Giα-protein by
26 %. However, Giα-mRNA levels and β-AR density were not altered.
Although in this group consistent tachyarrythmias occurred in the
contraction experiments a decreased potency of Carb in the presence
of Iso was evident (pD2 6.9±0.1 vs 6.4±0.1). Ouab did not change any
of the parameters. Gsα-mRNA was similar in all groups. - The results
suggest: 1. Myocardial β-AR and Giα are differentially regulated. 2.
Upregulation but not downregulation of Giα might be due to altered
gene expression. 3. Alterations in the amount of Giα modulate receptor-dependent and -independent stimulatory and inhibitory signal
transduction in the adenylyl cyclase pathway. (Supported by the DFG.)

Abteilung Allgemeine Pharmakologie, Universitäts-Krankenhaus Eppendorf, Universität Hamburg, Martinistr. 52, W-2000 Hamburg 20,
FRG

92

ALTERATION OF β-ADRENOCEPTOR-COUPLED ADENYLYL CYCLA-
SE (AC) ACTIVITY IN THE ISCHAEMIC MYOCARDIUM-CONTRIBU-
TION OF G PROTEINS
L. Will-Shahab, *W. Rosenthal, W. Schulze, I. Küttner

An impairment of AC function has been shown to occur
in sarcolemmal preparations (SL) of porcine hearts exposed to global ischaemia. To examine the contribution
of G proteins to this phenomenon,cholera toxin (CT)-ca-
talyzed ADP-ribosylation of $G_s\alpha$ and pertussis toxin (PT)-
catalyzed ADP-ribosylation of $G_{o,i}\alpha$ proteins has been
investigated in SL of porcine hearts exposed to global
ischaemia for 15-45 min. ADP-ribosylation by CT of an
approximately 45 kDa polypeptide was 0.46 ± 0.06 and
ADP-ribosylation induced by PT of 39-41 kDa polypeptides was 4.77 ± 0.77 pmol/mg of protein in SL of non-
ischaemic myocardium. Whereas no change was observed
in CT-catalyzed ribosylation after 30 min of ischaemia,
there was a reduction in PT-catalyzed ADP-ribosylation
to 3.7 ± 0.35 pmol/mg of protein after 30 min of ischaemia. Prolongation of ischaemia to 45 min did not further
decline the ADP-ribosylation capacity. Quantitative immunoblotting of PT-sensitive G proteins suggests that the
reduction of ADP-ribosylation might be caused by diminu-
tion of α subunits of G_o, G_i-1, and G_i-2 which have
been identified as PT-substrates in SL of porcine hearts.
The loss of α subunits of G_i-2 seems to be related to
the observed abolition of inhibitory regulation of AC,
whereas the functional importance of the observed re-
duction/ loss of α subunits of G_o and G_i-1 remains to
be elucidated.

Institute of Cardiovascular Research, Berlin-Buch, and
*Institute of Pharmacology, Free University Berlin

93

IN VITRO TRANSCRIPTION ASSAYS WITH NUCLEI OF ADULT RAT HEARTS. EXPRESSION OF G-PROTEIN ALPHA SUBUNITS

F.U. Müller*, K.R. Boheler+, T. Eschenhagen*, W. Schmitz*, and H. Scholz*

To investigate the transcriptional activity of genes coding for G-protein α-subunits in adult rat hearts, in vitro transcription assays were performed in the presence of [32P]-UTP on isolated ventricular nuclei (Zahradka et al., Exp Cell Res 185: 8-20, 1989). Hybridization efficiencies were measured using specific [3H]-cRNAs and background signals to the bacterial vector pGEM-2 lacking insert were used to determine the nonspecific binding. After purification, the radiolabeled nascent ventricular transcripts were hybridized to membrane bound cDNAs specific for the Giα-2 and Gsα subunits. After membrane washing under stringent conditions, the hybridization signals were quantified by dual label szintillation counting and by standardization to a hybridization efficiency of 100% after substraction of nonspecific binding.

In control hearts, the incorporation into nascent transcripts for Giα-2 and Gsα was 38±4 ppm (n=7, SEM) and 50±7 ppm (n=6, SEM) respectively, hybridization efficiencies were 10-15%. Nonspecific binding was 3±1 ppm (n=15, SEM) demonstrating the signal specificity for the G-protein subunits. Incubation in the presence of 1 μg/ml α-amanitin decreased total [32P] incorporation and abolished the signals for Giα-2 and Gsα. At this concentration, α-amanitin is a selective inhibitor of RNA-polymerase II, the enzyme responsible for transcribing nascent mRNAs.

These results demonstrate that radiolabel incorporation into transcripts for Giα-2 and Gsα can be determined in adult heart tissue using nuclear run-on assays. This technique will therefore allow a detailed analysis of the transcriptional regulation of G-proteins. (Supported by the DFG.)

*Abteilung Allgemeine Pharmakologie, Universitäts-Krankenhaus Eppendorf, Universität Hamburg, Martinistraße 52, W-2000 Hamburg 20, FRG
+INSERM U127, Hôpital Lariboisière, 41 Boulevard de la Chapelle, F-75010 Paris, France

94

Giα-1 EXPRESSION IN THE HUMAN THYROID IS REGULATED BY TSH: LOSS OF REGULATION IN THYROID NEOPLASIAS

E. Selzer*&, A. Schifferer*, M. Hermann*, B. Grubeck-Loebenstein*, and M. Freissmuth*&

The molecular mechanisms underlying the development of thyroid autonomous adenomas are still poorly understood, although abnormalities in G protein function and in the adenylyl cyclase system have been implicated. In membranes prepared from autonomous adenomas, basal adenylyl cyclase activities were significantly reduced when compared with the control membranes from the paired, undiseased tissue (10.5±1.65 vs 20.28±1.68 pmol cAMP.min⁻¹.mg⁻¹ protein; n=14). Levels of the stimulatory G protein subunit Gsα were comparable in membranes derived from these tumors with the control membranes as assessed by cyc- reconstitution assays and Western blotting using a Gsα-specific antibody. Pertussis toxin labelling of these membranes revealed significant differences in the expression pattern of inhibitory G proteins (Giα) between the diseased and normal membranes derived from patients with hyperfunctioning autonomous adenoma, but not in membranes derived from normothyreotic patients. By using antibodies with distinct specifities for different Giα subtypes, we show that thyroid membranes derived from the neoplastic tissue contain abundant levels of Giα-1 while this protein is barely detectable in membranes from the corresponding extranodular tissue. In primary cell culture, normal human thyroid cells do not express Giα-1 unless TSH (thyroid stimulating hormone) is added to the culture medium. In thyroid cells derived from autonomous adenomas, Giα-1 levels are not regulated by TSH. We conclude that the expression of Giα-1 in the normal thyroid is under tight control of TSH. This control is lost in autonomous adenoma such that Giα-1 is apparently expressed constitutively. Since signal transduction via Gi proteins can promote cell proliferation, the constitutive expression of Giα-1 in thyroid adenomas may be causally related to autonomous growth and/or endocrine activity.

Institutes of Pharmacology& and Experimental Pathology, Vienna University, Währinger Straße 13a; A-1090 Vienna, Austria
Department of Surgery*, Kaiserin-Elisabeth-Spital, Huglgasse; A-1150 Vienna, Austria

95

G-PROTEIN ACTIVATION BY COMPLEMENT C5-DERIVED CHEMOTACTIC PEPTIDES IN HUMAN GRANULOCYTE PLASMA MEMBRANES: A COMPARISON BETWEEN NATIVE AND RECOMBINANT HUMAN C5A, AND THEIR des ARG CONGENERS

R. Kupper, S. Bischoff*, C.A. Dahinden*, and P. Gierschik

Human C5a is a 74 residue glycopolypeptide generated from the fifth component of human complement during complement activation. The native molecule is a potent anaphylatoxin and chemoattractant for neutrophils. Circulating C5a is rapidly converted to the less potent C5a_des Arg by a carboxypeptidase B-like enzyme present in serum and plasma. The ability of low concentrations of C5a_des Arg to stimulate chemotaxis is markedly enhanced by the serum protein Gc globulin (vitamin D binding protein), which interacts with the carbohydrate chain of C5a_des Arg, and by deglycosylation. To analyze the role of the C-terminal arginine and the carbohydrate chain of human C5a in modulating the biological activities of the peptide at the molecular level, we have examined the ability of both native and recombinant (i.e. carbohydrate-free) C5a, and their des Arg congeners to elicit G-protein activation in human neutrophil plasma membranes by measuring their effects on [35S]GTP[S] binding to these membranes. Both native and recombinant C5a led to a marked (up to 5.5-fold) stimulation of [35S]GTP[S] binding to the membranes (EC50 ≈ 1 nM). The des Arg peptides were at least 100-fold less potent. Native and recombinant chemoattractants were equally potent in both cases. Furthermore, Gc globulin (100 nM) did not alter the ability of the native and recombinant C5a and C5a_des Arg peptides to stimulate [35S]GTP[S] binding. Taken together, our results demonstrate (a) that the low biological activity of C5a_des Arg observed in vivo is due to the low potency of the des Arg peptide to elicit G-protein activation and (b) that modulation of agonist potency is unlikely to be the mechanism by which Gc globulin or deglycosylation alter the biological activities of C5a_des Arg.

Pharmakologisches Institut, Universität Heidelberg, Im Neuenheimer Feld 366, 6900 Heidelberg, FRG, and *Institut für Klinische Immunologie, Universität Bern, Schweiz

96

RECOMBINATION OF THE GRANULOCYTE-ACTIVATING SIGNAL TRANSDUCTION PATHWAY IN XENOPUS LAEVIS OOCYTES.

P. Schultz, P. Stannek, K.H. Jakobs, and P. Gierschik

Many granulocyte stimuli regulate neutrophil functions by interacting with specific cell surface receptors which are coupled via G-protein(s) to stimulation of phospholipase C. To characterize the signal transduction mechanisms initiated by these receptors at the molecular level, we have cloned the cDNAs for the formyl peptide and the complement C5a receptors, and studied the receptor expression following the microinjection of receptor cRNA into Xenopus laevis oocytes. Receptor activity was determined electrophysiologically by measuring opening of [Ca²⁺]i-dependent Cl-channels, which is triggered by receptor-mediated formation of InsP3. Injection of pure formyl peptide or C5a-receptor cRNA did not lead to agonist-dependent changes in membrane current. In contrast, marked alterations of membrane currents were observed when the receptor cRNAs were supplemented with poly(A)+ RNA from undifferentiated human leukemia (HL-60) cells (HL-60ud mRNA), which is devoid of mRNA coding for the two receptors. Binding studies using the radiolabelled formyl peptide N-formyl-norleucyl-leucyl-phenylalanyl-norleucyl-[125I]tyrosyl-lysine revealed that HL-60ud mRNA was not required for formyl peptide receptor expression in the injected oocytes. Fractionation of HL-60ud mRNA on methylmercuric hydroxide-containing agarose gels showed that the mRNA required to complement formyl peptide-dependent signal transduction in oocytes had a size of ≈ 3.5 kb. These results strongly suggest that both the formyl peptide and the C5a receptor require a specific factor(s) lacking in Xenopus oocytes but present in undifferentiated HL-60 cells to activate the second messenger pathway in the injected oocytes. Identification of this factor will provide important information about the molecular mechanisms by which G-protein-coupled granulocyte-activating receptors stimulate phospholipase C.

Pharmakologisches Institut, Universität Heidelberg, Im Neuenheimer Feld 366, 6900 Heidelberg, FRG

97

ACTIVATION BY HISTAMINE AND A FLUOROPHENYLHISTAMINE OF HL-60 CELLS THROUGH PERTUSSIS TOXIN-SENSITIVE G-PROTEINS: HISTAMINE BUT NOT THE FLUOROPHENYLHISTAMINE ACT VIA H_1-RECEPTORS
R. Seifert

HL-60 leukemic cells possess histamine H_2-receptors which play a role in the inhibition of N-formyl-L-methionyl-L-leucyl-L-phenylalanine (fMet-Leu-Phe)-stimulated superoxide anion (O_2^-) formation, but the functional role of H_1-receptors is obscure. We studied the effects of fMet-Leu-Phe, histamine and the potent and selective H_1-agonist, 2-[2-(3-fluoro-phenyl)-4-imidazolyl]ethanamine (fluorophenylhistamine 1) (Zingel et al. (1990) Eur J Med Chem 25:673-680), on cytosolic Ca^{2+} ($[Ca^{2+}]_i$ and O_2^- formation in dibutyryl cAMP-differentiated HL-60 cells. fMet-Leu-Phe, histamine and 1 increased $[Ca^{2+}]_i$ with an EC_{50} of 3 nM, 5 µM and 50 µM, respectively. Pertussis toxin (PTX) abolished the increase in $[Ca^{2+}]_i$ induced by 1 and reduced the effects of fMet-Leu-Phe and histamine. H_1-Antagonists inhibited the rise in $[Ca^{2+}]_i$ induced by histamine in the potency order clemastine > chlorpheniramine > diphenhydramine, whereas the H_2-antagonist, famotidine, was without effect. Diphenhydramine and famotidine did not affect the stimulatory effect of 1 on $[Ca^{2+}]_i$. The histamine- but the compound 1-induced rise in $[Ca^{2+}]_i$ was desensitized in a homologous manner. Histamine did not desensitize for 1 and vice versa. Compound 1 activated O_2^- formation with an EC_{50} of 0.65 mM and a maximum at 1-2 mM, but histamine was inactive. PTX abolished fMet-Leu-Phe- and 1-induced O_2^- formation. Our data suggest the following: (I) In dibutyryl cAMP-differentiated HL-60 cells, histamine increases $[Ca^{2+}]_i$ through H_1-receptors coupled to PTX-sensitive guanine nucleotide-binding proteins (G-proteins). (II) H_1-Receptors do not play a role in the activation of O_2^- formation. (III) Fluorophenylhistamine 1 increases $[Ca^{2+}]_i$ and activates O_2^- formation through a receptor agonist-like mechanism which is unrelated to H_1-receptors but involves PTX-sensitive G-proteins.

Institut für Pharmakologie, Freie Universität Berlin, Thielallee 69/73, D-1000 Berlin 33, F.R.G.

98

ISOZYME-SPECIFIC STIMULATION OF PHOSPHOLIPASE C BY G-PROTEIN $\beta\gamma$-SUBUNITS.   M. Camps,   E. Strohmaier, D. Sidiropoulos, K.H. Jakobs, and P. Gierschik

We have recently demonstrated that human HL-60 granulocytes contain a soluble phospholipase C that is stimulated by both an endogenous soluble GTP-binding protein, and by exogenous G-protein $\beta\gamma$-subunits purified from retinal transducin ($\beta\gamma_t$). Stimulation of phospholipase C by $\beta\gamma_t$ was not due to activation of phospholipase A_2 and required the free $\beta\gamma$-dimer rather than the holomeric G-protein. We now report that $\beta\gamma_t$ also stimulates soluble phospholipase C from human and bovine peripheral neutrophils, as well as membrane-bound, detergent-solubilized phospholipase C from HL-60 cells. Stimulation of soluble HL-60 phospholipase C is not restricted to $\beta\gamma_t$, but is also observed with highly purified $\beta\gamma$-subunits from bovine brain. Partial purification of the soluble HL-60 phospholipase C on Fast Q-Sepharose revealed the existence of at least two distinct isoforms of the enzyme, designated QI and QII. $\beta\gamma_t$ (2 µM) led to a marked (≈ 12-fold) stimulation of only one of these phospholipase C isozymes (QII). The inability of $\beta\gamma_t$ to stimulate QI-phospholipase C was not due to the presence of a putative $\beta\gamma_t$-inactivating protein present in this preparation, since $\beta\gamma_t$ was equally potent in supporting the pertussis toxin-mediated [^{32}P]ADP-ribosylation of exogenous α_t added to either QI or QII. Taken together, our results demonstrate that both soluble and membraneous phospholipase C of cultured and peripheral granulocytes are markedly stimulated by retinal and/or non-retinal G-protein $\beta\gamma$-subunits. However, stimulation of phospholipase C is isozyme-specific. Thus, two classes of phospholipase C enzymes can be discriminated in granulocytes, those that are $\beta\gamma$-sensitive, and those that are resistant to stimulation by the $\beta\gamma$-dimer.

Pharmakologisches Institut, Universität Heidelberg, Im Neuenheimer Feld 366, 6900 Heidelberg, FRG

99

DISSOCIATION OF PHYTOHEMAGGLUTININ (PHA)-INDUCED INOSITOL PHOSPHATE (IP) GENERATION AND Ca^{++} INCREASES IN HUMAN LYMPHOCYTES (MNL)
M.C. Michel, L.J.H. van Tits, O.-E. Brodde

Two of the earliest biochemical events in the activation of resting MNL by mitogens such as PHA are the generation of IP and increases in intracellular Ca^{++}. We have investigated whether these two processes might be causally related as they are in many other model systems. Cooling from 37 to 25° reduced the PHA-stimulated IP generation (determined as formation of [^{3}H]IP from [^{3}H]inositol) by more than 80% but induced only minor changes in Ca^{++} increases (determined with the fluorescent indicator Fura-2). Prostaglandin E_2 (100 µM) inhibited PHA-stimulated IP generation completely but Ca^{++} increases by only 75%. Increases in extracellular Ca^{++} from 0.2 to 2.6 mM reduced PHA-stimulated IP generation by ≈50% but did not alter Ca^{++} increases. Since more PHA is necessary to increase Ca^{++} than to stimulate IP generation, these data suggest that IP generation cannot be the major stimulus for PHA-induced Ca^{++} increases in human MNL. In contrast, chelation of extracellular Ca^{++} abolished both Ca^{++} increases and IP generation and the Ca^{++} ionophore ionomycin stimulated IP generation with the same concentration-response characteristics as Ca^{++} increases. We conclude that the relationships between IP generation and intracellular Ca^{++} in PHA-stimulated human MNL differ from those in many other receptor systems.

Dept. Medicine, University of Essen, Hufelandstr. 55, D-4300 Essen, FRG

100

QUANTITATIVE MASS ANALYSIS OF MULTIPLE INOSITOL POLYPHOSPHATES IN THE HUMAN T-CELL LINE JURKAT UPON T-CELL RECEPTOR-MEDIATED STIMULATION
A.H. Guse and F. Emmrich

The formation of inositol polyphosphates was measured in quiescent and CD3-stimulated human Jurkat T-cells using a recently developed anion-exchange-HPLC separation method in connection with a post-column derivatization procedure (Mayr, G.W. (1988) Biochem. J. 254, 585-591). Besides the well known compounds inositol 1,4,5-trisphosphate (Ins(1,4,5)P3), Ins(1,3,4)P3 and Ins(1,3,4,5)P4, three novel InsP4 isomers were found in Jurkat T-cells. Two of these isomers were identified as Ins(1,3,4,6)P4 and Ins(3,4,5,6)P4. While the basal levels of all InsP3- and InsP4-isomers and of Ins(1,2,3,4,6)P5 were in the range of 27 to 115 pmol/10^9 cells (except for Ins(3,4,5,6)P4), the intracellular concentrations of InsP6 and two distinct InsP5 isomers with the configuration Ins(1,2,4,5,6)P5 and Ins(1,3,4,5,6)P5 were two orders of magnitude higher. Upon stimulation with the anti-CD3 antibody OKT3 (10 µg/ml) characteristic changes in the concentrations of all inositol phosphates were observed. While all InsP3-InsP4- and two InsP5-isomers and InsP6 increased with stimulation, the concentration of Ins(1,2,4,5,6)P5 decreased significantly. We consider that besides the calcium-mobilizing Ins(1,4,5)P3 other inositol phosphates may be involved in intracellular signalling because of their turnover in response to stimulation. Also, the drastic decrease of Ins(1,2,4,5,6)P5 after stimulation indicates a possible role as a metabolic precursor for other inositol polyphosphates.

Max-Planck-Society, Clinical Research Unit for Rheumatology/Immunology, Schwabachanlage 10, D-8520 Erlangen, F.R.G.

101

EFFECTS OF LITHIUM ON ENDOGENOUS LEVELS OF INOSITOL PHOSHATES IN RAT BRAIN MEASURED BY ION CHROMATOGRAPHY

P.A. Baumann and P. Wicki

Endogenous inositol phosphates have so far mostly been measured by means of GC/MS (inositol monophosphates) or radio ligand binding assays ($Ins(1,4,5)P_3$). Although the possibility of using ion chromatography has been published in 1988 by Smith et al. (J. Chromatogr. 439, 83-92), this method has not yet become widely known. As an example to demonstrate advantages and problems of this new method the effects of acute lithium treatment in rat brain on the inositol phosphates were studied. A DIONEX series 4000i ion chromatograph equipped either with a DIONEX CarboPac PA1 column and a pulsed amperometric detector (for the measurement of inositol monophosphates (IP_1)), or with a DIONEX IonPac AS5A-5µ column, followed by an anion micromembrane suppressor and a conductivity detector (for the measurement of inositol bis- (IP_2), tris- (IP_3) and tetrakisphosphates (IP_4)) was used. The method of killing the animals, as well as tissue extraction (neutral or acid) and sample preparation on DEAE-Sephadex columns turned out to greatly influence the inositol phosphate levels measured. LiCl subcutaneously administered markedly enhanced the IP_1 levels at doses of 1 mEq and above within 4 hours. In rat whole brain 3 mEq LiCl s.c., leading to a concentration of 1.3-1.4 mEq LiCl in serum, Ins(1)P was increased by 374 percent, Ins(4)P by 198 percent and also Ins(2)P was marginally increased by 33 percent. The effect of this dose of lithium varied from one brain area to another. Whereas Ins(1)P was preferentially increased in cortex, hippocampus and c. striatum, Ins(4)P was the preferred target in talamus, hypothalamus, cerebellum and pons-medulla, suggesting differences in IP_3 metabolism in different types of neurons. Whereas prominent effects of lithium on IP_1 levels were seen, this was not the case with IP_2, IP_3 and IP_4. Problems occurred particularly with the measurements of IP_2, IP_3 and IP_4. The column used was not optimal for the separation of IP_2 isomers. Because of the fast turnover of IP_3 and binding of IP_3 and IP_4 to glass, microwave killing and neutral extraction in plastic tubes should be performed for the measurement of IP_3 and IP_4.

Research Department, Pharmaceuticals Division, Ciba-Geigy Ltd., CH-4002 Basle, Switzerland

102

AGE RELATED ALTERATION IN PHOSPHOINOSITIDE HYDROLYSIS

M. Sugawa and H. Coper

The present work describes alterations in phosphoinositide breakdown occurring in rat brain tissue. These biochemical alterations can be correlated with the molecular events underlying aging. The understanding of the relationship between receptor/G-protein/inositol phosphates has advanced at a remarkable rate. It has been postulated that the phosphoinositide (PI) cascade plays an important role in the process of brain development (Moon, K.H., Lee, S.Y., and Rhee, S.G. Biochem. Biophys. Res. Commun. 164: 370-374, 1989). In contrast, there has been a dearth of studies about changes in the PI response during aging. The pivotal aim of the in-vitro studies described here is to gain insight into the aging related effect of the conversion of phosphatidylinositol-4,5-bisphosphate (PIP_2) to inositol phosphates, and of the endogeneous inositol 1,4,5-trisphosphate (IP_3) concentration in the CNS of rats. For this purpose, female Wistar rats of different age were investigated, i.e., young adult (about 2 months) and very old (approx. 40 months) exbreeders. According to previous results (Schulze, G., Coper, H., and Fähndrich, Ch. Neurochem. Int. 17: 281-289, 1990), 29-month-old animals are the 50% survivors of an original population, therefore senescence begins with this age. Our data show that: (1.) The endogeneous 1,4,5-trisphosphate concentration in the old striatal tissue (approx. 40 month-old rats) is significantly higher than in young one (approx. 2 month-old rats); (2.) No age-related alteration in PI hydrolysis is observed in the rat forebrain; (3.) Higher basal PI hydrolysis is monitored in old striatum than in young one for an incubation time of up to 40 min; (4.) Dopamine (1 µM) decreases PI hydrolysis in the rat striatum. A conceivable explanation is that the activation of striatal DA-2 receptors leads to the inhibition of phosphoinositide breakdown. This signal transduction pathway is more pronounced in the old rat striatum.

Dept. Neuropsychopharmacology, Universitätsklinikum Rudolf Virchow, Free University, Ulmenallee 30, W-1000 Berlin 19, FRG

103

STIMULATION AND INHIBITION OF EXOCYTOSIS FROM PERMEABILIZED BOVINE ADRENAL CHROMAFFIN CELLS BY GUANINE NUCLEOTIDES.

G. Ahnert-Hilger

In bovine adrenal chromaffin cells permeabilized by either alphatoxin or streptolysin O (SLO) guanine nucleotides differently modulated exocytosis.
1. In alphatoxin-treated cells (permeable for molecules up to 3kDa) guanyl-5'-yl imidodiphosphate (GMPPNHP) activated the Ca^{2+}-stimulated exocytosis. Preteatment of the cells with pertussis toxin or increasing the free Ca^{2+}-concentration over 50 µM, prevented the activation of the Ca^{2+}-stimulated exocytosis by GMPPNHP.
2. In SLO-treated cells (permeable for proteins up to 150 kDa) different G-protein alpha subunits (Giα, Goα) escaped the cells and were detected in the extracellular solution by various antibodies. GMPPNHP failed to stimulate Ca^{2+}-dependent exocytosis under these conditions.
3. In contrast to GMPPNHP, guanosine 5'-(3-o-thio)triphosphate (GTPyS) inhibited the Ca^{2+}-induced exocytosis from cells permeabilized by either pore-forming toxin. The effect was resistant to pertussis toxin.
4. A heterotrimeric G-protein which is lost during permeabilization with SLO may be responsible for the GMPPNHP-induced activation of the Ca^{2+}-stimulated exocytosis. The inhibitory effect of GTPyS may be mediated by other GTP-binding proteins which are not lost following permeabilization with SLO.

Institut für Neuropsychopharmakologie der Freien Universität Berlin, Ulmenalle 30

104

INFLUENCE OF PROTEIN KINASE C ON THE CONTRACTILITY OF THE ISOLATED MOUSE VAS DEFERENS

H. Brasch

An activation of protein kinase C (PKC) can increase (vascular preparations, uterus) or attenuate (trachea, ileum) the contractile force of different types of smooth muscle. In the present study the influence of the PKC stimulator phorbol-12 myristate-13 acetate (PMA) on contractions of the isolated mouse vas deferens was investigated.

Vasa were incubated in Krebs solution (2.54 mM $CaCl_2$; 32 °C) and contractions were elicited by either noradrenaline or bethanechol. The maximum force of contraction obtained with noradrenaline (12 ± 0.7 mN; EC_{50} 22 µM) was reduced by 21 %, 42 % and 63 % in the presence of 1, 10 and 30 µM PMA, respectively and the EC_{50} of noradrenaline was doubled. The same concentrations of PMA reduced the maximum force obtained with bethanechol (6 ± 0.5 mN; EC_{50} 119 µM) by 15 %, 23 % and 47 % and caused a small increase of the EC_{50}. Phorbol-12 myristate-13 acetate-4-0-methylether (PME), a compound which does not stimulate PKC, was ineffective in both cases.

In vasa incubated in calcium free, depolarizing solution (80 mM KCl; 0.11 mM EDTA) contractions could be elicited by addition of $CaCl_2$ (0.25 - 4 mM). The maximum response to calcium (18 ± 0.6 mM) was reduced by 28 % and 51 % in the presence of 10 and 30 µM PMA and by 55 % in the presence of 0.03 µM verapamil. PME (30 µM) and ryanodine (1 µM), an alkaloid which depletes intracellular calcium stores, were ineffective. The relaxant effect of verapamil could be antagonized by the calcium ionophore A 23187 (0.5 µM). The effect of PMA was not influenced by the ionophore, but was greatly attenuated in vasa preincubated with 1 µM ouabain for 1 h.

It is concluded that an activation of PKC by PMA reduces the contractility of the mouse vas. An increased calcium extrusion from the smooth muscle cells is a possible explanation and may be caused either by a stimulation of the Na^+/Ca^{2+} exchanger or indirectly by a stimulation of the Na^+-K^+-ATP'ase.

Institut für Pharmakologie der Medizinischen Universität zu Lübeck, Ratzeburger Allee 160, 2400 Lübeck, FRG.

105

A NEW ALPHA-SUBUNIT OF SOLUBLE GUANYLYL CYCLASE
D. Koesling, Ch. Harteneck, B. Wedel, E. Böhme, G. Schultz

Soluble guanylyl cyclase purified from bovine lung consists of two subunits designated α_1 and β_1 with apparent M_r of 73 and 70 kDa, respectively, on SDS PAGE gels. Molecular cloning of this enzyme resulted in calculated molecular masses of 77.5 and 70.5 for the α_1- and the β_1-subunits, respectively. A second β-subunit (β_2) has been cloned from rat kidney (P.S.T. Yuen et al., Biochemistry 29, 10872-10878, 1990). Comparison of the amino acid sequences shows high homologies in the C-terminal parts of the subunits (for review see D. Koesling et al., FASEB J., in press). Here, we report on another subunit of soluble guanylyl cyclase, which was identified using the polymerase chain reaction with oligonucleotides corresponding to the amino acids conserved between all guanylyl cyclases. A full length clone was isolated from an human fetal brain library. The new subunit has a calculated molecular mass of 81.7 kDa and shows the highest degree of homology towards the a-subunit and is, therefore, likely to represent an isoform of α-subunits (α_2-subunit). This assumption is supported by expression experiments, which show that the new subunit can form a catalytically active guanylyl cyclase when coexpressed with the β_1-subunit but not with the α_1-subunit.

Institut für Pharmakologie, Freie Universität Berlin, Thiel-allee 67-73, D-1000 Berlin 33

106

EXPRESSION OF cGMP-DEPENDENT PROTEIN KINASE (cGK) ISOZYMES Iα AND Iß IN COS-7 AND CHO CELLS
P.Ruth, W.Landgraf, B.May, A.Keilbach, F.Hofmann

Iα- and Iß cGK, which differ only in their first 100 amino acids, were transiently and permanently expressed by transfection of the cloned cDNAs into COS-7 and CHO cells, respectively. Cytosolic extracts from transfected COS-7 cells containing the recombinant Iα- or Iß cGK were used to study the biochemical characteristics of the isozymes. The recombinant Iα and Iß cGK were halfmaximally activated at 0.1 and 1.3 μM cGMP and 0.3 and 12 μM 8-Br-cGMP, respectively. The recombinant Iα cGK bound 2 mol cGMP/mol subunit to a high (site 1) and low (site 2) affinity cGMP binding site. The exchange rates were 0.009 min^{-1} for site 1 and 3.7 min^{-1} for site 2. In contrast, the recombinant Iß cGK bound 2 mol cGMP/mol subunit only to two low affinity binding sites (site 2) with k_{-1} values of 0.92 and 4.8 min^{-1}. These results suggest that a change from the Iα amino-terminal domain to that of Iß increases the apparent K_A value for cGMP 10-fold by altering the binding properties of binding site 1.
To study the physiological role of the cGK the cDNA of the Iα isozyme was permanently introduced in CHO cells which lack endogenous cGK. The transfected cDNA sequence for the cGK could be amplified in these cells, resulting in a concentration of 15 pmol holoenzyme/mg cytosolic protein. The calcium transients upon depolarization of the cGK-expressing cells and the non-transfected cells were investigated.

Inst.f.Pharmakologie und Toxikologie der Techn. Universität, Biedersteiner Str.29,W-8 München 40

107

INHIBITION OF PLATELET FUNCTIONS BY SELECTIVE ACTI-VATORS OF CYCLIC NUCLEOTIDE DEPENDENT PROTEIN KINASES
Elke Butt, Jörg Geiger, Christine Nolte und Ulrich Walter

Many platelet activators increase the activity of phospholipase C resulting in an increase of cytosolic Ca^{++}, activation of myosin light chain kinase and protein kinase C. cAMP and cGMP elevating agents like PG-I$_2$ and EDRF inhibit these effects of platelet aggregation. We have investigated some of these effects using new cyclic nucleotide analogs.
8-para-chlorophenylthio-cGMP (8-pCPT-cGMP) is shown to be a cell membrane permeable, non-hydrolysable selective activator of the cGMP-dependent protein kinase (cGK) with no apparent effect on cPDE's whereas Sp-5,6-dichloro-1-ß-D-ribofuranosyl-benzimidazole-3',5'-monophosphorothioate (Sp-5,6-DCl-cBiMPS) is a very lipophilic and stable cAMP-dependent protein kinase (cAK) activator.
In intact human platelets, nitrovasodilators and 8-pCPT-cGMP caused cGK-mediated protein phosphorylation whereas PG-I$_2$ and Sp-5,6-DCl-cBiMPS caused cAK-mediated protein phospho-rylation. Quantitative data are given for the phosphorylation of a 46/50 kDa protein (VASP), a substrate for both kinases in response to cAMP as well as cGMP elevating platelet inhibitors. 8-pCPT-cGMP (0.5 mM) inhibited the aggregation induced by agonists such as thrombin. Furthermore the analog inhibited the ADP-induced calcium mobilization in intact human platelets. Similar effects were obtained with 0.1 mM Sp-5,6-DCl-cBiMPS. The results suggest that the cGK and the cAK mediate the effects of nitrovasodilators and PG-I$_2$, respectively, and inhibit the activation and ADP-induced calcium mobilization in intact human platelets.

Universitätsklinik Würzburg, Labor für Klin. Biochemie, Josef-Schneider Str. 2, D-8700 Würzburg

108

SYNTHETIC LIPOPEPTIDES INDUCE TYROSINE PHOSPHORYLATION IN DIFFERENTIATED HL-60 CELLS
S. Offermanns, R. Seifert, G. Schultz

Synthetic lipopeptide analogues of the N-terminus of bac-terial lipoprotein are effective activators of macropha-ges, neutrophils and lymphocytes. We studied the effect of the lipopeptide, N-palmitoyl-S-[2,3-bis(palmitoyloxy)-(2RS)-propyl]-(R)-cysteinyl-(S)-seryl-(S)-lysyl-(S)-ly-syl-(S)-lysyl-(S)-lysine (Pam$_3$Cys-Ser-(Lys)$_4$) on tyrosine phosphorylation in Bt$_2$cAMP-differentiated HL-60 cells using an anti-phosphotyrosine antibody. Pam$_3$Cys-Ser-(Lys)$_4$ concentration-dependently stimulated tyrosine phosphorylation of 100/110- and 60-kDa proteins and, to a lesser extent, of 50/53- and 70/75-kDa proteins. Halfmax-imal and maximal effects were observed at concentrations of 1-5 and 10-100 μg/ml, respectively. The lipopeptide-induced increase in phosphorylation was rapid and tran-sient with a peak response after 30-60 s. In HL-60 promy-elocytes, Pam$_3$Cys-Ser-(Lys)$_4$ had no effect on tyrosine phosphorylation. HL-60 cells differentiated with 1,25-di-hydroxyvitamin D$_3$ showed a similar but less pronounced response compared to Bt$_2$cAMP-differentiated cells. Lipo-peptide Isocarba-Pam$_3$Cys-Ser-(Lys)$_4$ was as potent as Pam$_3$Cys-Ser-(Lys)$_4$, whereas Carba-Pam$_3$Cys-Ser-(Lys)$_4$ and Pam$_3$Cys-Ser-Gly did not induce tyrosine phosphorylation. The chemotactic peptide, formyl-methionyl-leucyl-phenyl-alanine (fMLP) weakly stimulated tyrosine phosphorylation of the 100/110-kDa proteins. The effect of fMLP was abol-ished after treatment of cells with pertussis toxin (PT), whereas lipopeptide induced tyrosine phosphorylation was not affected by PT. Preincubation of cells with the tyro-sine kinase inhibitor, genistein, inhibited lipopeptide stimulation of tyrosine phosphorylation. These results show that tyrosine phosphorylation is an early event oc-curing in HL-60 cells activated by lipopeptides.
This work was supported by the DFG

Institut für Pharmakologie, Freie Universität Berlin, Thielallee 69/73, 1000 Berlin 33

109

THROMBIN INDUCES ACTIVATION OF pp60^{c-src} PROTEIN TYROSINE KINASE IN HUMAN PLATELETS

U. Liebenhoff and P. Presek

The cellular homologue of the transforming protein of Rous sarcoma virus, pp60^{c-src}, represents the prototype of a nonreceptor protein tyrosine kinase of unknown physiological function. Human platelets possess abundant levels of a structurally uniform type of pp60^{c-src}, which correlates with high levels of protein tyrosine phosphorylation in response to stimulation events. In order to find out the kinase responsible for the enhanced protein tyrosine phosphorylation, we observed that overall pp60^{c-src} kinase activity increases about 2-3 fold upon thrombin-stimulation in a time- and concentration dependent manner. Other agonists like phorbol 12-myristate 13-acetate (PMA), vasopressin, collagen, the calcium-ionophore A23187 and Ca^{2+} revealed a similar effect. These agonists provoke the initial response in platelet stimulation events and involve a rapid turnover of inositolphospholipids. In contrast, the elevation of c-AMP by prostaglandin E$_1$ does not affect pp60^{c-src} kinase activity. Activation is accompained by an increase in enzyme phosphorylation, mainly at Ser-12 indicating protein kinase C activation. By comparison c-AMP-elevating prostaglandin E$_1$ had no effect on the phosphorylation of Ser-12 and surprisingly of Ser-17, which is thought to be exclusively phosphorylated by A-kinase. These results show that pp60^{c-src} participates in platelet activation-related signal transduction pathways and might be responsible for the elevation of protein tyrosine phosphorylation in stimulated platelets.

Rudolf-Buchheim-Institut für Pharmakologie der Justus-Liebig-Universität Gießen, Frankfurter Str. 107, D-6300 Gießen

110

CHANGES IN PHOSPHODIESTERASE SUBTYPE PATTERN IN THE HEART BY 7-OXO-PROSTACYCLIN.

L. Luthardt, H. Tenor, S. Bartel, E.-G. Krause and L. Szekeres*

PGI$_2$ and 7-Oxo-prostacyclin (7-Oxo) are known to produce antiadrenergic and antiischemic effects appearing 1 to 2 days after a single administration. There is evidence that hearts of pretreated animals are less responsive to isoprenaline (ISO) in respect to rising cAMP and contractile force, although the ß-adrenoceptor-adenylyl cyclase system is uneffected. In these studies the phosphodiesterase (PDE) subtype distribution was studied in the cytosolic and particulate fractions of the heart. Rats were treated with 50 µg/kg i.m. 7-Oxo for 48 h. In pretreated, perfused heart preparations the rise in cAMP by 10 nM ISO was diminished to 30 % compared to controls (p .01). There was not any influence on the specific activity of cAMP-PDE either in the cytosolic and microsomal fractions. However, the cGMP hydrolysing activity was significantly increased in the particulate fraction (617 $\pm$ 39 versus 242 $\pm$ 14 fmol/min/mg in untreated rats). After solubilization (1 % TRITONx100; 0.1 % BRIJ 30, 1 µM pepstatin 4° for 12 h) the PDE I to IV of the 100000 x g supernatant were developed by a Mono-Q-FPLC column (Fa. Pharmacia). In comparison to controls the peak of Ca^{2+}-calmodulin-dependent PDE I was 2.4 times elevated, whereas PDE II was unchanged. This rise in PDE I after 7-Oxo may explain partly the observed antiadrenergic effect by rising the effective cAMP hydrolysis by PDE III activity known as inhibited by cGMP. Whether the synthesis of PDE I is controlled by eicosanoids is under study.

Institut für Herz-Kreislauf-Forschung, Robert-Rössle-Str. 10, O-1115 Berlin-Buch, und *Institut für Pharmakologie, Albert-Szent-Györgi Universität, Szeged, Ungarn

111

DIFFERENCES IN THE DISTRIBUTION OF PARTICULATE PHOSPHODIESTERASES III AND IV IN THE SARCOLEMMA AND SARCOPLASMIC RETICULUM OF THE HEART.

H. Tenor, G. Luthardt, S. Bartel, E.-G. Krause

There is evidence that simultaneous administration of phosphodiesterase (PDE) inhibitors like milrinone and rolipram, which attenuates cAMP hydrolyses by selectively inhibiting PDE III and PDE IV isotypes, respectively, induces more effective the inotropism of the rat heart than milrinone alone (M. Shahid and C.D. Nicholson, Naunyn-Schmiedeberg's Arch. Pharmacol. (1990) 342: 698-705). As the specific subcellular distribution of particulate PDEs activity is unknown, this study assesses this distribution between sarcolemma (SL) and sarcoplasmic reticulum (SR) enriched fractions. In the SL fraction both the rolipram, inhibited PDE (ROI-PDE, IV) activity and cGMP inhibited PDE (CGI-PDE, III) activity were found. After solubilization of the SL membrane beside a small amount of PDE II (cGMP activated subtype) mainly the CGI-PDE activity was found (Km (cAMP) = 0.53 µM; Ki (milrinone) = 3 µM) in the supernatant, whereas the ROI-PDE remained in the SL pellet fraction. Contrary, no ROI-PDE activity was observed in the SR fractions, which only contains activity of the CGI-PDE (IC50 (cGMP) = 1 µM; IC50 (Rolipram) $>$100 µM). Thus the synergistic actions of PDE inhibitors like milrinone and rolipram on myocardial cAMP concentration and on inotropic response(s) concerns mainly the SL membrane compartment, containing both PDE III and PDE IV.

Institut für Herz-Kreislauf-Forschung, Robert-Rössle-Str. 10, O-1115 Berlin

112

CALCIUM-SENSITIVITY MODULATION IN SAPONIN-PERMEABILIZED VASCULAR SMOOTH MUSCLE BY RECEPTOR AND G-PROTEIN STIMULATION, R. Fermum, D. Kosche, and K.-U. Möritz

Permeabilized smooth muscle has been used extensively for studying regulatory mechanisms of the contractile protein system. It offers the advantage that normally impermeant aqueous solutes can be introduced directly into the cytosol and the concentration of Ca can be precisely controlled by the use of chelating buffers. Using saponin-permeabilized coronary arteries, we examined whether receptor or GTP-binding protein mediated mechanisms may be retained after permeabilization, and wether they may modulate muscle tension without a change in cytoplasmic Ca.
Our results indicate that contractile signal transduction that follow surface receptor activation can be retained after saponin-skinning.
Furthermore, histaminic or muscarinic receptor stimulation, as well as G-protein activation by fluoride or GppNHp can modulate the response of the contractile apparatus to Ca without a change in cytosolic concentration.
Saponin-permeabilized smooth muscle retaining coupled surface receptors may be valuable for exploring relationships between membrane-associated signal transduction and regulatory mechanisms of the contractile apparatus.
Our results provide evidence that the magnitude of agonist-mediated vascular contraction may not be solely determined by the concentration of free Ca in the myofilament space. Additionally, an increase in the apparent Ca-sensitivity of the contractile apparatus, presumably mediated by protein kinase C, may be of physiological relevance.

Institut für Pharmakologie und Toxikologie, Universität Greifswald, Friedrich-Loeffler-Str. 23d, D-2200 Greifswald, FRG

113

IMMORTALIZATION OF A FETAL RAT BRAIN CELL LINE, WHICH EXPRESSES mRNA CODING FOR CORTICOTROPIN RELEASING FACTOR K. Mugele* and J. Spiess

Corticotropin releasing factor (CRF) is a 41 amino acid peptide, which plays a key role in mediating the mammalian stress response. CRF mRNA expression starts at day 16 of embryonal development of the rat; the peptide is found in the paraventricular nucleus of the adult hypothalamus as well as in other brain regions. In vitro studies using northern blotting techniques and in situ hybridization indicate that the biosynthesis of CRF is regulated on the transcriptional level. However, the lack of an appropriate neuronal cell system, which expresses its endogenous CRF gene has made an analysis of tissue specific regulation rather difficult.

We have succeeded in establishing a cell line from primary cultures of fetal rat brain by transfection of a DNA construct which contains the SV40 T antigen under the control of the CRF promoter. Clone H32 produces mRNA for CRF as well as for SV40 T antigen and exhibits neuronal properties as indicated by positive immunestaining with antibodies against neurofilaments and neuron specific enolase. Thus, the cell line provides a useful system for the investigation of transcriptional regulation of CRF at an early stage of neuronal development.

*Present address: Inst. f. Biochemie und Molekularbiologie der Freien Universität Berlin, Ehrenbergstr.26-28,1 Berlin 33, F.R.G.
Dep. of Molecular Neuroendocrinology, Max-Planck Inst. f. Exp. Medicine, Hermann-Rein-Str. 3, 3400 Göttingen, F.R.G.

114

CARDIOVASCULAR RENIN-ANGIOTENSIN SYSTEM IN HYPERTHYROID DOGS Lindsay Brown, Catherine Marchant, Andrew Hoey, Conrad Sernia

In dogs, we have shown that experimental hyperthyroidism leads to tachycardia without echocardiographic evidence of ventricular hypertrophy; ventricular β_1-adrenoceptor density was increased by 64% (Hoey et al, Naunyn-Schmiedebergs Arch Pharmacol 343: R60, 1991). This study has characterised the renin-angiotensin system in this model since changes in this system may be involved in the cardiac deterioration observed in hyperthyroidism. Hyperthyroidism (HT) was induced by daily injections of T_3 (1 mg/kg s.c. for 14 days, n=10); 10 control (C) dogs received saline injections. Plasma renin activity increased (p<0.05) dramatically from 1.6±0.2 to 9.8±2.8 ng angiotensin I (AI)/ml/h probably due to an increase in plasma renin concentration from 13.0±3.7 to 34.5±5.6 ng AI/ml/h. Plasma angiotensinogen decreased from 505±39 to 441±44 ng AI/ml, indicating either a decreased secretion or, more likely, an increased consumption. Angiotensin II receptors in the right atrium, left ventricle and thoracic aorta were characterised using ^{125}I-Sar^1,Ile^8-angiotensin II binding. All tissues showed a single high affinity binding site (K_a, (1.2±0.1) x10^9 1/mol). There was no significant change in receptor density in right atrium (C, 0.32±0.03; HT, 0.28±0.03 pmol/g tissue). However significant increases in receptor density were measured in the left ventricle (C, 0.33±0.06; HT, 0.75±0.12 pmol/g tissue) and thoracic aorta (C, 0.19±0.02; HT, 0.28±0.03 pmol/g tissue). We conclude that experimental hyperthyroidism in dogs stimulates the plasma activity of the renin-angiotensin system and upregulates angiotensin II receptors in left ventricle and thoracic aorta but not in the right atrium; these effects are additional to and may augment an upregulation of cardiac β_1-adrenoceptors.

Department of Physiology and Pharmacology
The University of Queensland, 4072, Australia.

115

INTERACTION OF SEVERAL SYNTHETIC AND ENDOGENOUS STEROIDS WITH CYTOCHROME P-450 OF PRIMARY RAT HEPATOCYTES
H. Lepper, G. Schmitz and R. Böcker

Recent investigations on human liver microsomes in vitro have shown, that several synthetic progestogenic steroids and the synthetic estrogenic compound ethinylestradiol (which is commonly used together with the progestogens in oral contraceptive formulations) preferentially inhibit the oxidation of nifedipine from its dihydropyridine-form to the pyridine-form (F.P. Guengerich,1990,Chem. Res. Toxicol.3,363-371; R.Böcker, H. Lepper,1991,Naunyn-Schmiedeberg's Arch. Pharmacol. 343, R 13, Nr. 52). This effect on isolated microsomes had to be investigated in an intact cell system with active phase I- and phase II-reactions. For these studies we used freshly prepared rat hepatocytes. As substrate for the nifedipine-oxidase we used a nifedipine analogous compound which has no substituent at the aryl moiety and has no Ca^{++}-antagonistic potency (and therefore doesn't interact with cellular reactions). We compared the effects of the synthetic progestogens Gestoden (GSD), Norethisteron (NET), Desogestrel (DES), 3-Keto-Desogestrel (3-KD), Levonorgestrel (LNG) and of the synthetic estrogen ethinylestradiol (EE) in concentrations ranging from 0µm-50µM on the formation of the pyridine-form of our substrate. The macrolide antibiotic troleandomycin (TAO), a well known mechanism-based inactivator of the isozymes of the cyt. P 450 IIIA-family, was used for comparison.

All synthetic steroids tested in our in-vitro system under pre-incubation- as under co-incubation-conditions for 30 resp. 60 minutes showed an inhibitory effect on the nifedipine-oxidase activity. At the highest conc. (50µM) of the preincubation experiments the inhibition was nearly identical for GSD, EE, LNG, NET and somewhat lower for 3-KD, DES and TAO. Additionally we investigated the influence of the 17α-Ethinyl group at the steroid-system on the inhibition of the nifedipine-oxidase activity.The comparison of steroids with a 17α-Ethinyl group like Norethisteron, 17α-Ethinyltestosteron and 17α-Ethinylestradiol with steroids which has no 17α-Ethinyl function like 19-Nortestosteron, Testosteron and Estradiol showed no inhibitory effect of the non-ethinylated progestogenic and estrogenic steroids on the nifedipine-oxidase activity while all tested progestogenic and estrogenic compounds with the 17α-Ethinyl function inhibited this enzyme.
It is concluded that the 17α-Ethinyl moiety is responsible for the inhibitory effect possibly due to the metabolism which can occur at this group by building a possible intermediate ketene structure.

Lehrstuhl für Toxikologie und Pharmakologie der Univ. Erlangen,
Universitätsstr. 22,
D-8520 Erlangen

116

DISPOSITION AND PHARMACOKINETICS OF ^{3}H-DEHYDROEPIANDROSTERONE IN THE RAT
H.G. Hillesheim, Petra Ritter and G. Hobe

DEHYDROEPIANDROSTERONE (DHEA), 3ß-Hydroxy-5-androsten-17-one, is a main secretory product of the human adrenal, and has been shown to have a number of diverse therapeutic effects in such different conditions as diabetes, obesity, autoimmunity and cancer when administered in rodents. Our knowledge concerning the metabolic fate of DHEA in rodents is poor. Using the tritium-labelled compound, the principal parameters of disposition and pharmacokinetics have been evaluated in the rat.

^{3}H-DHEA (dose 10 mg/kg body weight) was administered to female Sprague-Dawley rats by gastric tube or by intravenous injection, and the following parameters were estimated:

- Course of disappearance from plasma during 48 hours p.a.
- Rate of excretion (urine, feces)
- Biliary elimination in bile fistula animals, and reabsorption of biliary metabolites

DHEA is extensively metabolized and rapidly eliminated by the renal and by the fecale route. Biliary elimination is considerable and accounts for 56 % and 69 % of the administered dose in 7-9 hrs following enteral and i.v. administration, respectively. About 40 % of bile metabolites were found to undergo enterohepatic circulation prior to final excretion in accordance with the experimentally determined reabsorption rate.

The metabolite pattern of DHEA differs significantly from that found in man. Polar compounds obviously dominate, whereas the principal metabolites in man, etiocholanolone and androsterone, play a minor role.

Institute for Mircobiology and Experimental Therapy,
Beutenbergstraße 11, O-6900 Jena

117

CHARACTERIZATION OF THE SOLUBILIZED SULFONYLUREA RECEPTOR FROM HIT-CELLS USING A ^{125}I-GLIBENCLAMIDE ANALOG

B. Rumpel[1], M. Schwanstecher[2], and H. Laatsch[1].

An iodinated glibenclamide analog - N-{4-[ß-(2-hydroxy-5-[125]iodo-benzene carboxamido)ethyl]benzene sulfonyl}-N'-cyclohexylurea (1) - was synthesized in order to characterize the sulfonylurea receptor from HIT-cells by binding studies, photoaffinity labeling and autoradiographic detection. Microsomal membranes from HIT-cells were prepared in the presence of protease-inhibitors and were then solubilized using Triton X-100. An incubation mixture consisting of Tris-buffer, 1 and triton-extract (80 µg protein/ml) was incubated until equilibrium was reached (2h) and incubations were terminated by precipitation with polyethylene glycol and filtration through Whatman GF/C filters. Binding to the sulfonylurea receptor was examined by displacement of 1 (50 pmol/l) by the unlabeled analog, glibenclamide or glipizide. The radioligand bound to the solubilized sulfonylurea receptor was displaced with K_i values of 0.6 ± 0.1, 0.4 ± 0.06 or 4.5 ± 0.4 nmol/l (n=3), respectively. Hill coefficients close to one indicated a single class of binding sites. Calculation of the dissociation constant for binding of the analog to the solubilized receptor from the kinetics of association ($t_{1/2}$ = 20 min) and dissociation ($t_{1/2}$ = 53 min) gave a value of 0.2 nmol/l, which corresponded well to the value obtained from equilibrium binding experiments. By ultraviolet radiation the analog was covalently coupled to several membrane proteins. A 140 kd protein was the only one the photoaffinity labeling of which could be prevented by the addition of unlabeled glibenclamide (100 nmol/l). The results show that the synthesized [125]iodo glibenclamide analog 1 is a valuable tool for detection and characterization of the sulfonylurea receptor.

[1]Institut für Organische Chemie, Tammannstraße 2, D-3400 Göttingen; [2]Institut für Pharmakologie und Toxikologie, Robert-Koch Straße 40, D-3400 Göttingen

118

MG[2+]ATP REGULATES GLIBENCLAMIDE BINDING TO THE SOLUBILIZED SULFONYLUREA RECEPTOR FROM HIT-CELLS

M. Schwanstecher, S. Behrends and U. Panten.

It has been found that MgATP controls glibenclamide- and diazoxide-binding to membranes from pancreatic islets. To further examine the mechanism of this regulatory effect of MgATP on the binding properties of the sulfonylurea receptor, the effect of MgATP has been examined on binding of glibenclamide and diazoxide to the solubilized state of the receptor. Extraction of the receptor from membranes of the ß-cell line HIT-T15 was performed using Triton X-100. Optimizing the conditions for solubilization yielded an extraction-efficiency of 40 ± 3% (n=8) for the active form of the receptor. Specific binding of ^{3}H-glibenclamide to the solubilized receptor (K_D = 0.35 ± 0.01 nmol/l, B_{max} = 0.17 ± 0.03 pmol/mg protein, n=5) corresponded well to the specific binding to HIT-cell membranes (K_D = 0.22 ± 0.02 nmol/l, B_{max} = 0.42 ± 0.05 pmol/mg protein, n=8). Competition binding experiments revealed that the effect of MgATP on binding of glibenclamide and diazoxide to the solubilized receptor was similar to the effect of MgATP on binding of glibenclamide and diazoxide to membranes. MgATP (0.1 mmol/l) inhibited ^{3}H-glibenclamide binding to the solubilized receptor by 76 ± 4% (IC_{50} = 20 ± 3 µmol/l, n=4) and enhanced displacement of ^{3}H-glibenclamide by diazoxide significantly (IC_{50} = 220 ± 10 µmol/l, n=4). Exogenous alkaline phosphatase accelerated the reversal of MgATP-induced inhibition of [^{3}H]glibenclamide binding to the solubilized sulfonylurea receptor. It is concluded that the binding sites for MgATP and glibenclamide are located at strongly associated proteins or at the same protein which may be a kinase.

Institut für Pharmakologie und Toxikologie der Universität Robert-Koch Straße 40, D-3400 Göttingen

119

SOLUBILIZATION AND CHARACTERIZATION OF THE SULFONYLUREA RECEPTOR FROM BRAIN

M.Schwanstecher, U.Schaupp, and U.Panten

Solubilization of the sulfonylurea receptor in an active form from pig brain microsomes was reported recently (Bernardi et al. (1988), Proc Natl Acad Sci USA 85, 9816-20). The aim of this study was to solubilize the sulfonylurea receptor from rat brain and characterise the binding properties of the solubilized receptor. Membranes from rat brain were prepared in the presence of protease-inhibitors and were solubilized using Triton X-100. An incubation mixture consisting of Tris-buffer, [^{3}H]glibenclamide and triton-extract was incubated until equilibrium was reached (2h). Incubations were terminated by precipitation with polyethylene glycol and filtration through Whatman GF/C filters. Optimizing the conditions for solubilization yielded an extraction- efficiency of 53 ± 7 % (n=8). Specific binding of [^{3}H]glibenclamide to the solubilized receptor (K_D = 0.47 ± 0.11 nmol/l, B_{max} = 34 ± 6 fmol/mg protein, n=8) corresponded well with the specific binding to membranes from rat brain (K_D = 0.06 ± 0.01 nmol/l, B_{max} = 63 ± 5 fmol/mg protein, n=5). The kinetics of association and dissociation for glibenclamide binding were slower for the solubilized receptor than for the receptor in membranes. Competition binding experiments revealed that control of glibenclamide binding by MgATP was similar to that of the solubilized sulfonylurea receptor from HIT-cells. MgATP (0.3 mmol/l) inhibited [^{3}H]glibenclamide binding (0.2 nmol/l) to the solubilized rerceptor from rat brain by 89 ± 3% (IC_{50} = 41 ± 4 µmol/l, n=4). These findings show that the sulfonylurea receptor can be solubilized from rat brain with retention of its specific binding activity for glibenclamide and that modulation of binding properties by MgATP is not restricted to the solubilised receptor from HIT-cells.

Institut für Pharmakologie und Toxikologie der Universität Robert-Koch Straße 40, D-3400 Göttingen

120

INFLUENCES OF COMPONENTS OF THE RENIN-ANGIOTEN-SIN/KALLIKREIN-KININ-SYSTEM (RAS/KKS) ON THE FERTILITY POTENTIAL OF MAMMALIAN SEMEN

W.-E. Siems, G. Heder, A. Böttger and H. Hilse

It is well known , that high activities and concentrations of components of the RAS/KKS occur in the mammalian reproduction tract. On the other hand the functions of these enzymes and peptides are completely unknown until now. On the basis of activities of a number of enzymes we investigated whether the spermatological values and consequently the male fertility correlate with these peptidases.

Spermatological values were characterized microscopically, and the enzyme activities were measured with synthetic substrates. Computer aided correlations were calculated between the enzyme activities in seminal plasma resp. on spermatozoa and the spermatological values of mammalian semen samples. Such significant correlations exist for the carboxypeptidases angiotensin-converting enzyme- (ACE) resp. neutral metalloendopeptidase-(NEP) activities in a strong species specific manner in all examined semen samples. Furthermore significantly elevated enzyme activities were found directly bound on sperm cells in cases of pathologically reduced sperm motility in man and boar. It was shown, that exogenous bradykinin (Bk) is efficiently inactivated by ACE and NEP in semen samples. Finally, an influence of the ACE-inhibitor ramipril was found on the spermiogenesis in rats, in spite of a non-penetration of the blood-testis-barrier by this compound.

Our results are interpretable by a motility stimulating action of kinins on Bk-receptors on the mammalian spermatozoa.

Present address: Institute of Drug Research, D-O-1136 Berlin, Alfred-Kowalke-Straße 4, FRG

121

INFLUENCE OF SUBSTANCE P ON ETHANOL INTAKE IN RATS

J. OTT, D.J. RUSAKOV[*], V.V. MAKSIMOV[*], and V.V. ROSHANETS[*]

In search of new therapeutical possibilities against alcohol abuse and alkoholism we investigated Substance P (SP), a neuropeptide, which plays a role in regulation of adaptive processes and which is able to reduce certain stress-induced disturbances of adaptive functions.

We used two different animal models both involving free choice between ethanol (10 Vol %) and water. Under these free choice conditions rats have the possibility to learn ethanol taking, which is a basis for development of a "psychic" dependence.

As a first model we selected the ethanol-preferring rats after 8 month of free choice drinking conditions. Individual drinking behaviour was measured 10 days before and 10 days after SP administration (250 ug/kg; i.p.). SP, when injected once or once on 4 days, decreased the ethanol intake.

As a second model we used rats that had been stressed for 6 weeks in daily sessions (20 min; footshock, light, tone). SP (250 ug/kg; i.p.) was administered 2 weeks after the beginning of the stress period. The determination of the pain threshold showed that stress induced an analgesia and SP reduced this effect. During the 6 weeks under free choice conditions the individual drinking behaviour was measured before and after the SP injections. Stress induced the ethanol intake, whereas SP, when injected on 4 consecutive days, decreased this stress-induced ethanol intake.

Present address: Institute of Drug Research, Department of Adaptation and Addiction Research, Alfred-Kowalke-Str. 4, O-1136 Berlin, FRG

[*] All-Union Research Center on Medical and Biological Problems of Addiction of the USSR Ministry of Health, Laborotory of Pharmacology of Alcohol and Experimental Treatment of Alkoholism, Malyi Mogiltsevskij per. 3, 121921 Moskow, USSR

122

STRESS-LIKE ALTERATIONS IN OBESE RATS

W. Krause, I. Roske, J. Furkert, J. Proll[1], R. Noack[1], and P. Oehme

We investigated stress-related parameters in a model of chronically obese rats. Obesitas induced by post-natal hyperalimentation (suckling of only two newborn rats per nest) lasts for the whole lives of the animals. The postnatally hyperalimentated rats had also in our experiment significantly higher body weights and significantly more interscapular brown adipose tissue in comparison to controls.

In addition, we found out that 10 of the 16 investigated obese rats showed a so-called "gut dependence", i.e. naloxone contracted their ileum in vitro. This is typically seen in animals treated with opiates and in chronically stressed animals.

Other changes occurring in stressed animals are related to substance P (SP). SP is released during stress. After chronic stress the levels of SP-like immunoreactivity (SPLIR) are lower in many peripheral organs. In our obese rats we found in the brown adipose tissue a SPLIR decreased by 46 % in comparison to controls, whereas no significant changes were detectable in blood plasma.

In adrenal slices of the adipose rats the nicotine-evoked release of catecholamines was significantly lowered. This result confirms earlier findings about a decreased catecholamine turnover in adipose rats. It differs to that seen in stressed animals (increased release of catecholamines).

In summary, our results suggest alterations in the opioid system and other peptidergic systems of obese rats. Some of the changes are in accordance with those known from stressed animals.

Institute of Drug Research, Alfred-Kowalke-Str. 4, O-1136 Berlin, Germany
[1] Central Institute of Nutrition, Arthur-Scheunert-Allee 114-116, O-1505 Bergholz-Rehbrücke, Germany

123

EFFECTS OF SUBSTANCE P ON TRANSMITTER RELEASE IN DIFFERENT BRAIN REGIONS

K. Nieber[*], B. Neufang and R. Jackisch

The generally accepted view on central action of substance P (SP) is that it, like that in the periphery, is mediated by receptors recognizing the C-terminal part (which is similar to the C-terminal sequence of other tachykinins). However, extensive research has demonstrated that certain N-terminal SP fragments, although they lack tachykinin-like activity in smooth muscle, are able to reproduce many of the central effects of exogenous SP. Therefore we investigated the effects of the undecapeptide SP and its N-terminal tetrapeptide SP(1-4) on the spontaneous and electrically evoked release of ^{3}H-noradrenaline (NA), ^{3}H-acetylcholine (ACH) and ^{3}H-5-hydroxytryptamine (5-HT) in rabbit hippocampus slices and of ACh and ^{3}H-dpoamine (DA) in rabbit caudate nucleus slices. Neither the evoked ACh nor NA release in hippocampal slices were affected by SP and SP(1-4) in concentrations up to 1 µM, whereas the evoked 5-HT release was significantly decreased by SP and SP(1-4). The two peptides did not influence the basal ^{3}H-outflow in slices preincubated with ^{3}H-NA, ^{3}H-choline or ^{3}H-5-HT. On the other hand, the basal ^{3}H-outflow in rabbit caudate nucleus slices preincubated with ^{3}H-DA (but not with ^{3}H-choline) was significantly enhanced by these peptides. The evoked release of both DA and ACh in this tissue was not affected by SP and SP(1-4) in concentrations up to 1µM. It is concluded that SP participates in the modulation of central transmitter release as follows: facilitation of DA release, inhibiion of 5-HT release, but no effects on ACh and NA release. The finding that SP(1-4) is equipotent with SP supports the hypothesis that N-terminal metabolites of SP play a role in mediating central effects of SP. The data provide further evidence for binding sites specific for the N-terminal sequence of SP in brain structures and suggest that other receptors, in addition to the accepted neurokinine receptor types, have to be considered.

[*]Institute of Drug Research, Alfred-Kowalke-Str.4, O-1136 Berlin, FRG.
Institute of Pharmacology, University of Freiburg, Hermann-Herder-Str. 5, W-7800 Freiburg, FRG.

124

CENTRAL PEPTIDERGIC MECHANISMS OF CARDIOVASCULAR CONTROL: C- AND N-TERMINAL FRAGMENTS OF SUBSTANCE P

R. Richter, F. Qadri, C. Tschöpe, N. Jost, P. Oehme[*], Th. Unger

The neuropeptide substance P (SP(1-11)), and some of its C-and N-terminal fragments known to be co-localized with catecholamines in the brain, have been implicated in central cardiovascular responses.

To elucidate the interaction between these neuropeptides and catecholamines we investigated the effect of SP(1-11) (500 pmol,icv) on the catecholamine release (NA,A,DA) from the anterior hypothalamus (AH) in conscious Wistar rats using microdialysis and HPLC-ED. Furthermore, we compared the cardiovascular responses (mean arterial blood pressure (MAP) and heart rate (HR)) to SP(1-4)COOH, SP(1-4)NH2, SP(5-11) and SP(1-4) (all 5,50, 500 pmol, icv) with those to SP(1-11) in conscious rats.

(1) SP(1-11) induced a significant and selective decrease in NA and A release (p<0.05) from AH.

(2) SP(1-11) caused dose-dependently a long-lasting increase in MAP and HR (MAP:20 ± 1.8 mmHg; HR: 161 ± 11.9 bpm; 500 pmol; n=10). The HR response usually featured 2-3 stages of activation, which suggested consecutive interactions with different brain areas.

(3) N-terminal tetrapeptides were not active (SP(1-4)NH2), or showed little activity (SP(1-4)COOH) at the dose of 500 pmol.

(4) Both C-terminal fragments (SP(5-11) and SP(4-11)) induced dose-dependent cardiovascular responses. The results provide evidence that central cardiovascular effects of SP(1-11) are linked to the C-terminus of the neuropeptide. The inhibitory effect of SP(1-11) on NA and A release from the AH suggests an interaction of the peptide with catecholaminergic pathways in the forebrain.

Department of Pharmacology, University of Heidelberg, and [*] Institute of Drug Research, Berlin, FRG

125

CCK$_8$ RELATED C-TERMINAL TETRAPEPTIDES: AFFINITIES FOR CCK-A AND CCK-B RECEPTORS
R. Harhammer, U. Schäfer, P. Henklein, H. Repke and T. Ott

We describe here the binding of new tetrapeptides derived from the C-terminal sequence of CCK$_8$ (-Trp-Met-Asp-Phe-NH$_2$) to CCK-B receptors in guinea pig cortex and CCK-A receptors in rat pancreas. IPT 31/90 (Boc-Trp-Met-Asp-Phe-NH$_2$) was found to be selective for central CCK-B receptors (K$_i$=34 nM, ratio pancreas/ cortex: 288). IPT 35/90 (Suc-Trp-Leu-Asp-Phe-NH$_2$) exhibited also high affinity for cortical CCK-B receptors (K$_i$=58 nM) but it's selectivity for this type is nearly 50 times higher (K$_i$ ratio 15000) than that of IPT 31/90. It is concluded that replacement of the Boc-Trp-Met-by the Suc-Trp-Leu- fragment markedly enhances the ability of C-terminal tetrapeptides to discriminate between CCK-A and CCK-B receptors. Substitution of Gly, Phe, Ser, Ala or Pro for Leu resulted in less effective tetrapeptides. Replacement of the Leu by hydrophilic amino acids (Asp, Lys) resulted in tetrapeptides with low affinity for both CCK receptor types. The loss of the aromatic groups in positions of Trp or Phe of the C-terminal CCK$_8$ tetrapeptide caused strong reduction of the binding affinity for the CCK-B receptor, in the same way as the replacement of the negative charged amino acid Asp by Ala. These findings may us suppose that following chemical interactions of the CCK-B receptor with the C-terminal sequence of CCK$_8$ be of importance: hydrophobic interactions with the Trp and the Phe, hydrogen bond with the Asp and incorporation of the Met in a hydrophobic pocket.

Institute of Pharmacology and Toxicology,
Humboldt-University of Berlin,
Clara-Zetkin-Str. 94, O-1040 Berlin, FRG

126

DIFFERENTIAL EFFECTS OF DRUGS AFFECTING DOPAMIN-ERGIG NEUROTRANSMISSION ON THE CCK CONTENT IN DIFFERENT PARTS OF THE RAT NC. ACCUMBENS

K. Vick, R. Schade and T. Ott

CCK-octapeptide (CCK-8) is a neuropeptide belonging to the so-called gastrin/CCK-peptide family, having in common the last five C-terminal amino-acids. Like other "brain-gut" peptides, CCK-8 is found both in the gastrointestinal tract and brain. Since it is assumed that CCK-8 coexists with dopamine (DA) in a subset of mesolimbic neurons we investigated whether pharmacological modulation of dopaminergic neurons affects the CCK-like immunoreactivity (CCK-IR) in different brain structures.

Rats were pretreated with either γ -Butyrolactone (GBL) or reserpine. CCK-IR was measured with a RIA, using an antibody which recognizes the C-terminal sequence of CCK-8. Administration of 750 mg/kg GBL increased significantly the CCK level in Nc.acc. ant. after 10 minutes, while it was without effect in Nc. acc. post. Reserpine (5 mg/kg) decreased the CCK level in Nc. acc. ant after 4 h and subsequently led to an increase after 24 h. In Nc. acc. post. and Striatum we found no decrease after 4 h, but an increase after 24 h. In a separate immunhistochemical experiment it is shown, that CCK-IR is uneven distributed in the nuclei under investigation. The results will be discussed with respect to an interaction of DA and CCK at the synaptic level.

Institute of Pharmacology and Toxicology,
Department of Medicine of the Humboldt-
University Berlin

127

INFLUENCE OF CCK ON 8-OH-DPAT-INDUCED HYPERPHAGIA IN RATS
H. Fink and M. Boomgaarden

Multiple neurotransmitter mechanisms are involved in the control of feeding.
The neuropeptide CCK is suggested to act as a satiety signal in both the gastrointestinal tract and the brain. Furtheron, it is evident from experimental data that central 5-HT$_{1A}$ receptors play an important role in the regulation of feeding.
The present study was conducted to determine whether or not the effect of 8-hydroxy-2-(di-n-propylamino)tetralin hydrobromide (8-OH-DPAT) on food intake can be antagonized by CCK-8s, acting at both CCK-A and CCK-B receptors, and CCK-4 showing a high affinity for CCK-B receptors in the brain.
CCK-8s and CCK-4 in dose ranges of 1 to 25 µg/kg i.p. and 2 to 50 µg/kg i.p., respectively, did not influence food intake in freely feeding rats during light period. 8-OH-DPAT (0.3 mg/kg i.p.) induced a strong increase of food intake under these conditions.
CCK-8s (5 µg/kg) depressed strongly the hyperphagic effect of 8-OH-DPAT by 80 % . CCK-4 (2 µg/kg) depressed the effect of 8-OH-DPAT by 40 % .
The experiments provide evidence for a potential link between central 5-HT$_{1A}$ and CCK mechanisms in the control of feeding.

Institute of Pharmacology and Toxicology, Charite, Humboldt-University of Berlin, Clara-Zetkin-Straße 94, O-1080 Berlin, FRG.

128

ROLE OF CCK-A AND CCK-B RECEPTORS IN LOCOMOTOR ACTIVITY, THIGMOTACTIC SCANNING AND CONFLICT BEHAVIOR
Th. Barth, T. Ott and H. Fink

Two CCK receptor subtypes have been differentiated: CCK-A receptors, located in the periphery and the brain, exhibit a high affinity for CCK-8s and a lower affinity for CCK-4, whereas CCK-B sites, widely distributed in the brain, display a high affinity for both CCK-fragments.
The present study was designed to examine the role of the CCK receptor subtypes in mediating behavior in particular stimulus situations of rats. The effects of the systemically given CCK fragments, the CCK-A antagonist L 364,718 (3S(-)-N -(2,3-dihydro-1-methyl-2-oxo-5-phenyl-1-H-1,4-benzodiazepine-3-yl)-1H-indole-2-carboxamide) and the CCK-B antagonist L 365,260 (3R(+)-N-2,3-dihydro-1-methyl-2-oxo-5-phenyl-1H-1,4-benzodiazepine-3-yl)-N'-(3-methylphenyl) urea), were investigated on:
    - spontaneous locomotor activity (open field),
    - thigmotactic scanning (scanning along a wall)
    - conflict test adapted from that of Bodnoff, S.R. et al. [Psychopharmacol., 97 (1989), 277]
Locomotor activity was decreased by CCK-8s (5 µg/kg) by increasing the immobilization duration, and increased by L 364,718 (1 and 10 µg/kg), mainly by decreasing the immobilization duration. A strong increase of latency to move from the center toward the wall of an open field was induced by both L 364,718 (10 µg/kg) and L 365,260 (1 and 100 µg/kg).
CCK-4 (10 and 50 µg/kg) and L 364,718 (100 µg/kg) showed a pro-conflict effect, whereas L 365,260 (1 µg/kg) induced an anti-conflict effect.
It can be concluded that the locomotor effects are mediated by CCK-A receptors, and that both receptor subtypes are involved in expression of wall-facing and conflict behavior. It is suggested that these behavioral effects of CCK agonists/antagonists may contribute to their anxiogenic/ anxiolytic action.

Institute of Pharmacology and Toxicology, Humboldt-University of Berlin, Clara-Zetkin-Str. 94, O-1040 Berlin, FRG

129

C-TERMINAL CCK-SEQUENCE INDUCES ANTINOCICEPTION

Gericke M., R.Morgenstern and T.Ott

It is well known that Cholecystokinin octapeptide, a gastro-intestinal hormone, produced significant antinociception after i.c.v. administration in the acetic acid-induced writhing test in the mouse.

In recent studies it has been shown that the C-terminal tetrapeptide (CCK-4) and pentapeptide (pentagastrin) of CCK binds to central CCK binding sites (CCK-B receptors) with high selectivity.

We report here that CCK-4 and pentagastrin also induced antinociception in the acetic acid-induced writhing test in the mouse.

CCK-4 appeared to be more potent in inducing antinociception than CCK-8 and pentagastrin.

The effect was dose-dependent, however the dose-response curves for CCK-4 and pentagastrin were "U-shaped".

The specific CCK-B receptor antagonist L-365,260 (3R(+)-N-(2,3-dihydro-1-methyl-2-oxo-5-phenyl-1H-1,4benzodiazepin-3y-1)-N'-(3-methylphenyl)-urea) was more potent to antagonize the antinociceptive effect of CCK-4 and pentagastrin than the CCK-A receptor antagonist L-364,718 (devazepide).

When tested against the CCK-8-induced antinociception these antagonists were approximately equipotent.

Therefore we conclude that CCK-4- and pentagastrin- induced antinociception is mediated mainly via CCK-B receptors, whereas CCK-8-induced antinociception seems to be mediated via both CCK-A and CCK-B receptors.

Institute of Pharmacology and Toxicology,
HU Berlin
P.B. 140, O-1040 Berlin, F.R.G.

130

EFFECTS OF PERIPHERALLY ADMINISTERED DES-TYROSINE[1]-D-PHENYLALANINE[3]-β-CASOMORPHIN ON APOMORPHINE-INDUCED HYPOTHERMIA

H. Stark[1] and H-L. Rüthrich[2]

The intracerebroventricularly injected non-opiate-like peptide des-tyrosine[1]-D-phenylalanine[3]-β-casomorphin (DT-D-Phe[3]-βCM) has been found to attenuate the apomorphine-induced decrease of the brain temperature in rats. Previous experiments with this tetrapeptide, which seems to be related to the dopaminergic system, have been revealed its anticonvulsant and antidepressive components. The effects of this peptide are reflected in a bell-shaped dose-response curve.

The aim of the present work was to correlate the plasma concentration of this peptide with the effect on the brain temperature after subcutaneous and oral application.

Male Wistar rats were chronically implanted a steel cannula into the brain to easily and precisely measure the temperature by an electronic microprobe. Catheters were inserted in the femoral artery to collect blood samples. By this arrangement it was possible to compare the effects on brain temperature and the plasma concentration of drugs in freely moving rats. In contrast to the subcutaneous injection, the oral administration yielded a relatively stable plasma concentration of DT-D-Phe[3]-βCM, resulting in a longer lasting peptide effect on the body temperature.

Due to the pharmacokinetics in the plasma, the mode of application of DT-D-Phe[3]-βCM, which shows a bell-shaped dose-response curve, seems to play an important role for both the duration and the strength of its centrally elicited effects.

[1]Institute of Neurobiology and Brain Research, Brenneckestr. 6, O-3090 Magdeburg, Germany
[2]Institute for Pharmacology and Toxicology, Medical Academy Magdeburg, Leipziger Str. 44, O-3090 Magdeburg, Germany

131

EFFECTS OF [DES-TYR-D-PHE[3]]BETA-CASOMORPHIN (2-5) ON CORTICAL EEG POWER SPECTRA IN RATS

M. Diedrich, T. Wagner and W. Wetzel

[Des-Tyr-D-Phe[3]]beta-casomorphin (2-5) (BCH-325) is a peptide (Pro-D-Phe-Pro-Gly) with antidepressant-like actions tested in related animal models (e.g. Porsolt test, bulbectomy test). In the present experiments, the effects of BCH-325 on EEG power spectra were studied in rats. The effects were compared with control recordings following saline injections and with different psychotropic drugs (diazepam, haloperidol, amitriptyline, imipramine, amphetamine). Drugs were injected intraperitoneally and EEG power spectra were recorded during two hours post injectionem. The EEG was recorded from the parietal cortex of freely moving Wistar rats during the state of relaxed wakefulness. We found that the administration of BCH-325 resulted in small but significant effects on EEG power spectra. Most effects were found during the second hour post injectionem. The alpha-2 band and the beta-1 band were increased and the delta activity was decreased by the peptide. Our results show that the effects of [des-Tyr-D-Phe[3]] beta-casomorphin on EEG power spectra differ from those of typical antidepressants and other psychotropic drugs.

Institute of Neurobiology and Brain Research, Brenneckestr. 6, O-3090 Magdeburg, Germany.

132

Noradrenaline (NA) release in human cerebral cortex is mediated by N-methyl-D-aspartate (NMDA) and non-NMDA receptors

K. Fink[1], R. Schultheiß[2] and M. Göthert[1]

Human brain cortex slices were used to investigate whether NA release can be stimulated via NMDA and non-NMDA receptors, both of which may be activated in vivo by excitatory amino acids (EAA) such as L-glutamate. Slices were prepared from temporal cortex specimens which were dissected from patients undergoing neurosurgery. After preincubation with ^{3}H-NA the slices were superfused with Mg^{2+}-free (unless stated otherwise) Krebs-Henseleit (KH) solution. NMDA or kainic acid, added to the superfusion medium (containing Mg^{2+} in the experiments with kainic acid) for 2 min, stimulated ^{3}H overflow in a concentration-dependent manner. The NMDA (1mmol/l)-evoked overflow was almost abolished by tetrodotoxin (TTX 0.3μmol/l), 1.2 mmol/l Mg^{2+} or absence of Ca^{2+}. 2-Amino-5-phosphonopentanoic acid (100μmol/l), a competitive NMDA receptor antagonist, reduced the stimulatory effect of NMDA (1mmol/l) by 68% and dizocilpine (former MK-801; 100nmol/l), an antagonist at the phencyclidine (PCP) receptor within the NMDA-gated ion channel, reduced the stimulatory effect of NMDA (1mmol/l) by 83%. 7-Chlorokynurenic acid (100μmol/l), which is an antagonist at the glycine recognition site coupled to the NMDA receptor, inhibited the NMDA (1mmol/l)-evoked ^{3}H overflow by 94%. The kainic acid (1mmol/l)-evoked ^{3}H overflow from slices superfused with KH containing 1.2mmol/l Mg^{2+} was reduced in the presence of 6-cyano-7-nitroquinoxaline-2,3-dione (30μmol/l) by 77%, whereas the competitive NMDA receptor antagonist DL-(E)-2-amino-4-methyl-5-phosphono-3-pentanoic acid (CGP 37849; 30μmol/l) was ineffective. - It is concluded that in the human brain cortex NA release is stimulated via NMDA receptors and via non-NMDA receptors. Both EAA receptor subtypes identified in the human brain cortex resemble the corresponding receptors in rat brain cortex or hippocampus, with respect to their pharmacological properties.

[1]Inst. Pharmacol., University of Bonn, Reuterstraße 2b; [2]Clinic of Neurosurgery, University of Bonn, Sigmund-Freud-Straße 25, D-5300 Bonn 1, F.R.G.

133

AMINOOXYACETIC ACID PRODUCES EXCITOTOXIC LESIONS IN THE RAT SUBSTANTIA NIGRA W.A. Turski

An active metabolite of MPTP (1-methyl-4-phenyl-1,2, 3,6-tetrahydropyridine), MPP^+ (1-methyl-4-phenyl-pyridinium ion), is believed to induce the acute neuronal toxicity in dopaminergic neurons in the substantia nigra. The neurotoxic action of MPP^+ can be explained by a depletion of intracellular energy resources. The neurotoxic action of MPP^+ in the rat substantia nigra pars compacta can be blocked by N-methyl -D-aspartate (NMDA) antagonists, presumably due to lowering membrane potential and relief of the voltage dependent Mg^{2+} block of NMDA receptor channels by the toxin. Aminooxyacetic acid (AOAA) possesses neurotoxic potential in the rat striatum and its action may be explained by a depletion of intracellular energy resources or effects on kynurenic acid metabolism. Furthermore, the toxic action of AOAA in the rat striatum can be blocked by NMDA antagonists. In the present study, male Wistar rats were injected with AOAA, 0.25 - 2 umol, into the substantia nigra pars compacta and the brains were histologically examined after 24 h - 14 days. Morphological analysis showed that AOAA induced excitotoxic lesions in the rat substantia nigra resembling that produced by MPP^+. The neurotoxic action of AOAA in the nigra was blocked by the NMDA antagonist 2-amino-7-phosphono-heptanoic acid. These data suggest that AOAA may induce permanent neurotoxic lesion in the rat substantia nigra. Some similarities in the mechanisms of neurotoxic action of AOAA and MPP^+ can be suggested.

Department of Pharmacology, Medical School, Jaczews-kiego 8, PL-20-090 Lublin, Poland

134

EFFECTS OF SUBCHRONIC ADMINISTRATION OF PYRITINOL ON RECEPTOR DENSITY AND PHOSPHATIDYLINOSITOL-METABOLISM IN AGED MICE. H.Hartmann, S.A.Cohen, and W.E.Müller

Pyritinol is one of the nootropic drugs used to improve age related impairments of cognitive functions. In animal-models on different levels like behaviour, electrophysiology and distinct biochemical systems a positive impact of chronic pyritinol administration has been shown. In the cholinergic-system, pyritinol activated presynaptic mechanisms in aged rats. (e.g, ACh- release, ChA-transferase-activity). We investigated the influence of subchronic (15 days) pyritinol treatment on receptor density and phosphatidylinositol (PI)-hydrolysis as a marker for receptor function. Chronic treatment of aged mice (20-22 months) with pyritinol (200mg/kg;daily; p.o.) elevated NMDA-receptor density in the forebrain by about 20% with no change in receptor affinity. α2-receptor density was slightly decreased after drug administration, but differentiation of high-and low-affinity-receptor-state revealed a percentual increase in number of high-affinity-state receptors. No changes in receptor density were found at the muscarinic-, benzodiazepine- and the beta-receptor. Carbachol, pilocarpine and fluoride induced PI-hydrolysis was determined in dissociated neurons, inositol-1-phosphate (IP1) accumulation was standardized on total incorporation (IP1+lipids). Chronic pyritinol treatment increased carbachol-induced (0.01, 0.1, 1mM) PI-hydrolysis by about 30%, a slight but statistically not significant elevation was found after stimulation with pilocarpine or fluoride. Considering the striking importance of the cholinergic and glutamatergic system on cognition, these findings support our hypothesis that pyritinol, like other nootropics, has a modulating effect on receptor-effector-systems, in this way improving cognitive function.

Department of Psychopharmacology
Central Institute of Mental Health; D-6800 Mannheim (FRG)

135

ENZYMES METABOLIZING GLUTAMATE IN THE RAT BRAIN: BIOCHEMICAL AND HISTOCHEMICAL STUDIES WITH REFERENCE TO THE INFLUENCE OF ALUMINIUM AND OTHER METAL IONS

K. Richter[1], G. Poeggel[1], I. Torgner[2], E. Kvamme[2], F. Rothe[3] and H-G. Bernstein[1]

One of the main targets of the neurotoxin aluminium is obviously the glutamatergic system (Yokel et al., 1988, NeuroToxicology 9, 429-442). The metal is thought to decrease transmitter release from glutamatergic synapses. The influence of the toxin on glutamate-metabolizing enzymes is not known at present. We therefore studied the phosphate-activated glutaminase (PAG), aspartate aminotransferase (AAT) and glutamate dehydrogenase (GDH) with respect to a possible influence of aluminium and other metal ions. Biochemically, it was found that PAG-activity is strongly depressed by copper, zinc, and aluminium (chloride salt), whereas lithium and magnesium did not change the activity (in-vitro experiments). In in-vivo experiments GDH diminished by 18%, when aluminium hydroxide was injected subcutaneously. Aluminium chloride was without any effect. AAT was not changed by aluminium .The regional distribution and cellular localisation of the three enzymes was investigated by histochemical and immunocytochemical methods. We are about to prove, whether aluminium is able to influence the distribution pattern of the enzymes in the brain tissue.

[1]Institute of Neurobiology and Brain Research, Brenneckestr. 6, O-3090 Magdeburg, FRG, [2]Neurochem. Lab.,Univ. Oslo,[3]Inst. Biol., Med. Acad. Magdeburg.
This research was supported by a grant of the BMFT of FRG (Nr. 0319939A5).

136

PENTYLENETETRAZOL-INDUCED KINDLING IN RAT AND RELATED LONG-LASTING SUPPRESSION OF OFFENSIVE BEHAVIOUR
H.Kittner and M.Müller

Epileptic disorders are often associated with disturbances in cognitive functions and emotional reactions. Kindling as an important model of neuronal plasticity and epileptogenesis seems to be also an unique method for the study of long-lasting behavioural changes associated with epilepsy. Ethoexperimental animal models, e.g. the home-cage intruder test may be valuable in the study of neurobehavioural systems, including emotional states and they may provide an analog to human emotions and mental illness.
In the present investigation the offensive behaviour of pentylenetetrazol (PTZ)-kindled rats was examined in the home-cage intruder test. The offensive interactions (back biting,lateral attack, standing on top of, piloerection, chasing) between territorial residents and intruders were counted. In all trials a suppressed offensive behaviour was observed 24h, 1, 3, 5 week(s) after the last PTZ-induced kindled seizure. Animals without expression of myoclonic jerks or generalized seizures showed no reduction of offense.
In further experiments it was found that treatment with carbamazepine prior to each PTZ-application attenuated the prolonged behavioural changes. There was no correlation between anticonvulsant efficacy and improvement of behaviour.
The phenomenon of long-lasting lowered offensive behaviour in PTZ-kindled rats may provide a model for some kind of complex relationship between epilepsy and mental disorders.

Institute of Pharmacology and Toxicology, University Leipzig, Härtelstr. 16-18, O-7010 Leipzig

R 68

137

^{3}H-D-ASPARTATE RELEASE FROM HIPPOCAMPAL SLICES OF PENTYLENETETRAZOL-(PTZ)-KINDLED RATS

Schröder H., A.Becker and B.Lössner

Rats were kindled to three class 5 seizures by repeated application of pentylenetetrazol (PTZ - 45 mg/kg ip., 10 times for 20 days). After one stimulus-free week, in vitro the influence of L-glutamate on basal and K^+(48 mM)-stimulated ^{3}H-D-aspartate release was measured either in slices of hippocampus or in slices of area dentata and CA1 subregions. The K^+-stimulated ^{3}H-D-aspartate release from hippocampal slices as well as from its subregions was unchanged after PTZ-kindling compared to saline controls. The L-glutamate-induced increase of the K^+-stimulated ^{3}H-D-aspartate release from hippocampal slices of kindled rats was consistently greater than that measured in saline treated controls. Whilst L-glutamate-evoked basal ^{3}H-D-aspartate release from hippocampal slices of kindled rats appeared unchanged.
Testing the effect of NMDA, quisqualate and kainate on amino acid release from control hippocampal slices it could be shown that the L-glutamate-induced ^{3}H-D-aspartate release is mediated by quisqualate receptor activation.
From these data it is concluded that PTZ-induced kindling is accompanied by an enhanced glutamate release from hippocampus.

Address: Institute of Pharmacology and Toxicology, Medical Academy, Leipziger Str.44, D-(O)-3090 Magdeburg, BRD.

138

MODULATION OF THE SEIZURE THRESHOLD FOR EXCITATORY AMINO ACIDS IN MICE BY ANTIEPILEPTIC DRUGS AND CHEMOCONVULSANTS
K.G. Steppuhn and L. Turski

Clonic seizures induced by intracerebroventricular (i.c.v.) infusion of N-methyl-D-aspartate (NMDA), kainate (KA) and α-amino-3-hydroxy-5-tert-butyl-4-isoxazolepropionate (ATPA) were assessed in NMRI mice, 20-24 g in weight, to study anti- and proconvulsant action of antiepileptic drugs and chemoconvulsants. For triggering seizures, freely-moving mice were equipped with i.c.v. injection cannula connected by plastic tubing to Harvard pumps and NMDA, KA and ATPA were continuously infused in a concentration of 1 nmol/5 μl and a speed of 5 μl/min until clonic convulsions occurred. The NMDA antagonist CPP (10-50 mg/kg; 3-((±)-2-carboxypiperazin-4-yl)-propyl-1-phosphonate) selectively elevated the threshold for NMDA seizures, while the quisqualate antagonist NBQX (0.5-5 mg/kg; 2,3-dihydroxy-6-nitro-7-sylfamoyl-benzo(F)quinoxaline) selectively elevated the threshold for ATPA seizures. Systemic administration of diazepam (0.5-10 mg/kg) and midazolam (10-20 mg/kg) elevated the threshold for KA, but had no effect on ATPA and NMDA. Phenobarbital (10-40 mg/kg) and valproate (100-400 mg/kg) elevated the threshold for NMDA, KA and ATPA seizures. Ethosuximide (200-400 mg/kg) lowered the threshold for NMDA, but enhanced the threshold for ATPA and KA seizures, as also did trimethadione (100-400 mg/kg). Diphenylhydantoin (10-40 mg/kg) and carbamazepine (10-40 mg/kg) selectively elevated the threshold for ATPA convulsions. Pentylenetetrazol (50 mg/kg) lowered the threshold for KA, but had no effect on ATPA and NMDA seizures. DMCM (1 mg/kg; methyl-4-ethyl-6,7-dimethoxy-9H-pyrido-(3,4-b)-indol-3-carboxylate) lowered the threshold for KA and ATPA but not for NMDA seizures. Picrotoxin (1 mg/kg) lowered the threshold for KA, had no effect on NMDA, but elevated the threshold for ATPA. Pilocarpine (100 mg/kg) had no effect on KA and NMDA thresholds but elevated the threshold for ATPA. Bicuculline (1 mg/kg), 3-mercaptopropionate (12.5 mg/kg) and strychnine (0.2 mg/kg) had no effect on the threshold for seizures induced by excitatory amino acids. These data demonstrate that antiepileptic drugs and chemoconvulsants differentially affect the threshold for seizures triggered by excitatory amino acids.

Department of Neuropsychopharmacology, Research Laboratories of Schering AG, P.O.Box 65 03 11, W-1000 Berlin 65, Germany

139

CHRONIC CLONAZEPAM- BUT NOT PHENOBARBITAL-TREATMENT DEPRESSES PETIT MAL-LIKE SEIZURES IN RATS
R. Scherkl and Mechthild Voits

Clonazepam but not phenobarbital is effective in the treatment of human petit mal absences. In a rat model, however, petit mal-like spike wave activity in the electrocorticogramm was depressed after single doses of phenobarbital (2.5-10 mg/kg, Micheletti et al., Arzneim.-Forsch./Drug Res. 35, 483-485, 1985). So we decided to study the efficacy of both drugs in this model during chronic treatment.
Clonazepam treatment for 3 weeks with a dose regimen providing plasma concentrations in rats known as therapeutically active in man (0.5 mg/kg i.p. t.i.d., plasma concentrations about 100 ng/ml 30 min after injection) led to a significant reduction of number, mean duration and sum of duration of the spike wave discharges in the ECoG, which was recorded every day 15-45 min after the morning dose. During the 3 weeks of treatment there were no signs of development of tolerance, but increased ECoG activity during the week after cessation of treatment indicated physical dependence.
Chronic treatment with weekly increased doses of phenobarbital in drinking water (5, 10, 20 and 40 mg/kg/d) providing plasma levels of 4-6, 8-11, 18-20 and 32-35 μg/ml during ECoG recording time rather seemed to have an aggravating effect on spike wave activity in the ECoG.

Department of Pharmacology and Toxicology, School of Veterinary Medicine, Freie Universität Berlin, Koserstr. 20, W-1000 Berlin 33

140

ANTICONVULSANT AND RELATED EFFECTS OF U-54494A IN DIFFERENT SEIZURE TESTS
W. Fischer, R. Bodewei* and M. Müller

Several lines of evidence indicate that opioid systems are implicated in epileptogenic phenomena as well as endogenous seizure control mechanisms and different opioid compounds are known to have pro- or anticonvulsant activities.
For the benzamid U-54494A (±cis-3,4-dichloro-N-methyl-(-N-[2-(1-pyrrolidinyl)-cyclohexyl]benzamid), a kappa opioid receptor related substance, recently anticonvulsant properties were described. In the present study, the protective effects of this drug were investigated in three selected models of experimental epilepsy. In the maximal electroshock seizure test in mice U-54494A was effective with a potency somewhat lower than phenobarbital. The anticonvulsant activity could be partially antagonized by naloxone. In combination with phenobarbital synergistic effects were found. On the other hand, U-54494A reveals no significant effects in the pentylenetetrazol seizure threshold test. In rats with chronically implanted electrodes in the dorsal hippocampus, U-54494A reduced the duration of electrically evoked EEG afterdischarges in higher concentrations. In addition, with regard to the possible mode of action preliminary experiments on cultivated neonatal cardiomyocytes of the rat using a whole-cell voltage-clamp technique, show that U-54494A was capable to depress the rapid inward Na^+ current in a dose- and use-dependent manner.
In summary, the results presented demonstrate remarkable anticonvulsant effects for U-54494A in grand mal-analogous seizure tests. It is suggested that besides the kappa opioid receptor related actions modulations of Na^+ (Ca^{++}) membrane currents could contribute to the mechanisms of action.

*Institute for Cardiovascular Research, O-1115 Berlin-Buch
Institute of Pharmacology and Toxicology, University Leipzig, Härtelstraße 16-18, O-7010 Leipzig, F.R.G.

141

INFLUENCNE OF PIRACETAM ON THE HIGH AFFINITY Ca^{++}-ATPase IN NEURONAL STRUCTURES OF RAT BRAIN
M. Blaschke and H.-D. Fischer

The synaptosomal high affinity Ca^{++}-ATPase, essential for the regulation of intrasynaptosomal calcium homeostasis is dependent on intact protein-phospholipid interactions. Hypoxia, in vitro generated free radicals and detergents reduce the synaptosomal high affinity Ca^{++}-ATPase activity (Blaschke et al. (1988) Biomed. Biochim. Acta 47:887).

Also acute and chronic treatment of rats with piracetam results in a decrease of this synaptosomal ATPase activity, depending on the concentration of calcium. The effect on the enzyme activity induced by chronic piracetam treatment is observed for 40 d after the last drug application and normalized only after 70 d.

The results agree with the observation that piracetam accelerates phospholipid metabolism via phospholipase A_2 induction, which triggers the catabolism of peroxidized membrane structures (Woelk (1979) Arzneimittelforschung 29:615; Van Kuijk et al. (1987) Trends Biochem. Sci. 12:31).

We suppose,phospholipids will be structurally changed to entities, formed slowly and being very resistent to further peroxidation processes as well as catabolic mechanisms.

Institute of Pharmacology and Toxicology, Medical Academy "C.G. Carus" Dresden, Karl-Marx-Str. 3, 0-8080 Dresden

142

INFLUENCE OF CEREBROPROTECTIVE SUBSTANCES ON NEUROTOXIC EFFECTS OF HEXACHLOROPHENE IN VIVO AND IN VITRO
K.Andreas and C.Matthes

Hexachlorophene induces a cytotoxic brain oedema used as experimental model of brain damage. Because of the clinical importance the brain oedema is suited for testing of cerebroprotective substances. The primary target of hexachlorophene is the neuronal cell membrane. Therefore, nootropic substances were examined because of their membranotropic efficacy. Rats recieved orally hexachlorophene in liquid diet during three weeks. Thereafter, the irritation of the coordinative motor response observed in an especially developed test and the alteration of the water content were used to characterize the hexachlorophene-induced injuries and the cerebroprotective efficacy of the test substances. Under the influence of some nootropic substances with different mechanism of action the disturbed coordinative motor response was restored and the water content of the brain was normalized significantly earlier as in spontaneous remission. With the purpose of promotion of alternative methods and of comparison between in vivo and in vitro results the influence of hexachlorophene on different permanent cell lines and primary cultures of rat brain cells was examined. The hexachlorophene-induced effects were antagonized by nootropic substances also found effective in vivo.

Institute of Pharmakology and Toxikology, Medical Academy "Carl Gustav Carus", Fetscherstr.74, D/O-8019 Dresden, FRG

143

IMMUNOENZYMATIC DETERMINATION OF CALBINDIN CONTENT IN CYTOPLASMIC RAT BRAIN PROTEINS

R. Honza and N. Popov

In the course of our investigations on calcium-binding proteins of rat brain during adaptive states, an immunological assay for the determination of calbindin D28K was developed. Calbindin was purified from rat kidney to near homogeneity by a combination of ion exchange chromatography and preparative electrophoresis. A polyclonal antibody to calbindin was obtained by immunization of rabbits. The content of specific antibody was shown by immunoprecipitation of purified calbindin, immunoblotting and affinity chromatography. This antibody was suited for the development of an immunological determination of calbindin. However, the recent availability of a monoclonal antibody to calbindin was the reason to use this antibody in the assay. It is based on the competition of a limited amount of antibody between solid-phase bound calbindin and the calbindin contained in the sample. The antibody bound to the wells of a microtiter plate is determined by a HRP-conjugated antibody to mouse immunoglobulins and an o-phenylenediamine substrate reaction. The amount of calbindin in the sample proteins is calculated from a standard curve. Using this assay, the content of calbindin was determined in different rat brain regions.

Institute of Pharmacology and Toxicology, Medical Academy Magdeburg, O-3090 Magdeburg, Leipziger Strasse 44

144

THE EFFECT OF $GABA_B$ RECEPTOR AGONISTS ON BENZODIAZEPINE AND MORPHINE ABSTINENCE SYNDROME

L. Allikmets, A. Zharkovsky and G. Cebers

Both in our experiments and in several other studies it has been firmly established that the increase of potassium-dependent Ca^{++} influx via voltage sensitive calcium channels is involved in the development of withdrawal syndrome after chronic ethanol, barbiturate, benzodiazepine, and morphine treatment. Calcium channel antagonists nitrendipine, nifedipine, and verapamil are effective in suppressing most of the withdrawal symptoms in experimental animals. In the present study we compared the effects of $GABA_B$ receptor agonists (baclofen, phenibut) and nifedipine on the withdrawal symptoms of diazepam (10 mg/kg daily i.p., 30 days) and morphine given in increasing dosages 10 to 140 mg/kg twice daily i.p. for 28 days. In diazepam experiments the BDZ antagonist CGS 8216 (5 mg/kg i.p.) and morphine experiments an antagonist naloxone (2.5 mg/kg i.p.) were used to facilitate the abstinence syndrome 1-3 days after withdrawal. Baclofen (1-10 mg/kg i.p.), phenibut (50-100 mg/kg i.p.), and nifedipine (5-10 mg/kg) were injected 30 min before facilitating drugs 48 and 72 hrs after diazepam and morphine withdrawal. In the doses used baclofen and nifedipine were superior to phenibut in suppressing the withdrawal syndrome. The effect of $GABA_B$ receptor agonists is depending on their ability to suppress neuronal Ca^{++} influx.

Present address: Department of Pharmacology, Tartu University, Tartu, ESTONIA 202400.

145

PHYSICAL DEPENDENCE ON ETHANOL VS. REBOUND PHENOMENA IN AN ANIMAL MODEL OF ALCOHOLISM

A. HEYNE, G. SLODKOVSKA, J. WOLFFGRAMM

The withdrawal syndrome after cessation of chronic drug supply consists in different components. Some symptoms are inverse to the drug's own actions. Others reflect a general hypersensitivity and disturbances of physiological regulations. Such signs are indicating a physical dependence. It has often been assumed that rebound symptoms are not more than a partial aspect of physical dependence. However there is growing evidence that they may be two separate phenomena. The present investigation aims to detect such differences.

We have studied the withdrawal syndrome after ethanol (ETOH) in male Wistar rats (N = 46). Three experimental groups were formed; all the rats were housed in single cages. Rats of the first group were forced to drink ETOH solutions (5 and 20 Vol %) for 32 weeks (high intake: 3.2 g/kg/d, HI). Rats of the second group had the choice between water and ETOH for only 22 weeks (low intake: 1.2 g/kg/d, LI). The last group served as control (CO). All the rats were submitted to the same set of tests being performed daily from 4 days before withdrawal to 4 days after. The following parameters were measured: body weight, food consumption, fluid intake, body temperature, pain threshold, locomotion, social behavior (dyadicen-counters) and exploration.

Significant differences appeared between HI-rats and LI-rats. HI-rats revealed signs of withdrawal. A significant (p < 0.001) decrease of body weight (no changes in food and fluid intake) on the second day of abstinence and a slight hyperthermia (+ 0.3 °C, p < 0.05) from the first to the third day were found. The threshold of reaction to an electric foot shock was significantly lowered (p < 0.001) during the first three days of withdrawal. A decrease of locomotion, a decline in exploration and a loss of social interactions appeared mainly on the second day. CO-rats revealed slight monotonous trends but no sudden alterations.

LI-rats increased food and fluid intake during withdrawal without changing their body weight. Hyperthermia was slightly stronger (+ 0.5 °C) than in HI-rats. However, the effects on both pain threshold and behavior were inverse. During the previous days of ETOH supply the threshold was lower than that of controls; on the first day of abstinence it was significantly increased (p < 0.05), but rapidly recovered on the next days. In a similar way locomotion, exploration and social interactions were shortly enhanced during withdrawal.

These discrepancies between LI and HI indicated that LI had not developed a physical dependence but only an ETOH-specific rebound. In contrast, the long term high intake of ETOH in HI led to a physical dependence on the drug which superimposed with the rebound phenomena.

Dept. of Neuropsychopharmacology, Free University, Ulmenallee 30, 1000 Berlin 19

146

INFLUENCE OF A SINGLE DOSE OF HALOPERIDOL ON THE NEUROTRANSMITTER CONTENT IN DIFFERENT BRAIN AREAS OF THE MARMOSET (CALLITHRIX JACCHUS) ON POSTNATAL DAY 1

Rudolf Schwabe, Xenia Haun, Renate Thiel, Kerstin Rautenberg, Gerd Bochert, Ibrahim Chahoud, Diether Neubert

There are considerable species differences in the development of neurotransmitters and their receptors during the perinatal period. Since there are no data available regarding the development of neurotransmitters in the marmoset (Callithrix jacchus) we performed a study with newborn marmosets and determined the neurotransmitters dopamine and serotonin and their metabolites on day 1 postnatally. Since the marmosets can only raise two babies from triplets, the third will die. We took only the third baby of a litter for our study. 15 marmoset offspring were used to evaluate a possible disturbance of the transmitter content by drug treatment. Half of the group was treated with 1 mg haloperidol/kg body wt i.p. A specified period of time after injection the animals were decapitated and the brain was immediately dissected into different brain areas and homogenized. The determinations of the neurotransmitter content were carried out by HPLC using ELCD. In the striatum of newborn marmosets we obtained the following results (Mean ± SD):

| | Control | Concentration* after | |
		0.5 hours	1 hour
n=	7	4	4
DA	3377 ± 1272	3228 ± 942	1943 ± 960
Dopac	269 ± 88	771 ± 224	323 ± 37
HVA	1492 ± 527	2405 ± 656	1006 ± 339
5-HT	181 ± 36	105 ± 24	99 ± 71
HIAA	407 ± 155	466 ± 244	230 ± 105

* = ng/g wet tissue, DA = 3-Hydroxytyramine, Dopac=3,4-Dihydroxyphenyl-acetic acid, HVA=Homo-vanillic acid, 5-HT= Sero-tonin, HIAA = Hydroxyindoleacetic acid

In newborn marmosets haloperidol induced a significant increase in the dopac content half an hour after treatment.

Institut für Toxikologie und Embryopharamkologie, FU Berlin, Garystr. 5, D-1000 Berlin 33. Supported by grants from the Deutsche Forschungsgemeinschaft to the Sfb 174

147

THE EFFECT OF SOMAN AND ATROPINE ON GABA-LEVELS IN DIFFERENT BRAIN PARTS OF GUINEA PIGS

M.Wentz, F.Worek, W.Biederbick, I.Steidl, L.Szinicz

Topical application of GABA to distinct brain areas causes cardio-respiratory depression. The centrally acting, cholinomimetic agent soman (SO) also depresses respiration and circulation. To investigate interactions of the GABA-ergic and the cholinergic system, the GABA-content was measured in different brain regions of SO poisoned guinea pigs. Female Pirbright-White guinea pigs were anaesthetized with urethane (1.8 g/kg), the trachea was canulated and respiratory parameters were measured for 60 minutes. Guinea pigs received i.v. either SO (0.032 mg/kg = 2 x LD50), atropine (AT) (10mg/kg), SO + AT (two minutes after SO application) or saline (control). After decapitation the brains were dissected on ice into cortex, hippocampus, striatum, hypothalamus, cerebellum, and medulla. The brain parts were homogenized in water-ethanol-glacial acetic acid, centrifuged, and derivatized with dansylchloride. GABA was separated by isocratic HPLC and quantitated by UV-detection at 254 nm. SO caused a respiratory arrest within 4 min after drug application. Survival time was less than 10 min. In contrast all animals of the SO + AT group survived the full 60 min observation period. Respiratory and cardiovascular parameters of this group improved to 80 % of baseline. Compared to the control group, after SO application an increase of GABA was observed in all brain regions. In medulla oblongata, the GABA-content increased from 214±14 μg/g (control) significantly (p<0.05) to 293±35 μg/g (SO group).The SO+AT group showed a GABA-level of 215±11 μg/g.
The results presented might suggest that GABA is involved in respiratory depression caused by soman.

Institut für Pharmakologie und Toxikologie, Akademie des Sanitäts- und Gesundheitswesens der Bundeswehr, BSW, Ingolstädter Landstraße 100, D-8046 Garching, FRG

148

DISTINCT TARGETS FOR TETANUS AND BOTULINUM A NEUROTOXINS

H. Bigalke, P. Marxen, F. Bartels, and G. Ahnert-Hilger*

Adrenal chromaffin cells have been used with increasing frequency in the study of the mode of action of tetanus and botulinum neurotoxins since it was shown that both toxins can block exocytosis when injected directly into the soma of the cells (Penner et al., Nature 324: 76, 1986). The toxins were also effective when they diffused into permeabilized chromaffin cells (Ahnert-Hilger et al., FEBS Lett. 242: 245, 1989). In both cases the toxins crossed a disrupted cell membrane and subsequently blocked the Ca++-induced exocytosis. Intact chromaffin cells can be sensitized to tetanus and botulinum A neurotoxins by enriching their cell membranes with gangliosides (Marxen et al., Toxicon 27: 849, 1989). Consequently, the carbachol-stimulated catecholamine release is blocked. The block due to botulinum A neurotoxin, in contrast to that of tetanus toxin, can be partially restored by enhancing the stimulation with carbachol. For a more precise characterisation of the steps involved in exocytosis that are affected by the two neurotoxins, ganglioside pretreated chromaffin cells were exposed to tetanus and botulinum A toxins and then permeabilized by staphyloccocal α-toxin. The treatment with either toxin inhibited the Ca++-stimulated ³H-noradrenaline release from these cells. The inhibition was resistant to increasing concentrations of free Ca++. The phorbolester TPA increased the Ca++-stimulated ³H-noradrenaline release but had no effect on the inhibitory action of the neurotoxins. 5'guanylylimidodiphosphate, to a small extent, promoted the basal and the Ca++-induced exocytosis and also left the block of exocytosis unchanged. We conclude that tetanus and botulinum A neurotoxins act via distinct targets and that neither the activation of proteinkinase C nor that of G-Proteins play a role in the mechanisms of action of tetanus and botulinum toxins. Instead, both toxins unfold their crucial action late in the chain of events leading to exocytosis, i.e. beyond the increase in intracellular Ca++.

Department of Pharmacology and Toxicology, Medical School of Hannover, 3000 Hannover 61, Germany; *Department of Pharmacology, Freie Universität Berlin, 1000 Berlin, Germany

149
CHARACTERIZATION OF CORTICOSTEROID RECEPTORS IN NEOCORTICAL CELL CULTURES
H. Vedder, I. Weiß and J.M.H.M. Reul

Corticosteroids are crucially involved in the regulation of neuronal functions such as expression of neurotransmitter genes, electrical excitability and basal metabolic functions. These actions of corticosteroids in neurons and glial cells are mediated by high affinity binding molecules, the corticosteroid receptors. Up to now, corticosteroid receptors can be discriminated in 2 subtypes, the mineralo-corticoid-(type 1) and the glucocorticoid-(type 2) preferring binding sites.
We characterized these receptors with a whole cell binding assay in living cells derived from neocortical brain tissue of prenatal rats grown in culture under serum-free, defined conditions.
Our data show that corticosteroid receptors can be detected in neuronal and nonneuronal cell populations under our in vitro conditions using [³H]dexa-methasone as a specific radioligand. Receptors become detectable after 2 - 3 days and increase during the first two weeks of culture time. Further characterization of binding sites with RU 28362 (11ß,17ß-dihydroxy-6-methyl-17α-(1-propynyl)-androsta-1,4,6-trien-3-one), a highly specific ligand for the type 2 receptor, showed, that the majority of binding sites is of the glucocorticoid receptor type. Corticosteroid receptors could not only be detected in young cultures consisting mainly of neuronal cells, but also in cultures of 4 - 8 weeks of age with more than 90% of nonneuronal cells. In addition, analysis of mineralocorticoid-binding sites with [³H]aldosterone in the presence of RU 28362 revealed a small number of mineralocorticoid receptors in neuronal preparations.
Treatment of cells with corticosterone, the physiological glucocorticoid of the rat, induced a down-regulation of type 2 receptors, indicating the homologous regulation of these binding sites.
Thus, our data demonstrate that corticosteroid receptors can be specifically measured under in vitro conditions and support the use of our defined cultivation system for further pharmacological studies of these receptors in neocortical cells.

Max Planck Institute for Psychiatry, Clinical Institute, Kraepelinstr. 2, W-8000 Munich 40, Germany

150
CAFFEINE INTERACTS WITH PSYCHOTROPIC EFFECTS OF ERGOTAMINE AND WITH ERGOTAMINE TAKING OF MICE
J. WOLFFGRAMM, S.LUTTER

The suspicion has been uttered that addition of caffeine to analgesics and anti-migraine drugs might promote the risk of drug abuse. In an animal model of drug self-administration we could recently show that voluntary oral intake of paracetamol but not of acetylsalicylic acid is increased by caffeine. The present investigation deals with interactions between caffeine (C) and ergotamine (E), a combination which is frequently used in migraine therapy. Three experimental series were performed:
In the first series (N = 512) the effects of single and combined dosages of C (0, 10, 20, 30 mg/kg) and E (0, 1, 2, 3 mg/kg) on the behavior of female mice were tested in an elevated plus maze. The drugs were administered i.p. Additional test groups were chronically pretreated for two weeks with C (40 mg/kg/d), E (5 mg/kg/d), or E + C. The experiments revealed an excitatory action of C and a motor depression after E. In addition, E also caused a dose-dependent anxiogenic effect. Both sedation and anxiogenesis were weakened, suspended, or even reversed by addition of caffeine. The interaction was superadditive (i. e. doses of C which were nearly ineffective when given alone had a massive effect in combination with E), it was most expressed after concomitant chronic pretreatment with E + C. The second series (N = 64) concerned the "voluntary" intake of E, C and combination by mice and the third series its alteration by a forced chronic pretreatment for 3 weeks with E (5mg/kg/d), C (40 mg/kg/d) and combination. In series 2: The mice were not able to discriminate between C and water or between E and E + C only by the fluid's taste. Thus they were not able to detect C. On the other hand the consumption of E depended decisively on the fact whether C was simultaneously present or not. The experiment consisted in three periods of free drug access separated by two periods of forced abstinence (6 weeks, each). During the first and third period water, C (200 mg/l), E (25 mg/l) and C + E (200 and 25 mg/l, resp.) were offered. During the second period, they received only E (25 and 12.5 mg/l) apart from water. During both periods with C, the mice took more than twice as much E (0.7 mg/kg/d) as without C (0.25 mg/kg/d; p < 0.001). The third experimental series revealed a highly significant depression of voluntary intake of E by forced chronic pretreatment with E. No such effect appeared after combined pretreatment with E + C. At the end of the experiment these mice even revealed the highest preference for E with a further rising trend. The experiments support the hypothesis that concomitant excitatory and depressant actions lead to a superadditive interaction which may serve as a powerful central nervous reward. Possible aversive effects of the single compounds are overruled. Voluntary intake of such drugs involves a high risk of abuse and behavioral dependence. Supported by a grant of the BGA, Institut für Arzneimittel.
Dept. of Neuropsychopharmacology, Free University, Ulmenallee 30, 1000 Berlin 19

151
INVESTIGATIONS ON THE OPIOID-INDUCED CHANGES OF THE THERMOREGULATION IN MICE.
W. Burckart, A. Steffens, W. Klaus, K. Güttler

Albeit opioids are known to produce profound and complex changes in thermoregulation, few laboratories have investigated the effect systematically. The aim of the present investigation was to elucidate in more detail the thermoregulatory actions of some opioids.
NMRI mice were used in the experiments. In all tests the drugs were given subcutaneously. The animals were placed in a specially designed unrestraining chamber which was kept at constant normal (20° C = norm-T) or high (35° C = high-T) ambient temperature. Body temperature was measured by insertion of a lubricated thermistor probe into the rectum (control values: norm-T: 38.4 ± 0.1° C; high-T: 40.1 ± 0.1° C) at intervals of 10 min. At norm-T all opioids tested produced a significant hypothermia in higher doses. Approximative equianalgesic doses yielded following data in comparison to control: 40 mg/kg pethidine: -4.4° C, 60 mg/kg tramadol: -4.4° C, 20 mg/kg piritramide: -3.1° C, 20 mg/kg morphine: -1.5°C. These hypothermic effects of opioids are intensified by diltiazem (25 mg/kg). At high-T the thermoregulatory actions of opioids were qualitatively changed into hyper-thermic reactions (up to 42° C) with a drastic enhancement of toxicity resp. lethality. Tramadol showed the relative lowest increase of heat-induced toxicity of the opioids tested.
From these results we conclude that the marked influences of opioids on temperature regulation and vice versa could be of clinical relevance.

Institut für Pharmakologie der Universität zu Köln, Gleuelerstr. 24, 5000 Köln 41

152
COMPARATIVE STUDIES ON ANALGESIC AND CONSTIPATING OPIOID EFFECTS IN MICE.
A. Steffens, W. Burckart, W. Klaus, K. Güttler

Although the constipating action occurs as a troublesome side effect of all opioids in analgesic therapy, because it requires considerably less opioid e.g. morphine to affect the gut than to produce analgesia, there are only rare experimental data in order to quantify the constipating activity of opioids. Therefore, we have studied several opioids (morphine = MOR, piritramide = PIRI, pethidine =PETH, tramadol = TRAM and pentazocine = PENT) under standardized conditions. NMRI mice were used in the experiments. Analgesia was determined by the hot plate test (50 ± 0.5° C). Maximum exposure time was limited to 60 sec (= 100 %). Constipating effect in terms of inhibition of the gastrointestinal propulsion (pylorus to appendix) was ascertained by the modified charcoal meal test (no charcoal inside intestine = 100 % obstipation). All opioids examined were more active in the charcoal test than in the hot plate test with following rank order of potency: MOR > PIRI >> PENT > PETH = TRAM. Only PENT showed a ceiling-like reduced efficacy (maximum constipating and analgesic activity: 75 % resp. 35%). A certain selectivity of drug action becomes evident in the charcoal ED-50 to analgesia ED-50 ratios (MOR: 0.06, PIRI: 0.1, TRAM: 0.5, PETH: 0.6) and in the comparison of the constipating activity at approx. equianalgesic doses: MOR: 87 ± 3 %, PIRI: 78 ± 2 %, PENT: 70 ± 6 %, TRAM: 67 ± 6 % and PETH: 51 ± 3 %. From these results we conclude that pethidine and tramadol are opioids with lower constipating activity than the other opioids tested.
Institut für Pharmakologie der Universität zu Köln, Gleuelerstr. 24, 5000 Köln 41

153

INVESTIGATIONS ON OPIOID AND NON-OPIOID COMPONENTS IN TRAMADOL ANTINOCICEPTION
E. Friderichs, W. Reimann and N. Selve

Tramadol is a centrally acting analgesic with a low opioid receptor affinity. To explain its relatively strong analgesic efficacy, the involvement of a further, non opioid mechanism of action has to be assumed. Since pain models are differently sensitive towards opioid and non opioid actions, we investigated tramadol in various test systems and used naloxone antagonism to identify the opioid component in tramadol's antinociception. Tramadol inhibited the tail-flick reaction in mice with an ED_{50} of 28 mg/kg i.p.. The tramadol dose response curve was displaced dose dependently by 4.64-46.4 µg/kg i.v. naloxone, and Schild plot analysis showed pure competitive antagonism to tramadol and morphine with similar apparent pA_2-values(7.8 vs. 7.9). Phenylquinone-induced writhing in mice was inhibited by tramadol with an ED_{50} of 3.7 mg/kg p.o.. In contrast to morphine effects, writhing inhibition by tramadol was only partly (max = 37%) reduced by naloxone. In the rat Randall-Selitto test using vocalization as the nociceptive criterion tramadol was effective with an ED_{50} of 4.6 mg/kg i.v.. Naloxone 1 mg/kg i.v. reduced maximum effects of tramadol only by about 50 %. The rabbit tooth pulp was stimulated electrically until a lick/chew response occurred. Tramadol 10 mg/kg i.v. enhanced the threshold to about 40 % of the maximal possible effect (MPE); 1 mg/kg i.v. naloxone reduced the effect to about 10 % MPE. In the rat tail-flick model with intrathecal (i.t.) injection, tramadol and morphine prolonged tail-flick latencies. Naloxone 10 mg/kg i.p. antagonized the effects of 12 µg i.t. morphine but did not affect the effects of 12 µg i.t. tramadol. Antinociception by tramadol was, however, almost completely antagonized by either 1 mg/kg i.p. yohimbine or 1 mg/kg i.p. ritanserin. These results show that in various animal models antinociception by tramadol cannot entirely be ascribed to an opioid type of action. Other mechanisms involved may be activation of noradrenaline and serotonin pathways.

Grünenthal GmbH, Dept. Pharmacology, W-5100 Aachen, FRG

154

A SPECIFIC δ-OPIOID ANTAGONIST INHIBITS LOW Km GTPase ACTIVITY IN RAT BRAIN MEMBRANES
Zafiroula Georgoussi and Christine Zioudrou

A specific δ-opioid antagonist, Diallyl-G (N,N-Diallyl-Tyr-D-Leu-Gly-Tyr-Leu-OH) inhibited the low Km GTPase activity in rat brain membranes, in a concentration dependent manner in the presence of NaCl. Half-maximal inhibition was observed at 10 nM. Diallyl-G was shown to be twice as potent in inhibiting low Km GTPase activity in rat brain, than ICI 174864 another δ-opioid antagonist (Costa and Herz, Proc. Natl. Acad. Sci. U.S.A., 86:7321, 1989). On the other hand the δ-opioid agonists DADLE and DSLET stimulated the low Km GTPase activity in rat brain membranes. This stimulation was blocked in the presence of Diallyl-G.
The inhibitory effect of Diallyl-G was abolished when rat brain membranes were treated with N-ethylmaleimide or by ADP-ribosylation with pertussis toxin. Similarly the above treatment abolished the stimulatory effects of δ-opioid agonists. We also found that Diallyl-G and ICI 174864 behave as pure antagonists by reversing the inhibitory effect of DADLE on adenylate cyclase in NG 108-15 cells, with half-maximal concentrations in the range of 100 nM. These observations suggest that selective δ-opioid antagonists exhibit negative intrinsic activity on GTPase and possibly could interfere with the functional coupling between δ-opioid receptors and G-proteins. Although the type of responses that follows this inhibition remains to be elucidated, it underlies a new post-receptor mechanism mediated by GTP-binding proteins.

National Center for Scientific Research "Demokritos", Institute of Biology, 153 10 Aghia Paraskevi, Athens, Greece.

155

CHRONIC MORPHINE AND LIPOLYSIS EVOKED BY ADRENALINE AND MORPHINE. Patočková J., Příborský J., Tikal K., Mühlbachová E.

The lipolytic sensitivity towards opioids was described several times. Especially for morphine (Mühlbachová. Wenke: Arzneim.-Forsch. 1983, 33;128) and for enkephalines and endorphines (Nencini & Paroli: Pharmacol. Res. Com., 96: 1486-1498. 1981). This sensitivity is well pronounced in trimmed adipose tissue (AT) of rats as well as in trimmed AT of rabbits.

Isoprenaline as well as naloxon do not change the lipolytic activity of morphine in vitro (Mühlbachová et al., Arzeim.-Forsch. 1987, 37,394).The question aroused whether adrenergic (AR) and/or opioid receptors (OR) are responsible for mediating the adipokinetic response to opioids. If OR are, but not AR, then chronic administration of MO (10 days increasing i.m. doses) should impair the adipokinetik response to opioids, due to desensitation of OR, but the adrenergic lipolytic reactivity should remain intact.

The results of the study are only partially compatible with this hypothesis. The opioid reactivity in chronic treated young animals is fully preserved whereas in old rats it is abolished. The negative influence of chronic MO on adrenergically stimulated lipolysis in vitro needs further studies to be explained.

Present address: Dept. of Pharmacology, 3 rd Medical Faculty, Charles University, Legerova 63, 120 00 Praha 2, ČSFR

156

INVESTIGATION OF β-ENDORPHIN IMMUNOREACTIVITY IN VAGINAL DELIVERY AND ELECTIVE CESAREAN SECTION
M.Terzic, M.Jevremovic

Opioid peptide β-endorphin (β-EP) is cleaved from proopiomelanocortine (POMC) by influence of Corticotropin releasing factor (CRF). It increases pain threshold and influences pituitary hormones synthesis, especially during stressful situations. β-EP stimulates secretion of prolactin, growth hormone and vasopressin and inhibits synthesis of follicle-stimulating and luteinizing hormone, oxytocin, dopamine and gonadotropine releasing hormone (GRH). Its activity is decreased or almost lost by acetylation, that is absent in fetal period. The aim of this study was to investigate β-EP concentrations during normal vaginal delivery and elective cesarean section. We analysed this opioid peptide levels in peripheral blood samples of women in term vaginal delivery (n=20) and in those with elective cesarean section (n=15). β-EP concentrations were also determined in umbilical cord, amniotic fluid as well as in the placental compartment by use of radioimmunoassay techniques. Obtained results showed β-EP increases in vaginal delivery with peak at expulsion, while levels were significantly higher in placental compartment. In peripheral blood samples of women with elective cesarean section β-EP immunoreactivities were found to be increased six hours after surgery, while in umbilical cord and amniotic fluid concentrations were as those in vaginal delivery. We stress that β-EP concentrations in placental compartment were higher in vaginally delivered women than in operated. Presented data indicate that β-EP is incorporated in regulation and modulation of intrapartal and postoperative stress in mother and her fetus.

Gyn/Ob Clinic, Visegradska 26, 11000 Belgrade, Yu

157

IDENTIFICATION OF β-ENDORPHIN IMMUNOREACTIVITY IN HUMAN FETAL AND NEONATAL THYMUS

M.Jevremovic, M.Terzic, G.Kartaljevic, S.Filipovic

According to the contemporary opinion thymus is a part of hypothalamus-pituitary-thymus-gonadal axis and participates in the regulation and modulation of the endocrine reproductive functions in humans. Therefore we studied endocrine properties-β-endorphin (β-EP) concentrations in the human fetal and neonatal thymus. Thymic samples were obtained at autopsy immediately after spontaneous preterm labor (n=10) or at term delivery (n=5). Peripheral blood samples of nonpregnant healthy persons (n=8) and of healthy pregnant women with normal gestation during intrapartal period (n=15) were taken as controls. β-EP determination in thymic samples was based on concentration evaluation by using radioimmunoassay techniques and in peripheral blood by RIA Nichols Kits. We found that β-EP immunoreactivity increase in thymic samples with progression of gestation. Concentrations of β-EP in peripheral blood during expulsion were higher than in nonpregnant women, but at the same time lower than those in thymus. Obtained data could suggest that the identified increased β-EP production is most probably caused by intrapartal stress. As an alternative hypothesis we propose that β-EP of thymic origin represents an antireproductive factor throughout intrauterine and early neonatal life. To get a definitive insight in human reproduction, endocrinology of thymus requires further research.

Gyn/Ob Clinic, Visegradska 26, 11000 Belgrade, YU

158

PREJUNCTIONAL A_1 ADENOSINE RECEPTORS INHIBIT THE STIMULATION-EVOKED [^{3}H]-NORADRENALINE RELEASE ON RAT IRIS.

H. Fuder, A. Brink, M. Meincke, and U. Tauber

Adenosine receptors inhibit the exocytotic noradrenaline (NA) release in many tissues. To determine the type of receptor mediating inhibition of [^{3}H]NA overflow evoked by field stimulation (180 pulses at 3 Hz, α_2-autoreceptors, uptake$_{1+2}$ blocked) on the rat isolated iris, the inhibition by non-selective and selective adenosine receptor agonists was determined. All agonists tested supressed the evoked [^{3}H]NA overflow by 60-80% compared to controls in the absence of antagonists. The concentrations of halfmaximal inhibition (IC$_{50}$ in µmol/l) for adenosine (2.9), 5'-N-ethylcarboxamidoadenosine (NECA, 0.5), N^6-cyclohexyladenosine (CHA, 0.1), (-)-(R)-enantiomer of N^6-(2-phenylisopropyl)adenosine (R-PIA, 0.1), and N^6-cyclopentyladenosine (CPA, 0.01) were consistent with the relative potency at an A_1 receptor. The inhibition by the A_1 selective agonist CPA was determined in the absence and presence of the A_1 selective antagonist 8-cyclopentyl-1,3-dipropylxanthine (DPCPX). The evoked [^{3}H]NA overflow was enhanced (by 30-40%) by DPCPX 100 nmol/l indicating a small tonic inhibition of sympathetic neurotransmission by endogenous adenosine released from the iris. DPCPX 10 and 100 nmol/l shifted the CPA inhibition curve to the right significantly without suppressing the maximum (around 80%). From the shift, which was linearly related to the antagonist concentration, a -logK$_B$ of 9.5 was estimated. The high DPCPX affinity is indicative of an A_1 adenosine receptor responsible for the inhibition of sympathetic transmission on rat iris. (supported by DFG)

Pharmakologisches Institut der Universität Mainz Obere Zahlbacher Str. 67, D - W - 6500 Mainz, FRG

159

PHARMACOLOGICAL CHARACTERIZATION OF THE INHIBITORY PRESYNAPTIC HISTAMINE RECEPTORS ON THE SYMPATHETIC NERVES OF THE HUMAN SAPHENOUS VEIN

G.J. Molderings, G. Weißenborn, E. Schlicker and M. Göthert

The human saphenous vein was used to examine whether presynaptic histamine receptors are involved in inhibition of noradrenaline release, and, if so, to determine their pharmacological properties. Segments of this blood vessel were incubated with [^{3}H]noradrenaline 0.2 µmol/l and subsequently superfused with physiological salt solution containing desipramine and corticosterone. The overflow of tritium evoked by transmural electrical stimulation (2 Hz) was inhibited by histamine (0.1, 1, 10) and the H$_3$ receptor agonist R-(-)-α-methylhistamine (0.1, 1, 10; in parentheses concentrations in µmol/l producing significant inhibition). The histamine-induced inhibition of electrically evoked tritium overflow of similar magnitude in the presence of rauwolscine (3 µmol/l). S-(+)-α-methylhistamine (up to 10 µmol/l) as well as the H$_1$ and H$_2$ receptor agonists 2-(2-thiazolyl)ethylhistamine and dimaprit (each up to 30 µmol/l), respectively, were ineffective. The selective H$_3$-receptor antagonist thioperamide (0.3 µmol/l) abolished the inhibitory effect of histamine. Ranitidine (3 µmol/l) only slightly reduced and pheniramine (3 µmol/l) did not affect the histamine-induced inhibition of evoked tritium overflow.

In conclusion, the sympathetic nerves of the human saphenous vein are endowed with inhibitory presynaptic histamine receptors, which do not appear to belong to the H$_1$- or H$_2$-receptor class; however, the pharmacological properties of these receptors are compatible with the characteristics of the H$_3$ class.

Institut für Pharmakologie und Toxikologie, Universität Bonn, Reuterstr. 2b, D-5300 Bonn 1, FRG

160

INFLUENCE OF HYPOXIA AND DEPRIVATION OF GLUCOSE ON THE 3H-NORADRENALINE RELEASE IN RAT VAS DEFERENS

Richter, R., B. Sperlagh+, P. Oehme and E.S. Vizi+

Earlier studies have demonstrated that oxygen is consumed in the metabolism of glucose to yield energy which provides the fuel for neuronal and muscle functions. In this study, the effect of hypoxia and deprivation of glucose on the 3H-noradrenaline (3H-NA) release from the rat isolated vas deferens during resting conditions and field stimulation was studied. The results obtained were compared with those of contractile responses (twitch and tonic contraction).

In control experiments the 3H-NA release to three consecutive field stimulations was constant (s2/s1 and s3/s2:0.97 ± 0.05 and 0.82 ± 0.07, respectively) and Ca^{2+}-dependent.

When vas deferens was either subjected to hypoxia (95% N2/ 5% CO2 for 30 min) or glucose-free solution the 3H-NA release was found to be unchanged. However, co-exposure to hypoxia and glucose-free Krebs solution caused a significant increase in 3H-NA release from vas deferens (s2/s1: 20.00 ± 4.59). Deprivation of glucose and hypoxia did not influence the twitch phase of the contraction, while hypoxia strongly reduced the tonic contraction.

To conclude, the 3H-NA release from rat vas deferens can be stimulated only by concomitant exposure to the two stimuli. Apparently, the ATP-sensitive twitch response is unaffected by both hypoxia and deprivation of glucose, whereas the NA-sensitive tonic contraction was diminished by the reduction of oxygen supply.

Furthermore, the possibly protective effect of the neuropeptide substance P (SP(1-11)) (10^{-7} to 10^{-6} M) and of two SP derivatives on the stimulated 3H-NA release as well as the contractile responses was also investigated.

Institute of Drug Research, Berlin, FRG
+ Institute of Exptl. Medicine, Hungarian Acad.Sci., Budapest, Hungary

161

LONG TERM TREATMENT WITH PHORBOL ESTERS SUGGESTS A ROLE FOR PROTEIN KINASE C IN ENHANCEMENT OF NORADRENALINE RELEASE

I.F. Musgrave (1,3), S. Foucart (2), H. Majewski (1)

Protein kinase C is present in sympathetic nerve terminals and its activation enhances noradrenaline release during nerve stimulation (Musgrave IF & Majewski H, Naunyn-Schmiedeberg's Arch. Pharmacol. 339:48, 1989). The aim of this study was to investigate further the role of protein kinase C in sympathetic neurotransmission using down-regulation of protein kinase C. Mouse atria were incubated for 10 h in tissue culture medium, containing either vehicle or phorbol ester. After this incubation the atria were washed and incubated with $[^3H]$-noradrenaline and the overflow of radioactivity induced by electrical stimulation (S-I outflow; 5 or 10 Hz, 60 s) was measured. 4-ß-Phorbol dibutyrate (4-ß-PDB; 1.0 μM) enhanced noradrenaline release after atria were incubated for 10 h in either vehicle or 4-α-phorbol dibutyrate (1.0 μM), which does not activate protein kinase C. However, after 10 h incubation with 4-ß-PDB and subsequent washing, reapplication of 4-ß-PDB (1.0 μM) was without effect on noradrenaline release. These results suggest that 10 h incubation of mouse atria with 4-ß-PDB induces functional down-regulation of protein kinase C. At 5 Hz, the S-I outflow of radioactivity was unaffected by 4-ß-PDB preincubation (107 ± 5% of control) but the S-I outflow at 10 Hz was significantly attenuated (to 72 ± 7% of control). Similar results were seen when the protein kinase C inhibitor polymyxin B was used, instead of down-regulation. Together these results are consistent with the hypothesis that protein kinase C activation is necessary to support high output noradrenaline release.

(1) Prince Henry's Institute of Medical Research, PO Box 118, South Melbourne, Vic 3205, Australia.
(2) Department of Pharmacological and Physiological Sciences, University of Chicago, Chicago, Ill 60637, USA.
(3) Institut für Pharmakologie, Freie Universität Berlin, D-1000 Berlin 33, FRG (present address).

162

CONTRACTION OF THE RAT ISOLATED TRACHEAL MUSCLE IN THE ABSENCE AND PRESENCE OF THE EPITHELIUM

T. Reinheimer, D. Pohan, K. Racké and I. Wessler

A large body of experimental evidence has been amassed showing an important role of the airway epithelium in regulating the responsibility of the smooth muscle fibres. Particularly, the epithelium has been suggested to mediate an inhibitory action on contractility. In the present experiments a new model has been established, to record the contraction of the isolated tracheal muscle elicited indirectly by electrical stimulation of the innervating parasympathetic nerves (recurrent laryngeal nerves (RLN)). Tracheae together with their RLN were removed from rats and opened longitudinally by cutting the cartilaginous rings. In the respective experiments epithelium was removed mechanically. The tracheal muscle was incubated with a physiological salt solution and suspended under a tension of 10 mN. Contractions were recorded with a force-displacement transducer and displayed on a Wekagraph 280. RLN were stimulated (0.4 and 1 ms pulse width, 20 and 60 V, 15 and 30 Hz) for 10 s periods, i.e. 8 successive 10 s stimulations with 1 min intervals were repeated every 15 min (control experiments) or 40 min (experiments with tubocurarine (TC) or hexamethonium (HE)).
The amplitude of the contraction was positively related to the stimulation strength, 2000±1020 μN and 8500±2500 μN were recorded at the lowest and highest stimulation strength, respectively (n = 3). In epithelium-denuded tracheae contractions were reduced (respective values: 650±80 μN and 3200± 1300 μN; n = 3-5). Contractions declined by about 20 - 30% during a 180 min period in epithelium-denuded or intact tracheae and were abolished by 0.1 μM scopolamine or 0.3 μM tetrodotoxin. TC (300 μM) reduced contraction to about 20%, irrespective of the stimulation strength or of the presence or absence of the epithelium. Likewise, HE reduced contractions in the presence of the epithelium, but was without any inhibitory effect in epithelium-denuded tracheae. The present experiments show RLN-evoked contractions of the isolated tracheal muscle. Removal of the epithelium may affect transmission at the pre- or postganglionic parasympathetic synapses.

Supported by the Deutsche Forschungsgemeinschaft (We 1165/2-1).

Pharmakologisches Institut der Universität Mainz, Obere Zahlbacher Str. 67, 6500 Mainz.

163

MODE OF ACTION OF BOTULINUM TOXIN E ON THE TRANSMITTER RELEASE PROCESS AT THE MOUSE NEUROMUSCULAR JUNCTION

Linda Wieszt and Florian Dreyer

Of the seven immunologically different botulinal neurotoxins the mode of action of botulinum toxin A (BoTx A) and botulinum toxin B (BoTx B) on transmitter release at neuromuscular junctions has been intensively studied by electrophysiological methods (Gansel et al. Pflügers Arch. 409: 533, 1987). We studied now the ability of botulinum toxin E (BoTx E) to block the neuromuscular transmission at mouse motor nerve endings and compared its action with the well established effects of BoTx A and B. BoTx E seems to be the most potent toxin because at 37°C the poisoned endplates are characterized by an extremely low frequency of spontaneous miniature endplate potentials (about 0,4 /min) and a complete block of nerve stimulated transmitter release. Also the application of 100 μM 4-aminopyridine which is a potent K^+ channel blocker did not increase the nerve evoked transmitter release in contrast to BoTx A or B treated endplates. Only an additional reduction of temperature to 22°C led to an increase in response to nerve stimulation with a frequency of 30Hz or more. Similar to BoTx B the transmitter release started with a delay of 3 sec and was desynchronized. This is in contrast to BoTx A which did not change the short latency between nerve impulse and postsynaptic response. Preliminary double poisoning experiments with BoTx A and E suggest that at least BoTx A and E act at different sites in the chain of events that result in transmitter release.

Rudolf-Buchheim-Institut für Pharmakologie der Justus-Liebig-Universität Gießen, Frankfurter Str. 107, D-6300 Gießen

164

PROSTANOID-CHOLINERGIC INTERACTIONS IN THE REGULATION OF NORADRENALINE RELEASE FROM THE RAT ISOLATED TRACHEA.

G. Brunn, C. Langer, I. Wessler and K. Racké

The release of endogenous noradrenaline (NA) from the isolated rat trachea is inhibited by muscarine receptors (Racké et al. Br J Pharmacol 103:1213, 1991), but enhanced in the presence of indometacin (Racké et al. this journal, 343:R93, 1991). In the present study, an interaction between endogenous prostanoids and the muscarinic modulation of NA release was tested.
Rat isolated tracheae were incubated in 1.7 ml Krebs-HEPES solution (containing yohimbine, desipramine and tyrosine) and the release of NA was determined. Two periods of electrical field stimulation (S1, S2; 540 pulses at 3 Hz) were carried out.
In the absence of test drugs the first electrical stimulation (S1) evoked the release of 44 ± 3.9 pmol/g NA (n=22). Oxotremorine inhibited the evoked release of NA almost completely with an EC_{50} of 43 nmol/l. The non-selective muscarine receptor antagonist scopolamine (10-1000 nmol/l) antagonized the effect of oxotremorine in a manner suggesting a simple competitive interaction (slope of the Schild plot 0.95, pA_2 value 8.88). The M_2 selective muscarine receptor antagonist methoctramine (10-1000 nmol/l) antagonized the effect of oxotremorine in a manner suggesting the involvement of multiple muscarine receptor subtypes (slope of the Schild plot 0.4). In the presence of 3 μmol/l indometacin, the release of NA evoked by S1 was increased to 63 ± 4.4 pmol/g (n=18) and the EC_{50} value for the inhibitory effect of oxotremorine was enhanced to 140 nmol/l. However, in the presence of indometacin, methoctramine (10-1000 nmol/l) antagonized the effect of oxotremorine in manner suggesting a simple competitive interaction (slope of the Schild plot 0.96, pA_2 value 7.56).
In conclusion, noradrenergic nerve endings in the rat trachea are endowed with inhibitory muscarine receptors of the M_2 subtype. Moreover, muscarine receptors, different from the M_2 subtype, appear to activate an additional, inhibitory mechanism which involves the release of endogenous prostanoids.

Supported by the Deutsche Forschungsgemeinschaft (Ra 400/3-1)

Pharmakologisches Institut der Universität
Obere Zahlbacher Str. 67, D-6500 Mainz, F.R.G.

165

REFLEX REACTIONS AFTER INTRATRACHEAL INSTILLATION OF CARBON TETRACHLORIDE IN RATS W. Poelchen, A. Rabe and V. Görisch

In toxicological investigations of the action of foreign substances on the lower airways in our laboratory it was found that administration of carbon tetrachloride on the tracheobronchial mucosa of rats results in a sudden death of the animals.

To examine these reaction new experiments were carried out. In the present study, we found that very small volumes of liquid carbon tetrachloride (5 µl) cause an intermittent apnoea, bradycardia sometimes with transient cardiac arrest, and severe hypotension immediately after intratracheal instillation. In some instances the strength of the reflex response led to death of the animals. Also the inhalation of carbon tetrachloride vapor (4 breaths) or their inflation (1 cm^3) in the lower airways via tracheostoma showed similar but smaller and also immediate responses as follows : hypopnoea, bradycardia and hypotension. The acute changes in heart rate, blood pressure and breathing and their immediate set in suggest a stimulation of specific nerve endings in the mucosa of lower airways.

Further investigations are going on to determine the afferent nerve fibers by vagal cooling experiments for additional characterization of the reflex mechanism.

Institute of Pharmacology and Toxicology, University Leipzig, Härtelstr.16-18, O-7010 Leipzig

166

BRONCHOPROTECTIVE EFFECT OF ZARDAVERINE VERSUS THEOPHYLLINE IN RATS, H.G. Hoymann, U. Heinrich, R. Beume and U. Kilian

Zardaverine (Byk Gulden, Konstanz) is a new selective PDE III/IV inhibitor with potent bronchospasmolytic activity in guinea pigs (Kilian et al., in: Agents and actions, Birkhaeuser Verlag, Basel, 331-348, 1989). We recently compared the bronchodilating and bronchoprotective potency of zardaverine and the nonselective PDE inhibitor theophylline by measuring typical spontaneous and forced respiratory function parameters in anaesthetized rats using whole-body plethysmography. 60 female Wistar rats (240 g) were used in the experiment. Zardaverine (3, 10, 30 µmol/kg) and theophylline (30, 100, 300 µmol/kg), respectively, were given orally in 4 % Methocel/0.9 % saline solution after more than 15 h starving. 20 min after treatment the measurements were started. One week earlier, to obtain control values, measurements were performed 20 min after feeding the vehicle. When spontaneously breathing, the 30 µmol/kg zardaverine (300 µmol/kg theophylline) treated animals showed a 23 % (14 %, ns) decreased lung resistance and a 43 % (25 %) elevated dynamic compliance. There was no indication of a changed lung elasticity based on quasistatic compliance and therefore the increased dynamic compliance as well as the decreased resistance can only be caused by bronchodilation. In the acetylcholine challenge test treatment with only 10 µmol/kg zardaverine (but 300 µmol/kg theophylline) revealed a 37 % (28 %) lower resistance and 85 % (44 %) higher compliance. This indicates a better bronchoprotective effect of zardaverine which was also supported by Peak Flow, FEF_{50} and FEF_{25} measurement after challenge.

Fraunhofer Institute of Toxicology and Aerosol Research, Nikolai-Fuchs-Straße 1, D-3000 Hannover 61, FRG

167

FAECAL EXCRETION OF REPIRINAST AND ITS ACTIVE METABOLITE AFTER SINGLE ORAL DOSES OF REPIRINAST IN HEALTHY VOLUNTEERS
C.Ewald (1,2), D.Beermann (1), H.G.Schaefer (1), G.Ahr (1), J.Kuhlmann (1) and R.Süverkrüp (2)

Repirinast (R) is a synthetic disodium cromogly-cate like antiallergic agent, which is marketed for asthma treatment in Japan since 1987. After oral administration it is hydrolysed to its active metabolite BAY w 8199 (M).
To investigate the pharmacokinetics and tolerability, single oral doses of 150, 300 and 450 mg R and placebo were administered to 12 healthy male caucasian volunteers in a randomized double-blind crossover trial. Plasma, urine and faeces samples were collected until 72 hours after administration and analysed for both compounds using an HPLC/UV method.
The drug was well tolerated at all investigated dose levels. The unchanged drug could not be detected in plasma and urine. M plasma concentrations were highly variable between subjects. Mean peak levels (geom. mean) were found at 0.14, 0.19 and 0.24 mg/L after the 150, 300 and 450 mg dose, respectively. Excretion of M into urine amounted to 7-8 % of the doses. Faecal excretion of M accounted for 29, 31 and 18 % of the 150, 300 and 450 mg doses, respectively; recovery of unchanged R amounted to 13, 32 and 31 %, respectively. The absorption of R in GI tract may be determined by its low solubility in aqueous media.

(1) Bayer AG, Pharma Research Center, Inst. of Clin. Pharmacol., 5600 Wuppertal 1, FRG
(2) Inst. of Pharmaceutical Technology, University of Bonn, 5300 Bonn 1, FRG

168

PHARMACOKINETICS OF ENOXACIN IN SEVERE RENAL INSUF-FICIENCY
H.J.Deuber*,R.Metz,W.Schulz,H.Kraeft,P.Muth,F.Sörgel

This study was done to investigate pharmacokinetics of enoxacin in patients with severe renal impairment.
10 patients with GFR below 30ml/min received 400mg enoxacin orally once a day for 7 days. Single dose (sd) pharmacokinetics were studied on day 1 and multiple dose(md) pharmacokinetics were studied at steady state on day 7.

		Cmax µg/ml	Clren ml/min	fu %	AUC µg.h/ml
Enoxacin	sd	2.3+1.2	11.6+19.3	5.3+6.2	55.7+30.2
	md	4.5+1.6			74.1+29.7

The half-life of unchanged enoxacin in renal failure was 15.1+5.5 hours.In comparison with data from volunteers without renal insufficiency Clren and fu were reduced,AUC was increased for enoxacin.On the other hand the value for Cmax of enoxacin at steady state was very similar to the corresponding value in healthy volunteers: 4.5µg/ml.

Therefore the reduction of the enoxacin dose by 50% and administration of 400mg once daily seems adequate for dosing in patients with GFR values below 30ml/min.

III.Med.Clinics,Municipal Hospital of Bamberg,and Institute of Nephrology and Osteology,Bamberg, Buger Straße 80,D-8600 Bamberg, FRG

169

BIOAVAILABILITY OF MINOCYCLINE VERSUS DOXYCYCLINE AND OXYTETRACYCLINE: EFFECT OF FOOD AND MILK

F.P. Meyer, H. Specht, B. Quednow

The intestinal application of tetracycline, oxytetracycline and doxycycline when taken at a time with food or milk is influenced in varied terms (Meyer et al., Zentr.bl. Pharm. Pharmakother. Lab.diagn. 127: 2-5, 1988; Meyer et al. Infection 17: 245-246, 1989). Therefore, we studied in a cross-over design in 11 volunteers (9 females, 2 males; aged 21-31 years; 50-80 kg) the influence of a standard meal (postprandial) and milk on the bioavailability of 200 mg minocycline-HCl (Klinomycin[R] film tablets 100, Lederle, Germany) in comparison to 9-hour food restriction period (preprandial). Blood samples were taken before and 0.5; 1; 1.5; 2; 2.5; 3; 4; 6; 8; 24 and 32 h p.a. Analysis: Fluorimetry modified as proposed by HALL (J. Pharm. Pharmac. 28: 420-423, 1976).

Minocycline 200 mg orally	Preprandial Water	Postprandial Water	Preprandial Milk
C_{max} (µg/ml)	3.4 ± 0.6	2.9 ± 0.6	2.2 ± 0.5
t_{max} (h)	2.2 ± 0.6	1.5 ± 1.8	2.6 ± 0.8
AUC (h µg/ml)	48.9 ± 7.5	42.0 ± 9.4	35.7 ± 9.3
$f_{minocycline}$	1	0.86	0.73
$f_{doxycycline}$	1	0.73	0.7
$f_{oxytetracycline}$	1	0.59	0.16

Compared to doxycycline and oxytetracycline, the absorption of minocycline was virtually not influenced by food (postprandial water) taken at the same time (86 % absorption). The maximum serum levels were reached even markedly earlier. However, tetracycline should not be administered together with milk.

Institute of Clinical Pharmacology, School of Medicine Leipziger Str.44, O-3090 Magdeburg, Germany

170

DIFFERENT EFFECT OF CISPLATIN, CARBOPLATIN AND TRANSPLATIN ON RAT RENAL CORTICAL GLUTATHIONE (GSH)-CONTENT IN VITRO AND IN VIVO

J. Hannemann, and K. Baumann

Glutathione (GSH) accounts for the majority of intracellular non protein sulfhydryl content of many cell types. It participates in detoxification of xenobiotics and in protection from free radical damage. In this study we examined the effect of cisplatin (CDDP), carboplatin (CBDCA) and transplatin (TDDP) on the GSH-content in rat kidneys in vivo and in rat renal cortical slices in vitro. In vitro: Slices were incubated in CDDP-, CBDCA- or TDDP-(0.42 or 1.67 mM) containing media (supplementary containing amino acids) for 0 - 180 min and were monitored for GSH-content (measured as non protein bound sulfhydryl groups). The GSH-content was markedly depleted by CDDP and TDDP in a time- and concentration dependent manner; CBDCA showed only a minor effect after 120 min (1.67 mM). In vivo: Rats were treated with single i.p. injections of CDDP (5 mg/kg BW), CBDCA (30 mg/kg BW) or TDDP (5 mg/kg BW). Rat renal cortical slices were prepared after 2, 5, 24, 48, 72 and 96 h and the GSH-content was determined. The GSH-levels were not altered by platinum-compound treatment, except for a slight but significant rise induced by CDDP after 48 h (116 % compared to 100 % in controls).
The results agree with previous studies showing only small in vitro and in vivo alterations induced by CBDCA. The in vitro results suggest, that GSH-depletion, caused by CDDP and TDDP may participate in platinum-compound related nephrotoxicity. The in vivo results do not confirm these results. The discrepancies between in vivo and in vitro results are probably not due to differences in platinum-compound concentrations. The in vivo effect of platinum-compounds on production and breakdown enzymes of glutathione might be a partial explanation.

Department of Cell Physiology, University of Hamburg, Grindelallee 117, W-2000 Hamburg 13, FRG

171

KINETICS AND DYNAMICS OF 4'-EPIDOXORUBICIN IN THE LOCOREGIONAL TUMOR CHEMOTHERAPY OF THE LIVER

U.Ulrich, H.Kelm, M.Matthias, and R.Preiss*

On 12 patients with the liver carcinoma or liver metastasization caused by colon carcinoma the kinetics and dynamics of 4'-epidoxorubicin (4'-ed), a steroisomere of doxorubicin, and of its main metabolite 4'-epidoxorubicinol (4'-ed-OH) were investigated after the locoregional administration of the anthracycline derivative into the Arteria hepatica. 4'-ed and 4'-ed-OH were measured in the systemic circulation by means of a HPLC-technique. In comparison to a bolus injection a 3 h-infusion led to 30-fold and to more than 10-fold lower C_{max} values for 4'-ed and 4'-ed-OH, respectively. Both the AUC of 4'-ed and 4'-ed-OH were also significantly lower in the systemic circulation after the 3 h-infusion than after the bolus injection. The formation rate of 4'-ed-OH was high. The main metabolites in the urine were the glucuronides of both 4'-ed and 4'-ed-OH. Under the conditions used 4'-ed shows the characteristics of a dose-dependent, non-linear pharmacokinetics. Some heavily metastasized patients show a saturated hepatic elimination process of 4'-ed and 4'-ed-OH also under the conditions of the 3 h-infusion of the antineoplastic drug. A good correlation was found between the liver-leaving amounts of both substances and the tumorstatic side effects. Hemodepression and nausea and vomiting were smaller after the 3 h-infusion of 4'-ed than after its bolus injection. From the therapeutic point of view a 3 h-infusion of 4'-ed should be preferred to a bolus injection in patients such as those underlying this study.

*Present address: Department of Clinical Pharmacology. University of Leipzig. Härtelstr. 16-18, O-7010 Leipzig, FRG

172

EFFECTS OF THE NOVEL DIHYDROPYRIDINE DERIVATIVE B859-35 ON THE HUMAN LEUKAEMIC CELL LINE K-562

M.P.R. Drozd and K. Gietzen

Recently we have shown that the dihydropyridine derivative B859-35 is a potent inhibitor of cell proliferation in a variety of cell lines (Gietzen K et al., Eur. J. Cancer 26: 922, 1990). However, the mechanism of the anti-proliferative action is not yet understood, although numerous effects of B859-35 on cellular functions have been observed thus far (e.g. blockade of L-type Ca^{2+} channels and α_1-adrenoceptors, modulation of K^+ channels, antagonism of calmodulin and protein kinase C, increase of cytoplasmic Ca^{2+} concentration in thymocytes).
Here we have examined, whether the B859-35-induced increase of cytoplasmic free Ca^{2+} is involved in inhibition of cell proliferation in K-562 leukaemia cells. K-562 cells are well suited for the measurement of intracellular free Ca^{2+} by the Quin-2 method since they grow in suspension and therefore need no treatment with trypsin which could influence membrane permeability. Growth of K-562 cells was inhibited by B859-35 as well as its (+)-enantiomer B859-34 with an IC_{50} value of 2 µM. At 10 µM B859-35, over 80% of the cells were killed by an overnight exposure, but cell viability was not affected by a 15 min exposure. Cytoplasmic free Ca^{2+} was increased markedly only at 10 µM of B859-35 within 8 min, the (+)-enantiomer B859-34 was even less effective. When tested at the same cell density as in the growth assay (10^5/ml) B859-35 provoked a rise in cytoplasmic free Ca^{2+} from a basal level of 70 nM to a final value of 130 nM. From the following facts the conclusion may be drawn that the B859-35-elicited Ca^{2+} increase in K-562 cells is not involved in cell killing: (a) unlike the elevation of cytoplasmic free Ca^{2+} growth inhibition is not stereoselective; (b) B859-35 exhibits higher potency to block cellular growth than to induce elevation of Ca^{2+}; (c) the Ca^{2+} rise in response to B859-35 does not indicate apoptosis, since it is markedly lower than the Ca^{2+} elevation observed in connection with programmed cell death; and (d) the Ca^{2+} rise does not reflect cell lysis, since it preceeds cell death.

Department of Pharmacology & Toxicology, University of Ulm, Albert-Einstein-Allee 11, W-7900 Ulm, Germany

173

ESTROGEN-RECEPTOR POSITIVE HUMAN BREAST CANCER CELLS DERIVED FROM STRAIN MCF-7 EXHIBIT ATYPICAL RESISTANCE TO TAMOXIFEN.

A. Reymann^, H. Arps^^, P. Röhlke°, S. Schmidt^^ and C. Woermann^

Antiestrogens induce remission in most cases of estrogen receptor positive breast carcinoma, but some 20 % are non-responders although the presence of estrogen receptors had been verified in ligand-binding studies or with specific antibodies aimed at the nuclear binding protein for estrogen (ER-ICA).

We characterized the tamoxifen(TAM)-resistant strain MCF-7LY2 as compared to wild type breast carcinoma cells MCF-7. Both cell lines were estrogen receptor positive in ER-ICA and binding studies; cell growth was stimulated by estrogen (10 nmol/l; 10 % charcoal-depleted fetal bovine serum). Unlike TAM-sensitive MCF-7 cells, resistant MCF-7LY2 cells proliferated unimpaired by antiestrogens (TAM or 3-hydroxy-TAM, 100 nmol/l). Accumulation of TAM was tested by 30 min incubation with radiolabelled substrate and centrifugation of cells through a silicone oil layer into trichloroacetic acid (10 % w/v). In MCF-7 cells, 45 % of the total TAM was extracted from the medium (100 nmol/l; 200 μl) into the cellular compartment (cytosolic space < 5 μl); 95 % of TAM was tightly bound to the acid precipitate of cellular matter after washing of the pellet. TAM uptake increased further when cell density was decreased in the assay, exhibiting a linear correlation of TAM content to the reciprocal of cell protein (pmol/mg protein, range: 21.5-215.8, r=0.86, n=17). In contrast, TAM content of antiestrogen-insensitive MCF-7LY2 was not significantly increased when fewer cells were employed in the assay. Studies at 8 nmol/l TAM verified these findings. However, in both MCF-7 and MCF-7LY2 tested at a given cell number, TAM content was proportional to the TAM concentration of the medium (8-1000 nmol/l).

Results are compatible with a) decreased affinity of (unspecific) TAM binding or b) the presence of a low-affinity extrusion system for TAM in estrogen-receptor positive, TAM-resistant MCF-7LY2 cells.

^Abteilung Allgemeine Pharmakologie, ^^Institut für Pathologie, °Universitäts-Frauenklinik, Universitäts-Krankenhaus Eppendorf, Universität Hamburg, Martinistraße 52, D-2000 Hamburg 20, FRG.

174

PHOSPHODIESTERASE-INHIBITORY EFFECTS AND BINDING OF NOVEL DIHYDRONAPHTHYRIDINE-TYPE CALCIUM ANTAGONISTS TO CARDIAC AND ARTERIAL MEMBRANES

G. Werner, C. Bornemann, L. Trutzenberg, U. Fricke

From recent studies on novel dihydronaphthyridine(DHN)-type calcium antagonists in porcine isolated coronary arteries and ventricular muscle, additional mechanisms, e.g. a phosphodiesterase(PDE)-inhibitory activity and/or a second binding site contributing to the action of these drugs has been suggested. Therefore, (a) the influence of three DHNs (Goe 5606, Goe 5438, and Goe 5584-A; Werner et al., Arch Pharmacol, 339:R47, 1989; gift from Gödecke AG, Freib., FRG) on the activity of a crude PDE and (b) binding of these compounds to microsomes of coronary arteries and ventricular muscle has been studied. Nisoldipine (NIS), theophylline (THEO) and nitrendipine (NTD), respectively, were used for reference. PDE-activity was determined by a two-step procedure as described by Bauer and Schwabe (Arch Pharmacol, 311:193,1980). Binding was followed according to Fricke (Brit J Pharmacol, 85:327,1985). DHNs-induced inhibition of the PDE was more pronounced in coronary arteries (IC_{50} values 15-108 μM) resulting in the following order of potencies: Goe 5584-A < Goe5438 < Goe 5606. Efficacy of the stereoisomeres was observed in the same concentration range (optical resolution by Gödecke AG). The IC_{50} of NIS (28 μM) was comparable to Goe 5438 (18 μM), that of THEO (210 μM) was similar to Goe 5584-A. In ventricular muscle the same rank order was obtained, IC_{50} values ranging from 29 μM (Goe 5606) to 346 μM (Goe 5584-A). Again NIS (IC_{50}=94 μM) was comparable to Goe 5438 (IC_{50}=98 μM) and THEO (IC_{50}=344 μM) to Goe 5584-A. Maximal PDE-inhibition at a concentration of 100 μM ranged from 32% (Goe 5584-A) to 86% (Goe 5606) in coronary arteries and from 22% (Goe 5584-A) to 74% (Goe 5606) in ventricular muscle. Half-maximal binding (K_i) of the DHNs to arterial membranes was observed in the low affinity concentration range only (0,8-92 μM; one-site model) and was comparable to NTD. A second low affinity binding site for the DHNs 2 orders of magnitude higher may be involved in coronary arteries. In cardiac membranes K_i values were determined as 20-35 μM for the DHNs and 0,2 μM for NTD. Inhibition of [^{3}H]-NTD binding was stereoselective. It is concluded that, PDE-inhibition and low affinity binding may contribute to the vasodilator activity of the DHNs studied.

Institut für Pharmakologie, Universität zu Köln, Gleuelerstr. 24, D-5000 Köln 41

175

INFLUENCE OF ENDOTHELIUM ON THE VASCULAR ACTIVITY OF 1,4-DIHYDROPYRIDINES

J.Günther, S.Dhein, W.Klaus, R.Rösen, U.Fricke

Recently a dependence of the vasorelaxing activity of 1,4-dihydropyridines (DHP) on endothelial function could be demonstrated (Kojda et al., Basic Res Cardiol. 85, 461, 1990).
In order to study the possible modulation of DHP-action by the endothelium derived relaxing factor (EDRF), we investigated (a) the vasorelaxation by nitrendipine (NTD) in various isolated porcine arteries and its dependence on endothelial function by using a specific inhibitor of the EDRF synthesis, L-N^G-nitro arginine (L-NNA, 3 μmol/l), and (b) the influence of NTD and the calcium agonist Bay K 8644 [(-)-S- resp. (+)-R-1,4-dihydro-2,6-dimethyl-3-nitro-4-(2-trifluormethylphenyl)-pyridino-5 carboxylate] on the formation of NO in coronary arteries.
Pretreatment of coronary, basilary and tail arteries with L-NNA resulted in a marked reduction of the NTD-induced vasorelaxation after precontraction with $PGF_{2\alpha}$ as compared to experiments in the absence of L-NNA.
The NO-release from coronary arteries during cumulative application of NTD resp. of the enantiomers of Bay K 8644 was determined by the transformation of oxyhemoglobin to methemoglobin by NO. Extinction was registered spectrophotometrically at 405 nm. Application of NTD resulted in a concentration dependent increase of extinction indicating an enhanced formation of NO. This could be suppressed by preincubation with L-NNA. Similar results were obtained with the Bay K 8644 enantiomeres [(+)-R-Bay K 8644 < (-)-S-Bay K 8644].
We conclude that (a) the vascular effects of different 1,4-DHP's may partially be mediated by an increased release of EDRF, and (b) the endothelial structures involved are unable to discriminate between calcium antagonistic and agonistic DHP-compounds.

Institut für Pharmakologie der Universität zu Köln Gleuelerstr.24, D-5000 Köln 41

176

SOME DERIVATIVES OF BAY K 8644 DISPLAY REDUCED CORONARY ACTIVITY.

R. RATKE, W. KLAUS, U. FRICKE

Facilitating the calcium inward current into cardiomyocytes and smooth muscle cells through voltage-dependent channels, calcium agonists of the 1,4-dihydropyridine (DHP) type would be of therapeutic interest if their vasoconstrictive activity could be abolished (SCHRAMM & TOWART, Life Sci. 37, 1845, 1985). In order to elucidate whether molecular variations of Bay K 8644 [(-)-S-1,4-dihydro-2,6-dimethyl-3-nitro-4-(2-trifluoromethylphenyl)-pyridine-5-carboxylate] result in derivatives which enhance myocardial force of contraction but are lacking any influence on the vascular tone, the actions of following DHPs have been studied on porcine right ventricular trabeculae and coronary arteries: Bay W 5037 [2-aminoethyl-N-(N'-methylpiperidinyl-4)-ester], Bay W 5434 [2-methylaminoethyl-ester] and 4-(1,4,5,6-tetrahydro-6-oxo-3-pyridazinyl)-benzylester derivatives with variation of the 4-phenyl-substitution: Bay T 5006 [2'-nitro], Bay T 5120 [2'-methoxy]. Porcine ventricular trabeculae were stimulated with 1 Hz in an oxygenated Krebs-Henseleit-solution (resting tension 5 mN; 30°C). Porcine right coronary artery segments were examined in the same solution after a test-contraction with 60 mmol/l KCl, washout and moderate depolarization by 15 mmol/l KCl (resting tension 20 mN; 37°C). All drugs were added cumulatively. In trabeculae muscles Bay W 5037 and Bay W 5434 displayed only a weak positive inotropic activity at low concentrations ($\leq 10^{-5}$ mol/l), whereas higher concentrations resulted in negative inotropic effects. Bay T 5006 (ED_{50} 1,8 ±0,4 x10^{-6} mol/l) and Bay T 5120 (ED_{50} 1,2 ±0,4 x10^{-5} mol/l) showed a lower affinity but higher activity than (-)-Bay K 8644. In coronary arteries Bay W 5037 and Bay T 5006 exhibited no detectible vasoconstriction. With Bay T 5120 and Bay W 5434 only 3,7 ±1,5 % respectively 10,8 ±2,3 % of the 60 mmol/l KCl-tone were obtained. Precontracted arteries (60 mmol/l KCl) were relaxed by Bay W 5434 only. Our results indicate that the pharmacological profile of calcium agonists can be modified. This may result from an increased cardioselectivity or from different affinities/activities of the optical enantiomeres.

Institut für Pharmakologie der Universität zu Köln, Gleuler Straße 24, W-5000 Köln 41

177

MEASUREMENTS OF FAST CALCIUM TRANSIENTS IN STIMULATED HEART VENTRICULAR CELLS WITH FURA 2.

A. Stampfl

Alteration of intracellular calcium homeostasis is considered a crucial toxic mechanism of chemicals. For studying this mechanism it is necessary to measure the intracellular Ca^{++} concentration in the same cell over a longer period. We used stimulated heart ventricular cells of adult guinea-pigs. The cells were loaded with the fluorescence dye Fura 2 for 10 min. The great advantage of using electrical stimulation is the possibility of repeated observation of fast Ca^{++} transients under control and experimental conditions in the same cell. The influence of substances can be observed as a change of the fast increase and decrease in Ca^{++} after the stimulation as well as during the rest. The Fura loaded cells were placed in a temperature controlled chamber (35° C; 0,5 ml) on a Zeiss IM 35 inverted fluorescence microscope. The chamber was perfused with a O_2 saturated modified Krebs Henseleit Buffer (1 ml/min) with or without the agent. The cells were alternatingly illuminated with two wavelengths (345/380 nm). The cell under observation was selected with an adjustable rectangular diaphragm. The measurement of the fluorescence was triggered with the stimulation pulse. Ca^{++} concentration was expressed by the ratio of the fluorescence from 345/380 nm excitation and therefore independent of bleaching. By our investigations of the influence on 0.3 mM Mn^{++} at 0.5 Hz stimulation frequency we found that 1 min after addition the Ca^{++} increased during the rest period. 4 min later the concentration on rest increased markedly while the maximum Ca^{++} value during action showed a small rise and the fast decrease was delayed. During the next 25 min the resting level reached 140 % of the control value and the decrease was prolonged by about 50%. These results can be explained by a retardation and diminishing of Ca^{++} sequestration. These findings agree with earlier investigations on papillary muscle (Vierling, Reiter, this journal 306,249-253,1979). The experiments show that this method is a useful sensitive tool for investigations on the mechanisms of toxicity of Mn^{++} and other agents.

Institut für Toxikologie, GSF-Forschungszentrum für Umwelt u. Gesundheit GmbH, Ingolstädter Landstr. 1, D-8042 Neuherberg

178

RELAXATION OF ARTERIES AND VEINS BY CALCIUM-ANTAGONISTS.

R.Rösen, W.Kaiser, W.Klaus.

'In vivo' calcium antagonists and organic nitrates act on different parts of the vessel tree. Whereas the calcium antagonists reduce the myocardial afterload by arterial dilatation the organic nitrates lower myocardial preload by predominant relaxation of the veins. We tried to verify this different behaviour of the arteries and veins in isolated vessel preparations. Helical strips of A. and V.fem. from rabbits isotonically mounted in Krebs-Henseleit buffer (preloaded with 0.7 resp. 0.2 g) and precontracted with 100 mmol/l KCl were submitted to cumulative concentration response curves with glyceryltrinitrate (GTN) or the calcium antagonists nifedipine (NIF), diltiazem (DIL) and verapamil (VER). As expected the veins were dilated at significant lower concentrations of GTN than the arteries (EC-50 A.fem. 3.4 umol/l; V.fem. 0.15 umol/l; A/V=22.7). In contrast to this there was no difference in the sensitivity of the arteries (EC-50 NIF: 5 nmol/l; DIL: 0.48 umol/l; VER: 0.15 umol/l) in comparison to the corresponding veins against the classical calcium antagonists (A/V NIF: 1.25; DIL: 1.6; VER: 1.0).

Conclusion: The blockade of potential sensitive calcium channels is no sufficient explanation for the observed differences in dilatation of arteries and veins 'in vivo'.

Institut für Pharmakologie der Universität zu Köln, Gleuelerstr.24, 5000 Köln 41

179

ACUTE EFFICACY AND DISTRIBUTION OF DILTIAZEM IS RELATED TO THE MYOCARDIAL INFARCTION SIZE IN RATS
R. Hrdina, D. Svoboda

Due to possible negative (-) inotropic effect and controversial results, an acceptance of calcium blockers (CB) in vasodilator therapy of chronic heart failure (CHF) has not been established. Severity of CHF plays, among others, an important role in efficacy of CB. In mild CHF CB have a positive effect, however, in severe CHF a harmful one was observed. The mechanism is not quite clear. The aim of this study was to ascertain some of the possible mechanisms affecting an acute ECG and hemodynamic efficacy of diltiazem (DZ; 0.5 mg/kg i.v.) in relation to the myocardial infarction (MI) size in rats (n=11). With an increase of MI size there was an attenuation of hypotensive and antianginal efficacy of DZ (r=-0.624; -0.614 resp.). A decrease in (-)chronotropic and vasodilating activity was also observed (N.S.). In relation to the limiting MI size (cca 32 % of left ventricle circumference) there were qualitative different changes of hemodynamic parameters: In MI<32 % an increase of stroke volume and cardiac output was observed, but opposite changes were noticed in MI>32 %. In addition, there was a(-)relation between MI size and concentration of DZ in myocardium and aorta (r=-0.496,N.S.; -0.640, p<0.05). A decrease in systolic function in larger MI could not be explained by higher concentrations of DZ in myocardium. A remodelling of ventricles plays possibly an important role in acute efficacy of DZ, because due to the increase of MI size a weight/volume ratio of the ventricles tends to be decreased (r=-0.586,N.S.). Thus (-)inotropic effect of DZ could be unmasked by ventricular dilatation (Jacob R, Basic Res. Cardiol., 83:521, 1988).

Address: Institute of Experimental Biopharmaceutics, Czechoslovak Academy of Sciences, Heyrovského 1203 Hradec Králové, Czechoslovakia

180

EFFECT OF NITRENDIPINE ON SOME CARDIOVASCULAR PARAMETERS AND AORTIC CONTRACTILE RESPONSE IN DOCA-HYPERTENSIVE RATS . M.EL-DAKHAKHNY , H.M.SAKR , M.G.MORSI AND M.M.MATTA.

The antihypertensive effect of Nitrendipine (N) was studied in DOCA-salt hypertensive rats. Long-term administration of (N;10mg/Kg.) daily for four weeks led to a significant decrease in SBP, starting at the end of the first week and was accompanied by an increase in heart rate,which was attenuated by the end of the fourth week. The relationship between α-adrenoreceptor and the sensitivity of contractile responses induced by Norepinephrine NE, phenylephrine PE and clonidine CL in presence of N was also investigated on isolated aortic strips from DOCA- and normotensive rats. N (10^{-5}) suppressed NE ,PE and CL induced responses both in DOCA- and normotensive rats only in presence of high doses of each agonist (starting from 10^{-7}M.).This may be due to decrease in the slow component of the contractile responses which depend mainly on extracellular Ca-influx. NE ,PE and CL elicited contractile responses with greater magnitude in aorta from DOCA-rats than normotensive rats . This may be due to increased vascular responsiveness to constrictor stimulation in hypertensive rats. It can be concluded that (N) is an effective antihypertensive agent which causes temporary increase in heart rate (eventually attenuated). The differential responses to NE,PE and CL in DOCA-and normal rats may be due to increased sensitivity of the post-synaptic α -adrenoreceptors in DOCA-hypertensive rats.

Pharmacology Department , Faculty of Medicine , Alexandria University , Alexandria , Egypt .

181

Ca- AND SEROTONIN-ANTAGONISTIC POTENCY OF LU 49938 - PHARMACOLOGICAL STUDIES IN RATS
Sabine Schult and Verena Baldinger

LU 49938, the (S)-enantiomer of a new phenylalkylamine derivative, combines Ca- and 5-HT$_2$-antagonistic properties (Kirchengast M. et al. Naunyn-Schmiedeberg's Arch Pharmacol 343 (Suppl) R64, 1991).
In perfused rat hindquarters serotonin antagonism of LU 49938 was shown to be several times stronger than Ca-antagonism, whereas Verapamil showed serotonin antagonism only at Ca-antagonistic dose levels.

	Rat hindquarters, ED50% (µg/preparation)	
	Ca-antagonism Inhibition of K-induced vasospasm	Serotonin-antagonism Inhibition of 5-HT$_2$-induced vasospasm
LU 49938	0.24	0.034
Verapamil	1.4	2.7

In the pithed rat marked inhibition of serotonin-induced blood pressure increase was demonstrated after i.v. and oral administration.
In anaesthetized rats LU 49938 lowered the blood pressure after i.v. administration and was 3 times more potent than Verapamil.
2 hours after oral administration LU 49938 caused a dose-dependent prolongation of the bleeding time in rats. The results indicate that LU 49938 has a higher serotonin-antagonistic potency than Verapamil which is of relevance not only to the vasculature but also to the bleeding time.

	5-HT$_2$-antagonism ED 50% (mg/kg)		BP decrease ED20% (mg/kg) i.v.	Prolongation of bleeding time ED 100% (mg/kg) p.o.
	i.v.	p.o.		
LU 49938	0.03	5.2	0.11	17.6
Verapamil	0.36	21.9	0.34	44.9

It has been shown that LU 49938 is a more potent blood pressure lowering agent than Verapamil and an effective inhibitor of serotonin-induced vasoconstriction and platelet aggregation.
Knoll AG, Research and Development, D-6700 Ludwigshafen

182

Receptor profile and vascular relaxing effects of LU 49938, a new phenylalkylamine with equipotent calcium and 5-HT$_2$ antagonistic properties
Liliane Unger and Manfred Raschack

LU 49938 ((S)-5-[N-methyl-N-(n-hexyl)] amino-2-isopropyl-2-(3.4.5-trimethoxyphenyl)-valeronitril-hydrochloride) was investigated in radioligand binding studies and in functional experiments in vascular smooth muscle.
High affinity binding both to the L-type calcium channel and to the serotonin 5-HT$_2$ receptor was demonstrated (displacement of (-)^{3}H-D888 and ^{3}H-ketanserin in heart and brain vesicles, respectively). Only medium affinity to the brain 5-HT$_{1A}$, 5-HT$_{1C}$ and dopamine D$_2$ receptor was found, and weak to no affinity to the other receptors tested (β$_1$, β$_2$, α$_1$, α$_2$, H$_1$, H$_2$, M, D$_1$, NMDA). In comparison to the binding profile of verapamil and gallopamil LU 49938 showed the highest affinity both to the L-type calcium channel and to the 5-HT$_2$ receptor.
LU 49938 relaxed K$^+$ precontracted (30 mmol/l) pig coronary rings and was 1.5 times more potent than verapamil. In K$^+$ depolarized (100 mmol/l) rat aortic strips LU 49938 inhibited contractions induced by Ca^{++} (0.5 mmol/l) and was 2.7 times more potent than verapamil and as active as gallopamil. Like the 5-HT$_2$ antagonist ketanserin, LU 49938 was an effective inhibitor of contractions induced by serotonin (10^{-6} mol/l). LU 49938 was at least as active as ketanserin and 5.5 times more effective than verapamil and gallopamil. Regarding the results with the (R) enantiomer LU 49939, a clear stereoselectivity is evident.
Summary of results:

	Receptor binding KI (nmol/l)		Antagonism in rat aorta IC50 % (nmol/l)	
	(-) ^{3}H-D888	^{3}H-Ketans.	Calcium	Serotonin
LU 49938	8	24	13	7.7
LU 49939	106	1500	200	890
Verapamil	41	177	35	42
Gallopamil	27	242	14	43
Ketanserin	> 1 000	0.4	> 500	8.6

Our results show that LU 49938 is a highly potent calcium and serotonin 5HT$_2$ antagonist. This promises therapeutic potential in hypertension and vasoconstriction, especially where there is increased serotonin sensitivity in pathologically modified vascular beds.

Knoll AG, Molecular Pharmacology and Screening, D-6700 Ludwigshafen

183

THE OVERADDITIVE ACTION OF W84 WITH MUSCARINIC ANTAGONISTS DEPENDS ON THE KIND OF ANTAGONIST
Inke Andresen & K. Mohr

The bisquaternary compound W84 (hexamethylene-bis-[dimethyl-(phthalimidopropyl)-ammonium bromide]) stabilizes complexes of [^{3}H]N-methylscopolamine ([^{3}H]NMS) with cardiac cholinoceptors, which indicates an allosteric action of W84 at M$_2$-cholinoceptors. Furthermore, W84 is known to elicit in combination with atropine an overadditive antidote effect against organophosphate intoxication in mice (Kords H et al., Eur. J. Pharmacol. 3:341, 1968), and to act in isolated guinea pig atria together with atropine overadditively antimuscarinic (Lüllmann H et al., Eur. J. Pharmacol. 6:241, 1969).
It was tested whether the overadditive antimuscarinic action depends on the antagonist applied together with W84. Antimuscarinic effects were revealed by the shift of the dose-response-curve for the negative inotropic effect of oxotremorine in isolated guinea pig left atria electrically stimulated at 3Hz.
The antimuscarinic effect of W84 (pA$_2$ 6.5) started to saturate at concentrations above 10µM, indicating a non-competitive action to be involved. In the combination experiments, 1µM - 1000µM of W84 were applied together with the antagonists at concentrations shifting the oxotremorine dose-response-curve by about 2 to 3 log-units. A shift of the oxotremorine dose-response-curve up to 10fold larger than expected was observed with the combination of W84 and the antagonists atropine, scopolamine, N-methylscopolamine, N-butylscopolamine, and dexetimide. In contrast, the combination of W84 with the M$_2$-selective antagonist AF-DX 384 did not yield an overadditive antimuscarinic effect. Apparently, the special features of the interaction of AF-DX 384 with M-cholinoceptors, which underlie its M$_2$-selectivity, render this antagonist resistent to the potentiating effect of W84.
In conclusion, the allosteric modulator of M-cholinoceptors, W84, acts overadditively antimuscarinic with most but not all M-cholinoceptor-antagonists. It may be anticipated that the same applies for the overadditive antidote effect of W84 with antimuscarinic drugs in organophosphate poisoning.

Abt. Pharmakologie, Universität Kiel, Hospitalstr. 4, 2300 Kiel

184

Characterization of the β-adrenoceptor blocking property of diprafenone in rats: stereoselective interaction, subtype specificity, and sensitization. C. Nanoff and W. Schütz

Due to their structural relationship to propranolol, propafenone and diprafenone display β-adrenoceptor blocking activity in addition to their class Ic-antiarrhythmic property. As demonstrated in membranes derived from rat ventricle (predominantly β$_1$-adrenoceptors) and rat lung tissue (predominantly β$_2$-adrenoceptors), the (-)-enantiomer of diprafenone was about four times more potent (K$_i$ 6.6 nmol/l) than the (+)-enantiomer in displacing [^{125}I]iodocyanopindolol (ICYP) binding. The K$_i$ values for all stereoisomers, racemic (+/-)-diprafenone, and 5-hydroxydiprafenone, the main metabolite of diprafenone in humans, were approximately 2.5-fold lower in lung than in ventricular membranes, suggesting very low β$_2$-selectivity for diprafenone. The regulatory effect of diprafenone on ventricular β-adrenoceptors was studied in vivo by prolonged intraperitoneal administration of the drug. Density of β-adrenoceptors was estimated by ICYP saturation binding after 2-day (4 and 20 mg/kg b.i.d.) and after 7-day treatment (4 mg/kg b.i.d.), respectively. For control purposes, different groups of animals were treated with propranolol (1.7 mg/kg b.i.d., intraperitoneally), isoprenaline (0.1 mg/kg/h via subcutaneously implanted osmotic minipumps) and vehicle (0.9% NaCl) only. Whereas propranolol and isoprenaline produced an increase (7-day treatment) and a decrease (2-day and 7-day treatment) in β-adrenoceptors, respectively, diprafenone did not produce any change in β-adrenoceptor number, irrespective of the dosage used and the duration of treatment. Furthermore, the concomitant administration of diprafenone and isoprenaline did not antagonize isoprenaline-induced down-regulation. We conclude that great fluctuations in the diprafenone plasma levels - due to its rapid metabolism - would prevent the developement of β-adrenoceptor upregulation.

Institute of Pharmacology, University of Vienna, Währinger Str. 13a, A-1090 Wien

185

DPI 201-106 AND BDF 9148 SHOW DIFFERENCES IN POSITIVE INOTROPIC RESPONSES AND ELECTRO-PHYSIOLOGICAL PROPERTIES IN CARDIAC PREPARATIONS FROM GUINEA-PIG AND RAT
A. Hoey, E. Wettwer, U. Ravens

DPI 201-106 (4-[3-(4-diphenylmethyl-1-piperazinyl)-2-hydroxypropoxy]-1H-indole-2-carbonitrile, DPI) and BDF 9148 (4-[3-(1-diphenylmethyl-azetidine-3-oxy)-2-hydroxypropoxy]-1H-indole-2-carbonitrile, BDF) are considered to induce their positive inotropic effects by inhibition of the inactivation of the cardiac Na current, I_{Na}, and thereby activating the Na/Ca exchanger. Both compounds enhance force of contraction in a similar magnitude and concentration range, however, DPI prolongs the action potential duration, APD, to a greater extent than BDF. We have studied the effects of DPI and BDF in isolated myocytes and papillary muscles in order to elucidate their mechanisms of action. In voltage clamped guinea-pig myocytes, both compounds produced a clear inhibition of the inactivation of I_{Na}. With low concentrations of BDF ($< 3~\mu M$), residual I_{Na} 100 ms after the depolarizing clamp step, was enhanced even more than with DPI, but the maximal effects were similar. The inhibitory effects of DPI and BDF on cardiac Ca current were also similar. DPI caused a reduction of the inward rectifier whereas BDF did not have this effect. We have also studied rat papillary muscles because this tissue has a high K conductance. In rat cardiac muscle, both compounds (0.01 - 10 μM) prolonged the APD, however, DPI had little positive inotropic effect. Our results suggest that the differences in prolongation of the APD induced by BDF and DPI are caused by an additional inhibitory effect of DPI on the inward rectifyer as can be simulated in a computer model of the action potential.

Department of Pharmacology, University of Essen, Hufelandstraße 55, 4300 Essen, FRG

186

THE EFFECTS OF ANTIARRHYTHMIC AGENTS ON CARDIAC POTASSIUM CURRENTS IN GUINEA-PIG VENTRICULAR MYOCYTES.
M. Grundke, E. Wettwer, U. Ravens.

In enzymatically isolated cardiac myocytes, we have compared the effects of the new antiarrhythmic agent E-4031 (1-[2-(6-methyl-2-pyridyl)-ethyl]-4-(4-methyl-sulfonyl-aminobenzoyl)-piperidine) on potassium currents with those of d-sotalol and quinidine. A single electrode voltage clamp method was used. E-4031 (1 μM) did not affect the inward rectifier which was inhibited by d-sotalol (100 μM) and quinidine (10 μM). For studying the effects of the drugs on the delayed rectifier, I_K, the sodium current was inactivated by a holding potential of -40 mV and calcium currents were blocked by Cd^{2+} (0.1 mM). The outward current at the end of depolarizing clamp steps was referred to as I_K (2 s were required for full activation), whereas the tail current, I_t, was referred to as the current amplitude upon return to the holding potential. d-Sotalol and quinidine depressed both I_K and I_t, however, E-4031 (0.1 μM) preferentially inhibited I_t. After wash-out of the compounds, only the effects of quinidine were reversible. Under control conditions, the current-voltage relation (I-V curve) of I_K showed an extra current component in the potential range between -20 and +20 mV, which was absent in the I-V curve of I_t. This particular component was inhibited by E-4031 and quinidine, but not by d-sotalol. For short clamp pulses (< 100 ms) to +50 mV, I_t was larger than I_K. The ratio I_t/I_K declined from a maximum of 4.12 ± 2.03 (mean ± SEM, n=13; duration of pulse 50 ms) to 0.85 ± 1.17 (n=3) after 5 minutes of exposure to E-4031 (0.1 μM). It is concluded that E-4031, d-sotalol and quinidine differentially affect potassium currents. This finding may have some significance with respect to the potential antiarrhythmic and proarrhythmic properties of these agents.

Department of Pharmacology, University of Essen, Hufelandstraße 55, 4300 Essen 1, FRG

187

MEANING OF I_{Na} FOR THE EPICARDIAL ACTIVATION PROCESS.
S.DHEIN, A.MÜLLER, W.KLAUS

The aim of our study was to examine the influence of a modulation of I_{Na} on velocity and pattern of the epicardial activation (EA) process. Therefore, an epicardial potential mapping (of 256 channels) in isolated perfused rabbit hearts (Langendorff-technique, perfused with Tyrode solution) was performed (according to Dhein et al., Basic Res. Cardiol. 85, 285-296, 1990). I_{Na} was modulated either by lidocain (LID; 2, 5, 10 $\mu mol/l$) or by DPI 201-106 (DPI; 0.1, 0.2, 0.3 $\mu mol/l$). Under this treatment self-similarity (SIM) of the activation patterns of various heart beats, velocity of EA, epicardial potential duration (EPD) and functional parameters as left ventricular pressure (LVP) and coronary flow (CF) were determined. LID resulted in in negative inotropy, slowing of EA and loss of SIM without significant alteration of EPD. In contrast, LVP was increased by DPI without influencing the quotient CF/LVP. But DPI also reduced SIM markedly and slowed EA as well as atrioventricular conduction. In contrast to LID, DPI prolonged EPD. In addition, computer simulations of action potential (AP) spreading in a monolayer of 40*40 Beeler-Reuter-cells were performed (for non-uniform and uniform anisotropic tissue, according to Lesh et al., Circ Res 65, 1426-1440, 1989). Influence of a 25 or 33 % I_{Na}-blockade was simulated. I_{Na}-blockade led to loss of SIM, AP-shortening, dispersion of AP-duration and conduction slowing. This was pronounced in non-uniform anisotropic tissue. From these results it is concluded that (a) any I_{Na}-modulation leads to loss of SIM and thereby is arrhythmogenic; (b) physical properties of the tissue may facilitate arrhythmogenesis via I_{Na}-modulation. (Supported by the DFG)

Institut für Pharmakologie, Universität zu Köln, Gleuelerstr.24, D-5000 Köln-41.

188

EVALUATING OF ADENOSINE RECEPTOR-MEDIATED REGU-LATION OF FUNCTIONAL PARAMETERS OF ISOLATED GUINEA-PIG HEARTS.
K. Güttler, Th. Schumacher, W. Klaus

In order to clarify the possible contribution of adenosine receptor (AR) - mediated effects to myocardial contractility, inotropic effects of several AR - ligands (adenosine = ADE, phenyl-theophylline = PTh, cyclopentyltheophylline = CPTh and theophylline = Th) were examined in isolated guinea pig hearts perfused according to the Langendorff technique at a constant pressure. Under these experimental conditions vaso-dilatation results in an increased myocardial contractile force, so-called "garden-hose-effect" (GHE), and therefore masks the pure drug action on the myocardium. By adequate pressure-flow adjustments the GHE-influence on myocardial contractility was determined and accordingly the pure inotropic drug action calculated (pINO). ADE (10^{-6} M) acts positive inotropic (+30%), because coronary flow is increased (+204 %), in reality the pure drug effect is negative inotropic (pINO: -36%). PTh an unspecific AR - antagonist shows in the lower concentration range (10^{-8}- 10^{-7} M) positive (pINO: +16 %) and at higher concentrations ($\geq 10^{-6}$ M) negative (pINO: -18%) inotropic effects. Th exerts negative (pINO: -16 %) resp. positive (pINO: +21 %) ino-tropic actions at 10^{-6} M resp. 10^{-3} M. CPTh a selective A_1-antagonist (10^{-6} M) elevates con-tractility (pINO: +14 %). ADE (10^{-6} M) pretreat-ment acts like an amplifier on AR antagonistic compounds (10^{-6} M) with these pINO-values: PTh: + 12 %, Th: + 41 %, CPTh: + 30 %. From these results we conclude that A_1 adenosine receptor antagonists possess a certain positive inotropic activity.
Institut für Pharmakologie der Universität zu Köln, Gleuelerstr. 24, 5000 Köln 41

189

IN VITRO DIFFERENTIATION OF PLURIPOTENT EMBRYONIC CARCINOMA (ECC) AND EMBRYONIC STEM CELLS (ESC) INTO CARDIAC MYOCYTES: DEVELOPMENTALLY CONTROLLED FORMATION OF HEART MUSCLE CELL-SPECIFIC CHARACTERS.
Anna M. Wobus and G. Wallukat+

Embryonic carcinoma and embryonic stem cells of the mouse are cultivated in hanging drops without (ESC D3 and Bl 17 cells) and with DMSO (ECC P19 cells) as differentiation inducer and develop into embryo-like structures, the so-called embryoid bodies resembling the egg cylinder stage. These embryoid bodies are plated onto gelatinized substrates where differentiated cell types of all three primary germ layers are growing out including spontaneously beating heart muscle cells.
At different times after plating the formation of adrenergic, cholinergic and digitoxine receptors as well as the presence of L-type calcium channels are measured by the chronotropic reactivity of heart cells in response to different agonists and antagonists or inhibitors and activators.
β_1- and α_1-adrenergic and cholinergic receptors and signal transduction signals and L-type calcium channels are present already in early differentiated myocytes whereas β_2-adrenergic and digitoxine receptors are functionally active only in terminally differentiated cardiac myocytes. There is no principal difference in the chronotropic reactivity of myocytes differentiating from ECC or ESC with the exception of a high sensitivity of myocytes which differentiated from ECC P19 cells after DMSO induction.

Institute of Genetics and Crop Plant Research,
0-4325 Gatersleben
+Institute of Cardiovascular Research,
0-1115 Berlin-Buch
FRG

190

PHOSPHODIESTERASE INHIBITION IN ISOLATED VENTRICULAR MYOCYTES AND MULTICELLULAR VENTRICULAR PREPARATIONS FROM GUINEA-PIG HEARTS
Th. Bethke, W. Schmitz, H. Scholz, B. Stein, K. Thomas, and H. Wenzlaff

In order to investigate whether in multicellular ventricular tissue preparations the cAMP phosphodiesterase (PDE) activities reflect the PDE in cardiomyocytes only, or in addition the PDE of other cell types (e.g. endothelial cells), we studied PDE activities in ventricular cardiac tissue and isolated ventricular cardiomyocytes from guinea pigs. In homogenates of ventricular cardiomyocytes four different soluble PDE activities could be separated by DEAE sepharose chromatography as similarly reported for PDE I-IV from multicellular ventricular tissue (Reeves et al., Biochem J 241: 535, 1987). In ventricular cardiac tissue as well as in isolated ventricular cardiomyocyte preparations cAMP PDE isoenzymes I-IV were comparable in terms of substrate affinities, Km values, the sodium acetate concentration at which they were eluted, and inhibition or stimulation by cGMP. However, Vmax was reduced by a factor of about 2 to 7 in cardiomyocytes. In order to investigate whether the PDE activities I-IV were similarly inhibited by PDE inhibitors in both preparations we studied the effects of 3-isobutyl-1-methyl-xanthine (IBMX), rolipram and UD-CG 212 Cl ((2-(4-hydroxyphenyl)-5-(5-methyl-3-oxo-4,5-dihydro-2H-6-pyridazinyl) benzimidazole HCl). UD-CG 212 Cl was a selective PDE III inhibitor in cardiomyocytes (IC50 0.3 μmol/l) and in multicellular ventricular tissue (IC50 0.1 μmol/l). Rolipram selectively inhibited PDE IV in cardiomyocytes (IC50 1.4 μmol/l) and in ventricular tissue (IC50 1.1 μmol/l) whereas IBMX was a nonselective PDE inhibitor in both preparations.
It is concluded that the PDE isoenzymes I-IV from multicellular ventricular tissue can be used as a representative system for investigating the PDE inhibiting properties of PDE inhibitors in the myocardium since comparable PDE isoenzymes I-IV exist in guinea-pig ventricular cardiomyocytes and multicellular ventricular tissue.

Abteilung Allgemeine Pharmakologie, Universitäts-Krankenhaus Eppendorf, Universität Hamburg, Martinistraße 52, W-2000 Hamburg 20, FRG

191

EFFECT OF ANGIOTENSIN CONVERTING ENZYME INHIBITION ON BRADYKININ METABOLISM BY HUMAN VASCULAR ENDOTHELIAL CELLS
M. Gräfe, C. Bossaller, K. Graf, W. Auch-Schwelk, C. R. Baumgarten, E. Fleck.

The role of angiotensin converting enzyme (ACE) on local bradykinin (Bk) metabolism was studied in cultures of human endothelial cells (HUVEC). To evaluate the specific ACE activity, other Bk degrading enzymes (neutral endopeptidase, aminopeptases, carboxypeptidases) were inhibited with phosphoramidon, amastatin, and MGTA. Bk concentrations (pg/ml) were measured after the addition of 10.000 pg/ml Bk at different timepoints with a Bk RIA (^{125}I Tyr-o-BK, detection limit 20 pg/ml immunoreactive Bk, cross reactivity to des-arg^9-Bk < 1%) in intact endothelial cells and cell homogenates. The ACE inhibitors lisinopril, ramiprilat, and captopril inhibited the Bk degradation in intact endothelial cells in a concentration-dependent manner with threshold effects at 10^{-10} M and maximal effects at 10^{-6} M (lisinopril and ramiprilat) and 10^{-5} M (captopril). The maximal concentration of the ACE inhibitors caused a > 90% inhibition of the Bk degrading activity (Bk half-life: 46±2 min without lisinopril, 386±52 min with lisinopril, n=21). In contrast, in endothelial cell homogenates only 60% of the Bk degrading activity could be attributed to the angiotensin converting enzyme (Bk half-life: 24±3 min vs 62±8 min, n=9).
The data demonstrate that endothelial cells in culture metabolize Bk. As judged from the effective reduction by ACE inhibitors, the Bk degrading activity can be attributed to angiotensin converting enzyme in intact endothelial cell cultures while other unknown enzymes may play a role in cell homogenates.

Department of Cardiology, German Heart Institute Berlin, Augustenburger Platz 1, D-1000 Berlin 65, FRG

192

ENDOTHELIUM DEPENDENT VASODILATATION WITH ACE INHIBITORS IN THE PRESENCE OF THRESHOLD CONCENTRATIONS OF BRADYKININ
C. Bossaller, W. Auch-Schwelk, M. Claus, K. Graf, M. Gräfe, H. Warnecke, S. Schüler, E. Fleck.

To study vasodilator mechanisms of ACE inhibitors bovine and human coronary arteries (from heart tranplantation patients) with intact endothelium were mounted in organ chambers for the recording of isometric tension. The arteries were precontracted with 10^{-6} M PGF$_{2\alpha}$ in the presence of 10^{-6} M indomethacin and stimulated with threshold concentrations of bradykinin (10^{-10} M) which caused relaxations of 15.2±6.4 % (n=12). The cummulative addition of ACE inhibitors produced further relaxations (in % of PGF$_{2\alpha}$ contractions):

	10^{-9} M	10^{-8} M	10^{-7} M	10^{-6} M
+ captopril	20.6±6.3	22.9±8.1	45.3±14.0*	66.4±9.5*
+ enaprilat	15.3±10.5	58.3±18.0*	76.5±5.1*	87.2±5.1*
+ lisinopril	26.2±8.3	81.8±12.2*	99.2±9.3*	99.3±4.0*

(x±SEM, n=6, *p<0.01 compared to control)
Similar results were obtained in human coronary arteries, although the tissue revealed a lower sensitivity to bradykinin. In contrast, the ACE inhibitors did not relax the arteries in the presence of threshold concentrations of other endothelium-dependent vasodilators including substance P, acetylcholine and ADP. Thus, in coronary arteries various ACE inhibitors evoke potent endothelium dependent relaxations in the presence of threshold concentrations of bradykinin. These effects are not explained by an inhibition of bradykinin degradation and reveal a new endothelial mechanism of ACE inhibitors.

Department of Cardiology, German Heart Institute Berlin, Augustenburger Platz 1, D-1000 Berlin 65, FRG

193

EFFECTS OF THE ENANTIOMERS OF SATERINONE ON THE PHOSPHODIESTERASE ISOENZYMES I - IV OF FAILING HUMAN HEARTS IN COMPARISON WITH THE RACEMATE
W. Zimmermann, C. Schmidt-Schumacher, and H. Scholz

Saterinone (SAT) in form of the racemate has been shown to be a selective phosphodiesterase (PDE) III inhibitor with positive inotropic and positive chronotropic effects (Brunkhorst et al., Arzneimittelforschung 38, 1293, 1988). As stereoisomers often exhibit differences in pharmacological activities we investigated the effects of the R(+)- and S(-)-enantiomers of SAT in comparison to the effects of the racemate on the PDE I-IV. The isoenzymes were separated chromatographically from ventricular tissue of human hearts with dilative cardiomyopathie (DCM). We also determined the inhibitory activities of the selective PDE III inhibitor milrinone (MIL) and the unselective compound 3-isobutyl-1-methyl-xanthine (IBMX).

cAMP PDE, IC50 (μmol/l)

Agent	I	II	III	IV	SF
SAT	38.5	40.3	0.02	0.03	1970
	(14.2-104.5)	(10.6-153.1)	(0.01-0.03)	(0.01-0.06)	
R(+)SAT	51.1	106.1	0.01	0.04	7860
	(28.3- 92.2)	(34.8-323.4)	(0.01-0.03)	(0.01-0.10)	
S(-)SAT	27.7	137.9	0.05	0.07	1656
	(13.1- 58.9)	(50.3-378.1)	(0.02-0.12)	(0.05-0.12)	
MIL	153.6	132.8	0.89	1.56	160.9
	(128.1-184.2)	(73.5-240.2)	(0.67-1.17)	(1.09-2.23)	
IBMX	14.8	22.1	4.02	7.16	4.59
	(12.0- 18.2)	(17.4- 28.0)	(2.97-5.44)	(2.68-19.1)	

n=5;geom.means(95 %confid.limit);SF=selectivity factor=$\bar{x}$(I,II)/III

It is concluded that the R(+)- and S(-)-enantiomers as well as the racemate of SAT are similarly selective and potent inhibitors of ventricular PDE III and IV of human hearts with DCM.

Abteilung Allgemeine Pharmakologie , Universitäts-Krankenhaus Eppendorf, Universität Hamburg, Martinistraße 52, W-2000 Hamburg 20, FRG

194

PHARMACOLOGICAL MODULATION OF THE MYOFIBRILLAR AND MYOSIN ATPase ACTIVITY FROM CARDIAC MUSCLE BY QUINOLINE DERIVATIVES AS INOTROPIC AGENTS
U. Hoffmann, Haike Leibiger

Quinoline derivatives have been identified as positiv inotropic agents in preparations of atrium from guinea pigs. The mode of mechanism is unknown. Therefore we studied the ATPase activity in myofibrils and myosin isolated from porcine heart under the influence of N-methoxy and N-hydroxyethyl substituted compounds.
The myofibrillar Ca^{2+}-dependent Mg^{2+}-ATPase was significantly decreased at $pCa > 5.6$. The degree of inhibition depends on the kind of the substitutes and its position and amounts to 70 %. The pD_2-values are in the range of 6.0-6.5 and do not differ from the control. The same is the case for the K_m-constants after LINEWEAVER-BURK or HANES. Because the V_{max}-constants are coincidentally diminished we postulate an un- or non-competitive inhibition. All calculated HILL-coefficients are n <1 and confirm several Ca^{2+}-binding places on the Troponin complex.
Also the Ca^{2+}-stimulated ATPase activity from desensitized myofibrils and the isolated myosin was decreased up to 50 % in preparations incubated with quinolines.
Discussing the mechanism we assume an allosterical attack of the quinoline compounds to the Troponin-C subunit of the regulatory proteins which induces a conformational change. Besides the Ca^{2+}-binding places on the myosin molecule should be directly influenced by the substances.

Department of Pharmacology, Ernst Moritz Arndt University Greifswald, F.-Loeffler-Str. 23 d, D- 2200 Greifswald, FRG

195

STUDIES ON THE COMPUTER-AIDED DEVELOPMENT OF A POSITIVE INOTROPIC SUBSTANCE   J. Tautz and H. Bercher

Heart failure is characterized by selective downregulation of β_1-adrenoceptors, reduced coupling to adenylate cyclase and reduced Ca^{++}-sensitivity of Troponin C. The aim of this study was to combine three principles of therapeutic intervention (upregulation of the number of β-adrenoceptors, inhibition of phosphodiesterases and resensitization of the myofilaments to Ca^{++}) in one substance with the help of computer-aided drug design.
We calculated for 18 β-adrenergic agonists and partial agonists as well as for 7 "pure" and 6 inhibitors of phosphodiesterase with Ca^{++}-sensitizing effects the molecular electrostatic potentials of their CNDO/2-minimum energy conformations in order to find out pharmacophoric structural elements for each component of action. Based on these results we synthesized a model substance B 76 (1-(4-benzimidazolyl-3-methoxy)-phenoxy-3-isopropylamino-propan-2-ol), which possesses electronic patterns of β-adrenergic partial agonists and phosphodiesterase-inhibitors/Ca^{++}-sensitizers. We investigated the positive inotropic effects of B 76 in isolated, electrically driven right ventricular papillary muscles of reserpinized guinea-pigs and compared them to those of isoproterenol (ISO) and milrinone (MIL). B 76 had an inotropic effect similar to that of MIL (EC_{50}: ISO: 11.6 nmol/l, MIL: 9.79 μmol/l, B 76: 19.2 μmol/l), but caused a greater maximum increase in force of contraction than MIL (ISO: 263 %, B 76: 219 %, MIL: 171 %). B 76 showed β-adrenoceptor antagonistic effects (pA_2: 5.82, slope of SCHILD-plot =0.92; tested vs. ISO). Therefore the theoretically developed substance B 76 possesses positive inotropic and partial β-adrenoceptor blocking effects.

Institute of Pharmacol. & Toxicol. of the E.-M.-A.-University, F.-Loefflerstr. 23 d, D-2200 Greifswald

196

CICLETANINE-DEPENDENT CORONARY DILATION MAY BE INHIBITED BY GLIBENCLAMIDE.
R.Rösen, J.Fuchs, B. Sigmund, W.Klaus

Vasodilation induced by cicletanine, a new antihypertensive drug, is thought to be mediated by stimulation of the prostacyclin-synthesis. We have tried to verify this hypothesis in Langendorff-perfused rabbit hearts. By cumulative application of cicletanine (1, 5, 10, 20 umol/l) only the highest concentration could induce a stable and significant increase in coronary flow (CF). By single application of this concentration to the hearts CF was enhanced by +13±3% (= +4.9±0.9 ml/min; n=8) an effect which may be completely washed out. Blockade of prostacyclin synthesis by pretreatment of the hearts with 1mmol/l acetylsalicylic acid did not inhibit the cicletanine-induced vasodilation, which in contrast seemed to be even higher (+22±5% = 6.8±1.1 ml/min). Inhibition of the EDRF-synthesis by scopolamine (1umol/l) or N^G-nitroarginine (10 umol/l) did not abolish the cicletanine induced increase in CF. However, after blockade of the ATP-dependent K^+-channels in the hearts with glibenclamide (1 umol/l) CF could not be enhanced any longer with cicletanine.
<u>Conclusion:</u> The direct coronary dilation with cicletanine is neither mediated by stimulation of prostacyclin- nor by increased EDRF-synthesis but seems to be related to K^+-channel opening.

Institut für Pharmakologie der Universität zu Köln, Gleuelerstr.24, 5000 Köln 41

197

SUBSTANCE P AND OPIOID PEPTIDES - RELATION TO THE GENETICALLY
CAUSED HYPERTENSION OF RATS

I. Roske, K. Nieber and R.Buske

Disturbances in the regulation of adaptive functions may be
caused genetically or epigenetically.
An importand parameter to indicate functional disturbances in
SHR is the increased blood pressure. SHR show a strong age
dependent increase of blood pressure compared with
normotensive WKY-rats. This finding is in agreement with an
increase of spontaneous NA release from adrenal gland slices
reported previously by our group. This may be caused by the
following facts:

- Coincided with this age dependent increase of blood
  pressure we found a distinct decrease of the endogenous SP
  content in the adrenals contrary to WKY rats of the same
  age and sex.
- Differences in alteration of endogenous SP content in
  adrenals between SHR and WKY we have found following acute
  stress (increase in WKY-rats, decrease in SHR).

These results support the supposition of a functionally
disturbed SP-system.
Furthermore, we detected also functional disturbances of the
endogenous opioid system in SHR. Contrary to WKY-rats in 4
weeks old SHR an endogenous opioid dependence exists.
SP applied prenatally on the 16th day of pregnancy prevents
the age dependent rise of blood pressure and the development
of endogenous opioid dependence of the offsprings.
SP (10 μM) added to the superfusion media normalizes the
increased spontaneous NA release from adrenal gland slices of
SHR to the baseline of normotensive WKY rats whereas the
spontaneous release of WKY-rats remains uneffected.

From these results we conclude that functional disturbances
of peptidergig systems - Substance P and opioids - may play
an important role in the pathophysiology of the genetically
caused hypertension.

Institute of Drug Research, Department of Adaptation and
Addiction Research, Alfred-Kowalke-Str. 4, O-1136 Berlin, FRG

198

**PRESYNAPTIC EFFECTS OF PROSTAGLANDINS ON
ADRENERGIC NEUROTRANSMISSION IN GUINEA PIG ATRIA IN
VITRO**

R. Beckmann, U. Knirk

Prejunctional, inhibitory effects of prostaglandins on noradrenaline
release have been described in various preparations and organs. Most
of the data suggest that this presynaptic inhibition is mediated by
PGE_2-sensitive EP receptors, probably of the EP_3 subtype.
Naturally occurring and synthetic prostaglandins were studied for
presynaptic inhibition of adrenergic neurotransmission using the
method of refractory period field stimulation (RPFS) of isolated right
atria (Haberey, 1982). The effects of different types of prostaglandins
were compared to characterize the prostanoid receptor(s) involved.
With IC_{50} values in the nanomolar range the E-type prostaglandins
and their derivatives were very potent inhibitors of RPFS-induced
increases of force of contraction. The order of potency regarding
presynaptic inhibition of adrenergic transmitter release was flunoprost
(EP_1, EP_3, FP) > sulprostone (EP_1, EP_3) > PGE_2 = nocloprost $(EP_1,$
$EP_3)$ > 6-keto-PGE_1. Cicaprost (IP) and etiprostone (FP) showed
some inhibitory effects in the micromolar range, whereas the stable
PGD_2-analogue ZK 110.841 (DP) was ineffective.
Presynaptic inhibition by sulprostone was not affected by the specific
EP_1-antagonist AH 6809.
Conclusion: The data presented suggest that presynaptic inhibition of
adrenergic neurotransmission in guinea pig atria by prostanoids may
be mediated by EP receptors of the EP_3 subtype.

Research Laboratories of Schering AG, Berlin, Germany, Müllerstr.
170-178, W-1000 Berlin 65

199

Na^+, K^+ ATPase INHIBITION BY THE GLYCOSIDES FROM CORONILLA
VARIA L.

M.Mráz[+], L.Opletal[++], M.Sovová[++], P.Drašar[+++], M.Havel[+++]

Coronilla varia L.- Fabaceae (Crownvetch) is a perennial plant
widely spread in Europe and cultivated in the USA. From the
seeds, the glycosides hyrcanoside (HY) and deglucohyrcanoside
(DHY) were isolated. According to literature only the antineoplastic effect of these substances has been studied so far.Be-
cause of their steroid character and the presence of the lacton
ring we have studied their possible cardiotonic properties.
The inhibition of Na^+, K^+ ATPase can be used as a test for cardiotonic activity. Precise and simple method for quantitative
estimatiOn of Na^+, K^+ ATPase activity is based on the uptake of
^{86}Rb into human erythrocytes in vitro. We used this method to
compare the inhibitory effect of Coronilla glycosides with that
of ouabain (OU) and digitoxin (DT).Both Coronilla glycosides
had remarkable Na^+, K^+ ATPase inhibiting activity, which lies
between that of OU and DT. Following IC_{50} (10^{-8}mol.1^{-1}) were
found: OU $3,07 \pm 0,27$, DHY $3,80 \pm 0,50$, HY $4,68 \pm 0,76$, DT $9,15 \pm 1,27$.
None of some other substances isolated from Crownvetch and
studied (daphnoretin, scopoletin, umbelliferone and epicate-
chin) showed any effect on ATPase activity, neither they in-
terfered with the inhibitory effect of the glycosides.

[+]Dept. of Pharmacology, 1st Medical School, Charles University,
Prague 2, Albertov 4, ČSFR
[++]Dept. of Pharmaceutical Botany, Fac. of Pharmacology, Charles
University, 501 65 Hradec Králové, ČSFR
[+++]Inst. of Organic Chemistry and Biochemistry ČSAV,Praha 6,

200

**EFFECTS OF SELECTED BIPYRIDINES ON THE
RELATION BETWEEN LEFT VENTRICULAR END-
DIASTOLIC PRESSURE AND STROKE VOLUME IN
ANESTHETIZED MINIPIGS**

B. Wiesner and E. Rohde

The instantaneous relation between preload and cardiac output
is given by the left ventricular (LV) function curve or FRANK
STARLING curve. In the basal state, e.g. unchanged contractily,
afterload and compliance, LV pump function is regulated only by
its preload. It is important to know how medical treatment can
influence this relation ship especially under pathophysiological
conditions.
The aim of the study was to investigate the effects of some new
cardiotonic compounds on LV function.

Left ventricular pressure and aortic blood flow velocity were
simultaneously measured in anesthetized minipigs. Enddiastolic
pressure and stroke volume were evaluated by means of a
computer added analysis. The results are represented in a
vector-diagram, were the vector is characterized by specific
changes of both parameters after i.v. application of the new
cardiotonic compounds.

The effects of selected bipyridines in healthy minipigs and in
minipigs under drug induced heart failure were investigated and
compared. The results and the value of the applied method will
be discussed.

Institute of Drug Research
Dept. Pharmacology
Alfred-Kowalke-Strasse 4
O-1136 Berlin

201

HEMODYNAMIC EFFECTS OF 3-CYAN-2-MORPHOLINO-5-(PYRID-4-YL)-PYRIDINE UNDER CALCIUM CHANNEL BLOCKADE IN ANESTHETIZED MINIPIGS

E. Rohde and B. Wiesner

Hemodynamic effects of this new cardiotonic substance with vasodilating properties were studied under Ca^{2+} channel blockade (verapamil, nifedipine) in anesthetized instrumented minipigs.

After pretreatment with verapamil the compound (1.17 - 18.75 mol/kg i.v.) increased left ventricular contractility ($LVdp/dt_{max}$) between 42.9% - 58.5%. After pretreatment with nifedipine the substance induced a dose-dependend increase in $LVdp/dt_{max}$ between 11.1% - 47.8%. Under both conditions cardiac output was increased, total peripheral resistance and diastolic blood pressure were reduced. The substance caused a moderate increase in heart rate.

In comparison to control conditions increases in $LVdp/dt_{max}$ were less under Ca^{2+} channel blockade. It has been shown earlier that the mechanism of the inotropic action of this substance is a inhibition of phosphodiesterase III. The results suggest that an additional mechanism of inotropic action may be an alteration of the calcium channel activity.

Institute of Drug Research
Dept. Pharmacology
Alfred-Kowalke-Strasse 4
O-1136 Berlin

202

SEPARATION AND ANALYSIS OF COMPONENTS OF RELAXANT ACTION OF NICORANDIL

G. Pöch, S. Holzmann, Ch. Braida, W.R. Kukovetz

Evidence from our laboratory suggests that the relaxing action of nicorandil (NIC) consists of two components, guanylyl cyclase activation (increase in cGMP) and opening of K^+-channels (hyperpolarization). Thus, the action of NIC resembles both, "nitrocompounds" and K^+-channel activators [cromakalim (CROM), pinacidil (PIN)]. The aim of this investigation was to separate the two components by inhibition of K^+-channel activation (1μmol/l glibenclamide) and by inhibition of guanylyl cyclase activation (10μmol/l methylene blue), repectively, and to study whether the remaining component shows the same site of action as nitroprusside-Na (NP) and CROM or PIN. Dose response curves of NP, CROM, and PIN were established in isolated strips of bovine coronary arteries in the absence and presence of fixed concentrations between 3 and 100 μmol/l NIC. These studies were also carried out with the respective inhibitors and were evaluated as described recently with respect to dose-additive combinations which correspond to competitive synergism (Pöch et al. J Pharmacol Meth 24: 311-325; 1990). In the absence of the inhibitors, the combined effects of the activators (NP, CROM, PIN) with NIC were significantly greater than dose-additive. This difference between them was abolished by the respective inhibitors, i.e., the combined actions were no longer significantly overadditive. For instance, the combined effect of NP and NIC was significantly overadditive (p<0.001) in the absence of glibenclamide but not significantly different from additive (p≈0.99) in its presence. From these results it can be concluded that NIC shares the same site of action with "nitrocompounds" (NP, uncovered in the presence of glibenclamide), as well as with drugs acting at glibenclamide-sensitive K^+-channels (CROM and PIN, uncovered by methylene blue).

Inst. f. Pharmakodynamik. & Toxikol. A-8010 Graz, Univ.-Pl.2

203

EFFECT OF DICHLOROMETHANE ON THE ISOLATED HEART OF THE RAT

E.Rosenfeld, M.Weise, M.Klapperstück, P.Hoffmann.

Dichloromethane (DCM) is widely used for industrial purposes. Cardiovascular effects of DCM including events of sudden cardiac death following occupational exposure have been reported.

In the experiments the effect of DCM on the isolated heart (Langendorff model) was investigated. After an equilibration period of 15 min hearts were exposed to a Krebs-Henseleit-solution containing increasing amounts of DCM (0-25 mmol/l). The solvent was dosed via carbogen enriched with DCM-vapour. The concentrations of DCM in the solution were determined by gas chromatography.

Estimated parameters were: ECG, LVP, and coronary flow as well as lactate and K^+ efflux. Furthermore lactate, glycogen, and GSH contents were analysed in shock frozen heart tissue. The results demonstrate negative inotropic, chronotropic, and dromotropic effects of DCM and an alteration of biochemical parameters. Higher concentrations of DCM caused an asystolia with complete loss of any electrophysiological activity.

(Supported by the BMFT grant No. 01HK011/2)

Institute of Industrial Toxicology,
Faculty of Medicine
Martin-Luther-University Halle-Wittenberg
Franzosenweg 1a, Halle/S., O-4020 , Germany

204

INFLUENCE OF DICHLOROMETHANE-INDUCED CARBOXY-HEMOGLOBINEMIA ON ASPHYXIA-ARRHYTHMIAS IN RATS

S.Müller and P.Hoffmann

Previous studies in experimental animals and men showed that dichloromethane (DCM) is biotransformed in the organism to carbon monoxide (CO), mediated by the hepatic cytochrome P-450 enzyme system, resulting in increased carboxy-hemoglobin (COHb) levels.

After a single DCM-exposure (6.2 mmol/kg po, dissolved in Oleum pedum tauri) COHb in the blood rose to a maximum of 10% within 6h. The treatment of rats with ethanol (130 mmol/kg po) 18 h prior DCM-exposure resulted in increased COHb levels (15%). The control groups received the vehicle or ethanol only. Their COHb concentrations were ≤ 1%. We observed a COHb dependent reduction of venous pO_2 from 62 Torr in the control group to 50 Torr in the ethanol/DCM group. In urethane anesthetized (1 g/kg ip) rats the trachea was occluded for 1 min. The ECG was recorded by two needle electrodes applied subcutaneously at both sides of the chest (lead II). DCM induced-carboxyhemo-globinemia per se did neither produce arrhythmias nor influence cardiovascular parameters, with exception of a reduced heart rate. During asphyxia the arterial pO_2 decreased from 98 Torr to 28 Torr and the incidence of 2nd and 3rd degree AV-blocks was 100% in control animals. After asphyxia the arterial pO_2 increased and AV-blocks disappeared within 2 min. The appearance of spontanous respiration after asphyxia was belated in dependence on COHb-concentrations. The duration of AV conduction delay was prolonged. Our results demonstrate that dichloromethane-induced carboxy-hemoglobinemia aggravated the asphyxia-arrhythmias.

(supported by the BMFT grant No. 01HK011/2)

Institute of Industrial Toxicology, Martin Luther-University Halle,Franzosenweg 1a, O-4020 Halle, FRG

205

BDF 9148: COMPARISON OF ACTION POTENTIAL DURATION IN VITRO AND PROLONGATION OF Q-T INTERVAL IN ANESTHETIZED DOGS (TIME COURSE STUDY)

A. Raap, B.I. Armah, E. Hofferber, W. Stenzel and W. Blechacz

Prolongation of cardiac action potential duration (APD) is characterized by a lengthening of Q-T interval in the ECG in animals as in man. This mechanism of action has been described for naturally occuring and synthetic agents like DPI (Buggisch et al., Eur. J. Pharm., 118, 303, 1985). While shortened Q-Tc (frequency corrected Q-T) is without serious consequences, a long Q-Tc is associated with ventricular fibrillation. Thus for positive inotropic agents that affect the Na^+-channel in similar fashion as DPI (4(3-(1-diphenyl-methyl-piperazinyl)-2-hydroxy-propoxy)-1-H-indol-2-carbonitril) the clinical value can be limited by lengthening of Q-Tc in man. We investigated the time course effects of BDF 9148 (4(3-1-(diphenyl-methyl-azetidine-3-oxy)-2-hydroxy-propoxy)-1-H-indol-2-carbonitril) on left ventricular contraction, heart rate, myocardial O_2-consumption and Q-Tc in anesthetized dogs (closed chest) and the influence on APD in guinea pig papillary muscles (stimulation at 1 hz) in comparison to DPI. Doses of 0.1; 0.3; 1.0; 3.0 and 10 mg/kg i.v. gave equieffective increases in $LVdp/dt_{max}$, thus enabling an objective assessment of the other parameters. While there was no difference in myocardial O_2-consumption, DPI lowered heart rate and altered Q-Tc dramatically. As reported previously (Muster, D. and Raap, A., Naunyn-Schmiedeberg's Arch. Pharm., 341, R 51, 1990) BDF was without effect on Q-Tc at dp/dt_{max} peak change, but a very slight, transient increase was observed during the first min drug infusion. In contrast, there was a much more pronounced and sustained lengthening in Q-Tc under DPI. While BDF transiently prolonged cardiac APD in guinea pig papillary muscles - an initial prolongation was followed by an reversal of prolongation - DPI irreversibly prolonged APD.

Dept. of Pharmacology, BDF-Beiersdorf AG, Unnastr. 48, D-2000 Hamburg 20

206

HISTAMINE H_3 RECEPTOR-MEDIATED INHIBITION OF THE NEURO-GENIC VASOPRESSOR RESPONSE IN PITHED RATS

B. Malinowska and E. Schlicker

In pithed rats, electrical stimulation (0.5 Hz, 1 ms, 50 V; for 15 s) of the preganglionic sympathetic nerve fibres increased diastolic blood pressure by about 30 mm Hg. This response was almost completely (by about 90 %) abolished by prazosin 10 µmol/kg. The electrically induced increase in blood pressure was diminished by the H_3 receptor agonist R-(-)-α-methylhistamine 0.1, 1 and 10 µmol/kg by 15, 25 and 30 %, respectively. The effect of R-(-)-α-methylhistamine was attenuated by the H_3 receptor agonist thioperamide 1 µmol/kg but not affected by the H_1 receptor antagonist dimetindene 1 µmol/kg and the H_2 receptor antagonist ranitidine 10 µmol/kg. On the other hand, R-(-)-α-methylhistamine 0.01 - 10 µmol/kg did not influence the vasopressor response to exogenously added noradrenaline 1 nmol/kg (which increased diastolic blood pressure by about 25 mm Hg). However, R-(-)-α-methylhistamine itself, at a dose of 1 and 10 µmol/kg, induced an increase in blood pressure by 7.3 $\pm$ 1.5 and 27.4 $\pm$ 2.3 mm Hg, respectively; this effect was not affected by dimentindene, ranitidine and thioperamide. These results suggest that R-(-)-α-methylhistamine has a dual effect on blood pressure in pithed rats. The effect on the neurogenic vasopressor response is mediated via H_3 receptors, which are probably located presynaptically on the postganglionic sympathetic nerve fibres of the resistance vessels and activation of which reduces the release of noradrenaline. The mechanism of the direct vasopressor response to R-(-)-α-methylhistamine, which occurs in a higher dose range and is not mediated via H_1, H_2 or H_3 receptors, remains to be established.

Institut für Pharmakologie und Toxikologie, Universität Bonn, Reuterstraße 2 b, D-5300 Bonn 1, Germany
B.M. (permanent address: Zakład Farmakodynamiki, Akademia Medyczna, Białystok, Poland) is recipient of a research fellowship from the Alexander von Humboldt-Stiftung.

207

CARDIAC ELECTROPHYSIOLOGICAL EFFECTS OF AZELASTINE - A NEW SELECTIVE BLOCKER OF H_1 RECEPTORS

R. Stadler, H. Antoni, J. Weirich

Azelastine (4-(-chlorbenzyl)-2-(hexahydro-1-methyl-1H-azepin-4-yl)-1(2H)-phthalazinone- hydrochloride) is a selective H_1-receptor antagonist. In concentrations of about 10 times its therapeutic range, azelastine has been found to exert negative chronotropic effects in isolated rabbit and guinea pig atria. The present study was undertaken to analyse in some more detail the influence of azelastine on cardiac excitatory processes. Conventional microelectrode measurements were performed in sinus node and in isolated papillary muscles from rabbit right ventricle. In papillary muscles azelastine (10^{-6} mol/l in Tyrodes solution of 32°C) caused an increase in action potential duration of 56% (52-60%) accompanied by a slight reduction of the maximal rate of rise by 13% (10-16%) with the resting potential remaining unchanged. The reduction of V_{max} was frequency dependent with a rate constant of 0.1 AP^{-1} at 1 Hz, increasing up to 0.13 at a higher concentration (3×10^{-6} mol/l). In slow response type action potentials elicited in high K^+ medium $K^+_o = 12$ mmol/l) azelastine reduced V_{max} by about 30% with little influence on the action potential duration. In the sinus node azelastine reduced the spontaneous beating frequency by about 50%, mainly by decreasing the slope of the slow diastolic depolarisation. It is concluded that azelastine exerts its additional electrophysiologic effects by an inhibitory influence on different types of ionic channels (mainly those for Ca^{++} an K^+).

Physiologisches Institut, Universität Freiburg, Hermann Herder Str. 7, D-7800 Freiburg

208

GLYCERYL TRINITRATE (GTN)-INDUCED VASORELAXATION: MODULATION BY THE ENDOTHELIUM

H. Osswald, K. Stieler, and J. Werringloer*

Several investigators have shown that GTN-induced relaxation of arteries is enhanced when the vascular endothelium was removed (Alheid U et al., Br.J.Pharmac.92:237,1987; Dinerman JL et al., Am. J.Physiol.260:H698,1991). Also sodium nitroprusside-induced relaxations were enhanced when the endothelium was destroyed (Pohl U, Busse R, Am.J.Physiol.252:H307,1987). The present experiments were carried out to study further the GTN-endothelium interactions.

Methods: Segments (appr. 3 mm in length) from the aorta of Sprague-Dawley rats (300-350 g body weight) were dissected and mounted in an organ bath (Schuler, Hugo Sachs, Hugstetten FRG) filled with Krebs-Henseleit solution and gassed with carbogen at 37°C. Tension of the vascular rings preloaded with 10 mN was recorded isometrically. After precontraction of the rings with noradrenaline (0.3 µM) endothelium-dependent relaxation was tested by adding acetylcholine (0.1 µM) to the bath which produced a 90 % relaxation.

Results: In a paired fashion 4 rings with intact endothelium were precontracted and subsequently relaxed by GTN. Thereafter, endothelium was removed, and following 120 min equilibration, a GTN dose response curve was established. GTN-EC_{50} was 7 nM in the presence but 45 nM in the absence of endothelium. In the next series of unpaired experiments we found in rings with intact endothelium at 3 nM GTN a 39.5 ± 3.0 % relaxation (n=9; SEM) with an EC_{50} of 4.5 nM, whereas denuded rings relaxed by 36.9 ± 5.2 % (n=7) at 30 nM GTN with an EC_{50} of 45 nM. This latter value is in good agreement with the literature but the ten-fold higher potency of GTN in the presence of endothelium is clearly in contrast to the above cited references.

Conclusion: We assume that modulation by the endothelium of the GTN-induced relaxation has clinical relevance for GTN dosing and tolerance, but we cannot offer a conclusive explanation for the different results concerning GTN and endothelium interaction.

Departments of Pharmacology and *Toxicology, Univ. Tübingen, FRG

209

USE OF CHICK EMBRYO ECG FOR CARDIOTOXICITY
TESTING

U.Haacke and P.Hoffmann

To obtain ECGs from the chick embryo, we used
2 needle electrodes inserted opposite on the
"equator" of fertilized eggs of Lohmann White on
the 15th day of incubation. The bipolar waves are
not a regular ECG, because of the irregular
orientation of the embryo inside the egg, but on
principle allow to determine the heart rate.
Registration was done by an electroencephalo-
graph. Experiments showed a high dependence of
heart rate on temperature, so all further
experiments were carried out in the incubator
with 37°C. To eliminate the artifacts caused by
embryo movements, we produced a relaxation by
injection of 2.5 mg pentobarbital per egg. All
injections were made into the air sac of
fertilized eggs and ECGs recorded 10 min after
each drug injection. The following drugs were
tested and evaluated by two-tailed STUDENT's
t-test: epinephrine (0,1 mg/egg), acetylcholine
(5 mg), digoxin (0.05 mg) and metoprololtartrate
(0,25 mg). Epinephrine led to tachycardia and the
others to bradycardia. The values of heart rate
were also decreased by dichloromethane (0.01 ml).
30 minutes after injection asystolia was
observed. The dichloromethane LD_{50} was estimated
to be 0.018 ml per egg.
In conclusion the method may be used as an
alternative for experiments on cardiotoxicity.

(Supported by the BMFT grant No. 01 HK 011/2)

Institute of Industrial Toxicology
Martin-Luther-University Halle-Wittenberg
O-4020 Halle, Franzosenweg 1a,
FRG

210

INTERACTION OF LOCAL ANESTHETICS WITH VASCULAR
ALPHA-ADRENOCEPTORS. F. Kehlbach, E. Knoll-Köhler

The knowledge of possible interactions between
epinephrine and local anesthetics at the
pharmacodynamic and/or pharmacokinetic level is a
prerequisite for establishing an optimal dose ratio
between epinephrine and the different local
anesthetic substances in local anesthetic
solutions. To evaluate the possibility of
interactions at vascular α-adrenoceptors,
competition binding experiments were carried out
with local anesthetics and α-adrenoceptor
antagonists at membranes of thoracal aorta of the
pig. The densities of the α_1- and α_2-adrenoceptors
and the K_D-values were determined with ^{3}H-prazosin
(B_{max} = 45.7 ± 8.50 fmoles/mg protein, K_D = 0.27 ±
0.060 nmoles/L, n = 9) and with ^{3}H-rauwolscine
(B_{max} = 59.9 ± 6.66 fmoles/mg protein, K_D = 5.23 ±
1.382 nmoles/L, n = 7). The inhibition constants
(K_i) of lidocaine (4.6 ± 1.57 x 10^{-4} and 3.5 ± 1.89
x 10^{-4} moles/L, n = 4) and articaine (4.8 ± 0.11 x
10^{-4} and 2.5 ± 0.83 x 10^{-4} moles/L, n = 4) were not
significantly different for the α_1- and α_2-
adrenoceptors. For tetracaine, however, a high (K_i
= 4.5 ± 1.74 x 10^{-8} moles/L) and a low affinity
binding site (K_i = 8.4 ± 2.96 x 10^{-5} moles/L) of a
ratio of 32 : 68 was found at the α_1-adrenoceptor.
All values are given as mean ± SD.
These results show that local anesthetics in doses
appropriate to block nerve conduction (75-150
mmoles/L) do compete with the co-injected
epinephrine at the vascular α-adrenoceptors at the
application site.

Address: Freie Universität, Institut für Pharmakologie, Thiellallee 69-73, W-1000 Berlin 33,
Germany

211

ACTIVATION (PROLIFERATION) OF MYOCARDIAL PEROXISOMES BY
SEVERAL AGENTS.

J. Zipper

In recent years it has become clear that mammals peroxisomes
fulfil a number of essential function and that dysfunction or
absence of this organelles can have serious clinical consequences. Thus today peroxisomes are very interesting objects in
view of many aspects. There are important open questions
specially in respect of the role of peroxisomes in the heart. The
present study was designed to assess the influence of several
agents upon the activity of myocardial peroxisomes by quantitative electron microscopic investigations.
Ethanol and Erucic Acid (substrates for peroxisomal enzymes),
HL 41 / Na-salt of 1-Benzyl-3-(1-carboxy-1-methyl-ethoxy)-4-
methyl-pyrazole (a hypolipidemic agent), Adriamycin and Isoproterenol (cardiotoxic substances), Milrinone and IWF-122-14 /
3-Cyano-2-morpholino-5-(4-pyridinyl)-pyridine (cardiotonic
drugs) were administered to male rats for 5 wks. (Ethanol, by
drinking water), 3 wks. (Erucic Acid, 1.3 g/d, p.o.), 3 wks.
(Adriamycin, 10 x 2 mg/kg, i.p.), 2 wks. (HL 41 5 x 10^{-4} M/kg/d,
p.o.), 2 wks. (Milrinone and IWF-122-14, 5 x 10^{-5} M/kg/d, p.o.),
1 wk. (Isoproterenol, 4 x 25 mg/kg, s.c.).
In all cases a significant activiation effect could be observed.
The increase of peroxisome number compared to the control
(100 %) was: 318 % (Isoproterenol), 238 % (IWF-122-14), 230 %
(Adriamycin), 224 % (Erucic Acid), 209 % (Milrinone), 196 %
(HL- 41), 195 % (Ethanol).
These results are very interesting mainly in regard to Adriamycin, Isoproterenol and the cardiotonic drugs. The mechanism
and the significance of this effects are not clear. However, it
seems to be possible that an increase of the activity of catalase
and other peroxisomal enzymes associated with peroxisome proliferation represents a protective response of the heart.

Institute of Drug Research, Alfred-Kowalke-Str. 4,

O - 1136 Berlin, FRG

212

COMPARISON OF THREE PEPTIDERGIC INHIBITORS OF PLATELET AGGREGATION:
RGDS, THE CARBOXYTERMINAL DUODECAPEPTIDE OF THE FIBRINOGEN GAMMA-
CHAIN, AND THE SNAKE VENOM ECHSTATIN.

Peter F.J. Verhallen, Karl-Heinz Schönberg, Berthold Baldus, Karl-Heinz
Thierauch[1], Herman Graf[1], Frank Misselwitz[2].

A new generation inhibitors of platelet aggregation is currently under investigation in various laboratories. These inhibitors are peptidergic in nature and interfere with the binding of fibrinogen to its platelet receptor (glycoprotein IIb/IIIa).
To evaluate the concept in more detail we investigated three prototype fibrinogen receptor-antagonists: RGDS, the C-terminal duodecapeptide of the fibrinogen gamma-chain (HHLGGAKQAGDV, Fibgam), and the snake venom
polypeptide Echistatin. These prototypes were compared in various respects:
(1) platelet aggregation in platelet-rich plasma and plasma-free medium;
(2) desaggregation of preformed platelet aggregates; (3) platelet release reaction; (4) thrombin generation in platelet-rich plasma; (5) their in-vitro antithrombotic efficacy was compared with prostacyclin-analogues and aspirin;
(6) attachment of endothelial cells to fibronectin-coated and collagen-coated
surfaces; (7) adhesion of polymorphonuclear neutrophils to endothelial cells
under static conditions in vitro.
The following results were obtained: (1) echistatin inhibited platelet aggregation independent of fibrinogen concentration, in contrast to RGDS and Fibgam;
(2) RGDS and echistatin were able to desaggregate preformed aggregates
when added within 15 minutes after aggregate formation; (3) RGDS and
echistatin inhibited the platelet release reaction; (4) thrombin generation in
platelet-rich plasma was inhibited by RGDS and not Fibgam; (5) the in-vitro
antithrombotic efficacy of all fibrinogen receptor-antagonists was independent
of stimulus strength, in contrast to prostacyclin-analogues and aspirin;
(6) attachment of endothelial cells to fibronectin-coated surfaces was inhibited
by RGDS and echistatin, but not by Fibgam; (7) adhesion of polymorphonuclear neutrophils to endothelial cells was inhibited by Fibgam. Taken together these results indicate that different fibrinogen receptor-antagonists may
share the same antithrombotic principle, but will differ in various other respects
which may be hazardous (like detachment of endothelial cells and inhibition of
haemostasis leading to increased bleeding times) or beneficial (like inhibition
of neutrophil adhesion).

Cardiovascular Pharmacology and [1]Biochemical Pharmacology, Research
Laboratories Schering AG, P.O.Box 650311, W-1000 Berlin 28, Germany. [2]Central
Institute for Cardiovascular Research, Academy of Sciences, Wiltbergstr. 50, O-
1115 Berlin , Germany.

213

FUNCTIONAL ACTIVITY OF HUMAN VASCULAR TISSUE AFTER CRYOPRESERVATION. E. Müller-Schweinitzer

Despite the relevance of human isolated tissue for drug development, it's use is still very much the exception rather than the rule. The major reason for this is, that the supply of fresh human material is both irregular and unpredictable. We have developed a simple and reliable technique for storing isolated blood vessels for pharmacological studies.
Segments of freshly obtained blood vessels (15-20 mm) are placed in 2 ml liquid nitrogen storage ampoules filled with foetal calf serum containing 1.8 M DMSO (dimethylsulphoxide) as a cryoprotecting agent. The ampoules are slowly frozen to -70°C and placed after 3-20 hr into liquid nitrogen (-196°C) where they are stored until use. Before being used, the samples are rapidly thawed by placing the ampoules for 2.5 min in a 37°C water bath. The organs are then rinsed in a dish containing Krebs-Henseleit solution at 37°C and cut into rings for isometric recording.
Comparative studies on frozen/thawed and unfrozen blood vessels revealed some reduction of the maximal force development but even after several months of storage at -196°C main biochemical properties and uptake mechanisms are well preserved. Moreover, the experiments demonstrated that after thawing of frozen stored human veins and arteries of different vascular beds the affinities of various agonists and antagonists are well preserved suggesting that freezing of human blood vessels yields an excellent cryopreservation of this tissue for subsequent pharmacological studies.
Hence, this technique offers clear potential for ensuring the supply of human vascular material for pharmacological studies.

Preclinical Research, Sandoz Pharma A.G., CH-4002 Basel, Switzerland

214

EXPERIENCES WITH THE EMIT-CYCLOSPORINE - ASSAY FOR THE THERAPEUTIC DRUG MONITORING
K. Göhler and H. Hüller

Although the clinical usefulness of the immunosuppressive drug Cyclosporine-A is well established, its relatively low therapeutic index and a wide interindividual difference in response to given doses require a therapeutic drug monitoring. Most authors prefer specific methods, which determine the concentration of the parent drug in whole blood.
Since May 1991, the Institute of Clinical Pharmacology of the Humboldt-University Berlin carries out the therapeutic drug monitoring of Cyclosporine for patients after kidney, liver and heart transplantation with the EMIT-Cyclosporine-Assay (SYVA-Diagnostica) on the COBAS MIRA S analyzer (Hoffmann La Roche). This method allows the specific determination of the parent drug in whole blood. Analytical recovery varied from 94 to 106 %. The coefficients of inter- and intraassay variation with twolevel controls (100 and 400 ng/ml) were lower 7 %. Correlation of EMIT-Cyclosporine-assay patient samples values with those of RIA (Sandimmun-Kit, Sandoz) yielded the following correlation parameters: slope: 0.96, y-intercept: 8.7 and r= 0.978 (n= 98).
The EMIT-Cyclosporine-assay is a precise and rapid method for quantitating Cyclosporine in whole blood samples for therapeutic drug monitoring.

Institute of Clinical Pharmacology, Department of Medicine (Charité), Humboldt-University, Schumannstraße 20-21, O-1040 Berlin

215

INTERINDIVIDUAL VARIABILITY AND INTRAINDIVIDUAL STABILITY OF THE CYCLOSPORIN-METABOLITE RATIO
H.G. Trautsch-Förster, J. Brockmöller*, S. Unger, D. Scholz, I. Mai

During immunosuppressive therapy with cyclosporin A (CsA), the concentrations of CsA metabolites often exceed those of the parent compound in blood and tissues. To date, there is only limited information available about the long-term intraindividual variation of the cyclosporin-metabolite ratio. The proportion of CsA metabolites may be of toxicological and immunological impact and obviously complicates CsA therapeutic drug monitoring.

Ratios between CsA and its metabolites from 32 consecutive, clinical stable renal transplant patients on triple therapy (CsA, azathioprine, and steroids) were determined by radioimmunoassay, using an assay specific for the parent drug and a second assay, which quantifies the sum of CsA and its metabolites. The thus determined metabolite-drug ratio showed a wide interindividual variance (95-%-conf. limits: 1.9 - 5.1). Intraindividually, however, the drug-metabolite ratios were remarkedly constant over a period of 9 months. High ratios were significantly correlated with serum bilirubin concentrations and gamma-glutamyltransferase activity between 3 and 9 months after transplantation. In contrast, the drug-metabolite ratios showed no correlation with the administered CsA doses or with serum creatinine concentrations.

The observed high interindividual differences of the cyclosporine-metabolite ratios may be due to differences in metabolic activities or to variability in the biliary excretion capacity. These mechanisms and their clinical relevance have to be further investigated.

Institute of Clinical Pharmacology, Department of Medicine, Charité, Humboldt-University, Schumannstraße 20-22, O-1040 Berlin, FRG, *Inst. of Clinical Pharmacology, Klinikum Steglitz, Free University Berlin.

216

DETERMINATION OF LIVER BLOOD FLOW AND INTRINSIC CLEARANCE IN LIVER TRANSPLANT RECIPIENTS USING CYCLOSPORINE KINETIC DATA.
W. Weber, M. Looby, J. Brockmöller, P. Neuhaus*, and I. Roots

Although monitoring of the liver function is particularly important following liver transplantation, coadministration of test substances for the determination of liver blood flow and intrinsic clearance is avoided for fear of toxicity. Using kinetic data following therapeutic administration of cyclosporine (Cya) in 10 liver transplant recipients, both of these parameters were determined.
The AUC ratio for the primary metabolite 17, determined after oral and intravenous administration of Cya, gives the absorbed dose fraction (fabs). A prerequisite for the validity of this calculation is the complete metabolism of Cya in the liver. The hepatic extraction ratio (EH) is calculated as the ratio of the systemically available dose fraction (fa), to gastrointestinally absorbed dose fraction. Combination of EH with the systemic clearance (Cl) allows the calculation of the intrinsic clearance (Cli) and the liver blood flow (QH).

Cya	median	95% CI	
fa	0.30	0.10-0.46	
fabs	0.45	0.16-0.78	
EH	0.41	0.30-0.50	
Cl	0.39	0.27-0.47	L/h/kg
Cli	0.66	0.41-0.76	L/h/kg
QH	1.07	0.42-1.53	L/h/kg

Institut für Klinische Pharmakologie, Hindenburgdamm 30, D-1000 Berlin 45, *Chirurgische Klinik, Klinikum Rudolf Virchow, Berlin 19

217

INTERACTION OF THE IMMUNOSUPPRESSANT FK506 WITH CYTOCHROME P-450 ISOENZYMES

S. Bauer[1,2], J. Brockmöller[1], W.-O. Bechstein[3], H. Hüller[2], I. Roots[1]

FK506 is a new immunosuppressant which is similar in its mechanism of action, but about 50 times more potent than the cyclic polypeptide cyclosporin A (CyA). From its macrolide structure, interactions especially with cytochrome P-450IIIA isoenzymes can be anticipated.

Methods: Interactions of FK506 were studied with liver microsomes prepared from rat liver after pretreatment with ß-naphthoflavone, phenobarbital, and dexamethasone (Dx) and with microsomes prepared from human liver. The interactions were evaluated by differential spectroscopic analysis and by coincubations of FK506 with CyA and 7-ethoxyresorufin (7-ER). FK506 was studied between 1.2 nM and 600 nM by spectroscopy and between 4.8 nM and 4.8 μM in the enzymatic coincubations with CyA and 7-ER. CyA concentrations were 2-21 μM and 7-ER was between 5 nM and 5 μM.

Results: FK-506 showed, like cyclosporin A, type I binding spectra in all incubations. Spectral affinity constants (K_s) of FK506 were with rat liver microsomes after pretreatment with Dx 8 nM, ranging between 7 and 9 nM (n=5 preparations) and were in the similar range with human liver microsomes between 8 and 30 nM (n=3 different liver samples). For comparison, also CyA and erythromycin were investigated. K_s of CyA was considerably higher than that of FK506 with values around 1.0 μM (range: 0.5 to 1.4 μM) with rat liver microsomes. Erythromycin showed an even higher affinity than FK506 to these microsomes with K_s values between 2.3 and 6 nM. Inhibition of CyA metabolism by FK506 was quantified by K_i values between 50 and 200 nM, as tested in three different preparations of rat liver microsomes after Dx pretreatment. In contrast, FK506 exhibited less pronounced inhibition on 7-ER deethylation in the concentrations described above. The clinically promising immunosuppressant FK506 is shown to be a relatively selective inhibitor of cytochrome P-450IIIA isoenzymes, allowing to predict drug interactions especially with compounds (including CyA) metabolized via this isoenzyme.

[1]Institut für Klinische Pharmakologie, Klinikum Steglitz, Freie Universität Berlin, [2]Institut für Klinische Pharmakologie, Charité, Humboldt-Universität, and [3]Chirurgische Klinik, Klinikum Rudolf Virchow, Berlin, FRG.

218

OMEPRAZOLE INDUCES CYTOCHROME P-450 IA2 ACTIVITY IN CARRIERS OF THE CYTOCHROME P-450 IIC DEFICIENCY

L. Rost, H. Brösicke*, J. Brockmöller, M. Scheffler, H. Helge*, I. Roots

Omeprazole is a most potent gastric acid inhibitor binding to the proton pump in gastric parietal cells. Diaz et al. (Gastroenterology 1990; 99: 737) reported an increase of cytochrome P-450 IA1 and IA2 isoenzyme activity in human hepatic cell cultures and microsomes after omeprazole treatment. Specific mRNA was also increased. This inductive effect may be comparable to that of cigarette smoking. Caffeine N3-demethylation is specifically mediated by the P-450 IA2 isoenzyme (Butler et al., Proc Natl Acad Sci, USA 1989; 86: 7696). Induction of P-450 IA2 enzymes in vivo should thus be evidenced with the [13]C-[N3-methyl]-caffeine breath test by monitoring [13]CO_2 as the end product.

Oral doses of 40 mg omeprazole were administered for 7 days to 10 healthy volunteers (5 f, 5 m; 18-82, median 64 ys.). The caffeine breath test with 3 mg/kg ^{13}C-caffeine p.o. was performed three times: before, at the 7th dose, and one week after termination of omeprazole administration. Breath samples were collected during 8 h on each test day. The excess of ^{13}C was measured by mass spectrometry. Omeprazole and metabolite kinetics were followed at the 7th day of dosage by reversed-phase HPLC. The volunteers comprised 4 poor (PM) and 6 extensive metabolizers (EM) of mephenytoin (characterizing cytochrome P-450 IIC), who are also PMs and EMs for omeprazole. Mean elimination ($\pm$SD) as reflected by $AUC_{(0-8h)}$ of [13]CO_2 in all volunteers was 22.9 $\pm$ 9.5 % before, 26.1 $\pm$ 8.2 % after the 7th dose, and 22.6 $\pm$ 8.8 % one week after termination of omeprazole administration. Taking each individual as his own control, changes under omeprazole treatment were -9.8, -0.9, +11.3, +11.3, +13.1, and +27.4 % in EMs. All PMs responded with increased [13]CO_2-exhalation of +12.8, +23.6, +59.7, and +62.8 %. Mean AUCs of omeprazole in PMs were 5 times higher than in EMs. The EM with the highest increase of [13]CO_2-exhalation had the highest AUC of omeprazole in the EM-group. The data suggest that high omeprazole levels are necessary for a noticeable enzyme induction; such levels are mainly attained in carriers of the cytochrome P-450 IIC deficiency.

Institute of Clinical Pharmacology, Klinikum Steglitz, Free University of Berlin, Hindenburgdamm 30, D-1000 Berlin 45, *Clinic of Paediatrics, Klinikum Rudolf Virchow.

219

DETERMINATION OF ARYLAMINE N-ACETYLTRANSFERASE GENOTYPE IN HUMANS.
N. Drakoulis, M. Beland and I. Roots

Human arylamine N-acetyltransferase (NAT) plays an important role in biotransformation of drugs and other xenobiotics including carcinogens and is subject to genetic polymorphism. Among the European population genetically slow and fast acetylators distribute about equally. Lately, a restriction fragment length polymorphism (RFLP) was found that indicates the NAT genotype (Ohsako et al., J. Biol. Chem. 265, 4630, 1990). This allowed the development of specific genotyping procedures in humans. Acetylator phenotype was evaluated by quantifying 5-acetylamino-6-formylamino-3-methyluracil and 1-methylxanthine in 5h urine after caffeine ingestion. For genotype determination oligonucleotide primers were synthesized according to published NAT cDNA-sequence (Grant et al., Nucl. Acid. Res. 17, 3978, 1989) to produce a gene-probe by polymerase chain reaction (PCR) using genomic DNA from mononuclear cells as starting material. The NAT polymorphism was determined after hybridization of KpnI digested patient DNA by Southern-blot. Allele specific PCR was applied to determine a rare point-mutation (G_{857} to A) reported recently (Ohsako et al., 1990). The NAT gene-probe hybridization revealed 10 RFLPs. Phenotypically fast acetylators are represented by 15/5.2 kb (a), 19/15/5.2 kb (b), 15/5.2/4.6 kb (c), 19/15/8/5.8 kb (d), 19/15/5.2/4.6 kb (e), and 19/17/8/5.2 kb (f) patterns. Phenotypically slow acetylators show a 19 kb band (g), or 15/4.6 kb (h), 19/15/4.6 kb (i), and 19/15/8/4.6 kb (j) combinations. Pattern (a) seems to represent the homozygous fast acetylator, (g) one and (h) another homozygous mutation causing impaired acetylation. The remaining combinations represent the heterozygous status of either slow (i) or fast acetylators (b, c) or other not yet characterized mutations (d, e, f, j). These results are in conformity with previous findings indicating the existence of at least two different ways of acetylation activity impairment (Grant et al., J. Clin. Invest. 85, 968, 1990). Among 169 persons screened 4.8 % were heterozygous for the G_{857} to A mutation. So far no correlation between this point mutation and NAT expression could be established. RFLP-patterns (a) to (j) clearly indicate the slow and fast acetylator genotype determinable from human blood samples or any other tissue.

Institut für Klinische Pharmakologie, Freie Universität Berlin, Hindenburgdamm 30, D-1000 Berlin 45

220

PROPAFENONE N-DEALKYLATION IS MEDIATED BY CYTOCHROME P450IIIA3/4

S. Botsch, P. Beaune*, M. Eichelbaum and H.K. Kroemer

Propafenone is widely used in the treatment of cardiac arrhythmias. The drug undergoes extensive biotransformation to the active metabolites 5-hydroxypropafenone and N-desalkylpropafenone. Formation of 5-hydroxypropafenone is known to be mediated by cytochrome P450IID6 which exhibits a genetic polymorphism in man. As a consequence, propafenone interacts with drugs that are substrates for cytochrome P450IID6 (eg: metoprolol, quinidine). Propafenone, however, also interacts with compounds the metabolism of which is not mediated via cytochrome P450IID6 indicating that propafenone binds to other P450 isozymes as well. The isozyme involved in formation of N-desalkylpropafenone has not been identified and the interaction potential deriving from this pathway is unknown.

In order to characterize the isozyme involved in formation of N-desalkylpropafenone, we prepared microsomes of 9 human livers and screened them for their activity to N-dealkylate propafenone. High performance liquid chromatography was used for quantification of N-desalkylpropafenone.

The rate of formation of N-desalkylpropafenone was correlated to the cytochrome P450IIIA3/4 content of the individual livers as quantified by Western blotting (r= 0.75, p< 0.05). Specific antibodies against cytochrome P450IIIA3/4 inhibited 61.4% $\pm$ 13% of the N-dealkylation of propafenone. A highly significant correlation was observed for V_{max} of N-dealkylation of propafenone and V_{max} of N-dealkylation of verapamil which is mediated by P450IIIA3/4 (r = 0.94, p< 0.01). Moreover, verapamil was a competitive inhibitor of N-desalkylpropafenone formation (k_i 75 μM).

These data indicate the N-dealkylation of propafenone to be catalyzed by cytochrome P450IIIA3/4. Therefore, propafenone has the potential to interact with other drugs which are substrates (lidocaine, nifedipine, cyclosporine) or inducers (rifampicin) for this isozyme.

Supported by the Deutsche Forschungsgemeinschaft (Kr 945/2-1) and the Robert-Bosch-Stiftung.

Dr. Margarete Fischer-Bosch-Institut für Klinische Pharmakologie, Auerbachstraße 112, 7000 Stuttgart 50, Germany; *Inserm U75, CHU Necker-Enfants-Malades, rue de Vaugirard, 75730 Paris, France.

221

MODEL SUBSTANCES IN CHARACTERISATION OF LIVER BIO-
TRANSFORMATION REACTIONS - INFLUENCE OF INDOMETHA-
CIN THERAPY ON PATIENTS WITH LIVER CHIRRHOSIS AND
PATIENTS WITH NORMAL LIVER FUNCTION
M. Hippius, A. Hoffmann, M. Krauß, J. Truckenbrodt,
M. Reinhardt, K. Penzold, M. Gassel, K. Abendroth

The known effects of indomethacin on the liver are
few, although it has been listed as a drug of fre-
quent clinical use with known hepatotoxic potential. Therefore studies were performed to determine
the influence of indomethacin therapy on biotransformation reactions characterized by model substances in patients with liver cirrhosis and patients
with normal liver function. Additionally indomethacin kinetics was studied in all patients.
A cocktail of model substances was used to characterise various liver enzymes. Metamizol and caffeine were used for phenobarbital and for 3-methyl-
cholanthrene inducible cytochrome-P-450, respectively. The acetylation and hydroxylation phenotypes
were characterised using sulfadimedine and debrisoquine. The investigations were carried out in both
groups before drug administration and after two
weeks treatment with indomethacin.
There are not differences between the kinetic parameters after oral administration of indomethacin
in these two groups. No differences could be demonstrated between the two groups in acetylation
and hydroxylation phenotypes.
Because there are no differences between the kinetic parameters of caffeine and 4-monomethylamino-
pyrine before and after oral administration of indomethacin, it is believed that the reduced demethylation of the liver is compensated by other metabolic pathways.
Department of Clinical Pharmacology and Clinic
Internal Medicine, Friedrich Schiller University,
Bachstraße 18,0-6900 Jena, FRG

222

GALANTHAMINE O-DEMETHYLATION IN MAN
R. Bachus, T. Thomsen, U. Bickel, and H. Kewitz
Introduction: Galanthamine (GAL), a tertiary amine, chemically related to codeine, is currently investigated for treatment of senile dementia of Alzheimer's type. The 2 metabolites of GAL known, a stereoisomer epigalanthamine (EPI) and a presumed ketone intermediate galanthaminone, have been found only in negligible amounts in plasma of healthy volunteers in a recent phase-I-trial [Bickel et al., Clin.Pharmacol.Ther., in press]. The cumulated excretion of EPI in urine up to 72 h after application of GAL did not exceed 2 % of the administered oral and i.v. doses, and galanthaminone was detected only sporadically.
Methods: To elucidate the biotransformation of GAL, ion-pair-HPLC and fluorescence detection was used for the simultaneous determination of GAL, EPI, galanthaminone, O-demethyl-Galanthamine (ODG), and their putative glucuronides, according to Svensson et al. [J.Chromatogr. 230, 427-432, 1982], in plasma and urine samples of healthy volunteers. ODG was identified using purified standards and its respective glucuronide after hydrolysis with 1 M hydrochloric acid for 1 h at 100°C and after incubation with ß-glucuronidase for 24 h at 37°C, respectively. In addition, in vitro glucuronidation of ODG in human liver microsomes was performed and the respective glucuronide served as an internal standard.
Results: The recovery of GAL and its 3 metabolites, ODG, ODG-glucuronide and EPI in urine samples collected during 12 h was about 50% of the given i.v. doses of 20,25,35 mg GAL hydrobromide. O-demethylation accounted for approximately 50% of the total urinary recovery, in contrast to EPI, which accounted for only 1%. UV-absorbance of ODG showed the typical bathochromic shift indicating a free phenolic group. Most of ODG in urine, however, was conjugated with glucuronic acid, which resulted in a loss of the respective shift. We conclude that the significant route of metabolism of GAL in man involves its O-demethylation and subsequent glucuronidation of its phenolic OH group. This is similar to the metabolism of codeine to morphine-3-glucuronide.
Institute of Clinical Pharmacology, Free University of Berlin, Klinikum Steglitz, Hindenburgdamm 30, D-1000 Berlin 45, Germany.

223

IN VITRO INHIBITION OF HUMAN CHOLINESTERASES BY
O-DEMETHYL-GALANTHAMINE
T. Thomsen, R. Bachus, U. Bickel, and H. Kewitz
Introduction: Galanthamine (GAL), an alkaloid of the snowdrop, is a competitive inhibitor of human acetylcholinesterase (AChE) and rather selective on AChE as opposed to butyrylcholinesterase (BuChE). Stereoselectivity of the inhibitory effect was shown recently [Thomsen et al., Eur.J. Clin.Pharmacol. 39, 603-605, 1990] by demonstrating that GAL was 130-times as potent as its 2 metabolites reported, the diastereomer epigalanthamine (EPI) and the ketone galanthaminone. Additional metabolites of GAL in man, O-demethyl-galanthamine (ODG) and its glucuronide, have been identified in a recent study [Bachus et al., in preparation].
Methods: A series of concentration response experiments was performed to elucidate the inhibition of cholinesterases by ODG in plasma and erythrocytes of 8 healthy volunteers, and in post-mortem brain frontal cortex tissue of 6 individuals. ODG was used in the range of 10 nmol/l to 0.5 mmol/l after an in vitro incubation for 60 min at 25°C. The enzyme activity was measured radiometrically as published earlier in more detail.
Results: The inhibitor concentrations (μmol/l) of ODG producing a half maximal effect (IC_{50}) compared with GAL were:

	BuChE (Plasma)	AChE (Erythr.)	AChE (Brain)
ODG	24	0.12	0.50
GAL	14.1	0.36	3.24

Compared to the parent compound, the metabolite ODG appears about half as effective on BuChE, but 3 times more efficient on AChE in erythrocytes and 6-7 times more efficient in brain.
Conclusions: The inhibitory effect of ODG on AChE is more pronounced and about 10 times more selective than that of GAL, but due to rapid glucuronidation it may not contribute very much in the inhibition of cholinesterase after application of GAL.
Institute of Clinical Pharmacology, Free University of Berlin, Klinikum Steglitz, Hindenburgdamm 30, D-1000 Berlin 45, Germany.

224

PHARMACODYNAMIC AND PHARMACOKINETIC INTERACTION OF NISOL-
DIPINE AND PROPRANOLOL DURING STEADY-STATE CONDITIONS
H.G. Adelmann, R. Heinig, J. Kuhlmann
In a single-dose interaction study with propranolol and
nisoldipine fast release tablet the AUC values as well as
C_{max} of both drugs were increased in the combination
(LEVINE et al, 1988). The aim of our study was to investigate a possible interaction between propranolol and the
controlled-release formulation of nisoldipine (coat-core).
The study was conducted in a threefold, randomized, non-
blind crossover design with 12 male healthy volunteers
(age 18 - 40). Target parameters were assessed in each
period after 5-day treatment to achieve steady-state conditions. Doses administered were: nisoldipine 20 mg o.d.
or/and propranolol 40 mg t.i.d. Parameters of interest
were: heart rate, non-invasive blood pressure, ECG, C_{max},
t_{max}, $AUC_{0-\infty}$, AUC_{0-24}, $t_{\frac{1}{2}}$.
Results: ECG parameters were not altered in monotherapy or
combination. Nisoldipine had no marked effect on heart
rate and blood pressure. Propranolol effected a significant decrease in heart rate but had no marked influence on
blood pressure. In combination the effect on heart rate
was comparable to that of the propranolol monotherapy;
blood pressure was not affected. Kinetic evaluations
demonstrated a slight decrease (-14 %) in mean AUC_{0-24} of
propranolol when nisoldipine was administered concomitantly. Mean AUC_{0-24} and C_{max} of nisoldipine at steady-state
gained a slight increase (+ 7 %) in the combination with
propranolol. Overall, there were large interindividual
differences.
Our study evaluated no clinically relevant pharmacodynamic
or pharmacokinetic interaction between propranolol and
nisoldipine coat-core.

Address: Bayer AG, Pharma Research Center, Institute of
Clinical Pharmacology, Aprather Weg, 5600 Wuppertal 1, FRG

225

PHARMACOKINETICS AND -DYNAMICS OF VERAPAMIL ISOMERS AFTER ADMINISTRATION OF IMMEDIATE- AND SUSTAINED-RELEASE RACEMIC VERAPAMIL DOSAGE FORMS

A. Aschoff[1], G. Bühler[1], G. Hahn[2], W. Möhrke[3], E. Mutschler[2], J. Rosenthal[1], H. Spahn-Langguth[2]

The racemic mixture of R-(+)- and S-(-)-verapamil (V) is used in hypertension, ischemic heart disease and some forms of cardiac arrhythmias. A stereoselective first-pass effect was revealed in studies with pseudoracemic V using deuterated derivatives. The effects of V on atrioventricular conduction are closely related to the respective enantiomer plasma concentrations, whereas the relationship of the hypotensive/antiischemic effect and pharmacokinetics remains controversial. In addition the main metabolite norverapamil (NV) contributes to the effects of V. Therefore, the aim of this study was to compare plasma levels of V and NV enantiomers with the effects on PQ intervals and blood pressure reduction in hypertensive patients after administration of immediate- (i.r.) and sustained-release (s.r.) dosage forms. Hypertensive patients received 160 mg i.r. and 240 mg s.r. V for seven days in a randomized order with a drug-free period of 1 week between the treatments. On the first and the seventh day blood pressure, PQ time and plasma concentrations of V and NV enantiomers were measured over 24 hours. In order to assay low concentrations of V and NV enantiomers a sensitive and specific HPLC method was developed using a chiral stationary phase. V and NV enantiomers as well as the internal standard S-(-)propranolol were well separated. The intraday coefficients of variation were less than 10% at concentrations of 5 ng/ml or more of each enantiomer. The detection limits were less than 2 ng/ml (signal to noise ratio 5:1). C_{max} and PQ_{max} were reduced after the administration of s.r. V. Blood pressure reduction was independent of the respective drug dosage form. The S/R ratio of concentrations of V and NV enantiomers were 0.27 (confidence interval 0.24-0.30) and 0.45 (confidence interval 0.36-0.53), respectively. These ratios were independent of the respective total plasma concentration and did not change with time, dosage form, or duration of treatment. Thus, it can be hypothesized that the stereoselectivity of the first-pass effect is independent of the input rate.

[1]Sektion Pharmakotherapie der Universität , D-7900 Ulm, [2]Pharmakologisches Institut für Naturwissenschaftler der Universität, D-6000 Frankfurt/Main, and [3]Röhm Pharma, D-6108 Weiterstadt

226

COMPARISON OF THE EFFECTS (IN VIVO AND IN VITRO) OF ATROPINE IN CHILDREN AND ADULTS AFTER P.O. AND I.M. ADMINISTRATION

*C Volz-Zang, *T Waldhäuser, *B Schulte, **MH El Gindi, **P Rademacher, **HW Gervais and *D Palm

The effects of 30 µg/kg p.o. and 20 µg/kg i.m. administration of atropine on heart rate and salivary flow were compared in premedicated children (n=15 per administration) and healthy adult volunteers (n=7; crossover). In parallel plasma samples were taken to detect the in vitro occupancy of cardiac M₂-cholinoceptors (pig) by the atropine concentration equivalents present in plasma as determined by a radioreceptor assay (RRA).

Oral administration of 30 µg/kg atropine caused a slight but not significant increase of heart rate in children and adults. After i.m. administration of 20 µg/kg atropine heart rate increased significantly (mean max. effect: +18±5 bpm/+22±4 bpm) in children and adults, respectively.

The reduction of salivary flow was comparable in maximum values between oral and i.m. administration (84.3%/87.5%). The almost complete inhibition of salivary flow might be explained by a lower vagal tone at salivary glands in comparison to the heart.

The insignificant heart rate increase after oral administration of 30 µg/kg atropine was accompanied with a receptor occupancy near the detection limit. The distinct heart rate increase after i.m. administration of 20 µg/kg atropine corresponded with a receptor occupancy up to 62%. Therefore the effect on heart rate can be explained by the in vitro receptor occupancy. Thus, 30 µg/kg atropine p.o. were not equipotent to 20 µg/kg atropine i.m. This might be explained by an uncertain absorption after oral administration of atropine.

*Zentrum der Pharmakologie, Univ. Klinikum, Theodor Stern-Kai 7, 6000 Frankfurt/M. 70
**Klinik f. Anästhesiologie, Univ. Klinikum, Mainz

227

THE CLINICAL RELEVANCE OF HEMORHEOLOGICAL PROPERTIES OF PENTOXIFYLLINE ON SKIN FLAP SURVIVAL.

H. Dassow*, H.A. Vogel, and R. Schmidt

The study was assigned to ascertain whether the skin flap survival is affected by the administration of pentoxifylline(PE). We investigated the effects of PE on various hemorheological (whole blood viscosity under low shear conditions=WBV, plasma viscosity=PV, platelet aggregation=PA, red cell aggregation =RCD, red cell deformability=RCD, hematocrit=HT) and hemostasiological (fibrinogen=FG) factors. Clinical efficiency was determined by assessing the dehiscence distance in relation to the whole wound edge distance, the skin flap temperature and transcutaneous pO_2. Included into the study were 28 patients with random skin flaps to close defects in different face areas (either sex, age range 37-87 y). The patients were treated for 10 days with PE (400 mg t.i.d.,p.o.) or a placebo (PL) beginning at the 3rd pre-operative and ending at the 7th post-operative day in a controlled double-blind randomized trial. The PL group shows an increase in his FG levels (+27.9%) associated with an increase in PV (+3.9%) and RCA (+27.6%) and further an elevation of WBV (+9.8-18.1%). The FG levels in those taking PE did not change. PA in this group is inhibited (-23.6%) compared with the pretreatment level. Further we observed a fall in HT (-4.6%) and WBV (-14.8-24.3%) in these patients. All differences described were statistically significant (p<0.05). Associated with the more favourable hemorheological conditions the patients in the PE group show a promoted wound healing as assessed by the estimation of the dehiscence distance (PE:2.6% v. PL:8.8%). Transcutaneous pO_2 and temperature measurements reflect the promotive PE effect on flap vitality.

*Present address: Department of Clinical Pharmacology,University of Leipzig. Härtelstr. 16-18, O-7010 Leipzig, FRG

228

DO CURRENT TREATMENT REGIMENS APPROPRIATELY COUNTERACT THE HEMODYNAMIC ALTERATIONS UNDERLYING HYPERTENSION?

G.H. Koch and L. Fransson

The pathophysiology of hypertension with respect to hemodynamics is mainly characterized by increasing vascular resistance (TPR), increasing impairment of left ventricular (LV) systolic and diastolic function, decreasing cardiac output (CO) and reduction of renal blood flow (RBF). Any rational therapy should hence primarily aim at lowering TPR and left ventricular strain and maintaining CO and RBF. This report summarizes a series of hemodynamic studies in different groups of grade 1-2 hypertensive patients aged 42 to 65 years conducted during recent years with the purpose of evaluating how appropriately different antihypertensive regimens counteract the underlying hemodynamic pathophysiologic mechanisms. Emphasis was laid on also studying LV filling pressures (LVFP).

The regimens evaluated were: Clonidine, selective and unselective β-adrenoceptor blockade (metoprolol, sotasol, bisoprolol), slow calcium (Ca) channel blockade (nifedipine), combined α/β blockade (labetalol), combinations of β-receptor blockade with a Ca-antagonist (metoprolol-nifedipine), with a non-Ca-antagonist vasodilator (oxprenolol-hydralazine), with a diuretic (sotasol-chlorthalidon), ACE inhibition (captopril). Both acute and long-term studies were performed, both at rest and during steady state bicycle ergometer exercise. Blood pressures were measured both in the systemic and pulmonary arteries using percutaneously inserted catheters, CO was determined by the Fick principle, RBF by PAH-clearance.

Irrespective of selectivity, β-blockade as the only regimen reduces CO and RBF and fails to lower TPR and LVFP; it thus does not appropriately counteract the pathophysiologic hemodynamic derangement. The hemodynamic profile of β-blockade is not substantially improved by adjunction of hydralazine or chlorthalidon. Ca-blockade alone reduces TPR but increases adrenergic and cardiac activity. Conversely, the combination of a β-receptor blocker with an appropriate vasodilator, in particular a Ca- or α-receptor antagonist, as well as ACE inhibitors, correct or improve the hemodynamic profile including the renal circulation. They also reduce or tend to reduce LVFP. The combination regimens have the advantage that, in general, significantly lower doses of the respective components are needed to achieve equivalent blood pressure reductions thus reducing the risk of serious side effects such as metabolic derangements.

Department of Physiology, Free University, Arnimallee 22, D-1000 Berlin, FRG, and Department of Clinical Physiology, Central Hospital, Karlskrona, Sweden

229

PHOSPHORYLATION OF C-PROTEIN, TROPONIN I AND PHOS-PHORYLASE IN FAILING HUMAN HEART.
S. Bartel, E.-G. Krause, B. Stein*, W. Schmitz* and H. Scholz*

In congestive heart failure the rise in cAMP and con-tractile force (CF) induced either by isoprenaline (ISO) or phosphodiesterase inhibitors (PDEI) are weakened. This reduction can be reversed by a combination of both drugs. We studied the effect of ISO (0.2 µmol/l) and pimobendan (PIMO; 100 µmol/l) on CF and the in vivo phosphorylation (PHOS) of C-protein (CP), troponin I (TNI), and phosphorylase (Pase) in ventricular trabecu-lae isolated from explants of failing human heart (n=5; NYHA III/IV). CF was elevated by ISO and PIMO by about 85 % and 41 %, resp., but by ISO + PIMO to about 160 % (p < .05). In vitro back-PHOS of CP and TNI by cAMP-dependent protein kinase (in untreated tissue: 29.8 ± 1.9 (n=10), and 66.5 ± 6 pmol P/mg tissue protein (n=9),resp.) was reduced by 25 % or 19 % (p< .05) by ISO or PIMO alone and was even more reduced by ISO + PIMO (42 %) indicating an enhanced PHOS in vivo. In contrast, Pase activity reflecting both cAMP and Ca^{2+}-mediated proces-ses was increased from an activity ratio (-AMP/+AMP) of 0.13 ± 0.02 (n=10) in untreated tissue to values of 0.31 ± 0.04 (n=5) and 0.34 ± 0.03 (n=5) after exposure either to ISO and ISO + PIMO, resp. (p< .05).
The data show the in vivo PHOS of myofibrillar proteins and the glycogenolytic enzyme, Pase, in human heart tissue. We conclude that the enhanced increase in cAMP by combination of ISO + PIMO is reflected by enhanced in vivo PHOS of TNI and CP and could account for the increased CF of the failing heart.

Inst. für Herz-Kreislauf-Forschung, Robert-Rössle-Str. 10 0-1115 Berlin; *Abt. Allgem. Pharmakologie, Universi-täts-Krankenhaus Eppendorf, Martinistr. 52, W-2000 Hamburg

230

DETERMINATION OF LIPOIC ACID IN HUMAN PLASMA.
J. Teichert[†], F. Baumann and R. Preiss

The classical method of determination of lipoic acid was based upon microbiological assay. A gas chromatographic and a high-performance liquid chromatographic analysis have been recently developed but not for determination of lipoic acid plasma levels. In the present investigations a high-performance liquid chromato-graphic method has been developed for the determination of total alpha-lipoic acid concentration in human plasma. The samples were extracted with n-hexane/chloroform after hydrolysis in concentrated hydrochloric acid under nitrogen atmosphere over 6 hours and finally injected on a Nucleosil C18 reversed-phase column.
Lipoic acid was determined by electrochemical detection. For calibration the pure substance as external standard was used. Recovery of lipoic acid was 30.9 ± 1.8% for the concentration ranges studied. Values of correlation coefficients for 3 standard curves were 0.998.
Plasma levels of measured 7 healthy volunteers (blood donors) range from 12.3 to 31.6 ng/ml. These data are consistent with published lipoic acid plasma concentrations obtained by other methods.
In equilibrium existing reduced dihydrolipoic acid is oxidized into lipoic acid during hydrolysis.

[†]Present address: Department of Clinical Pharmacology, Univer-sity of Leipzig, Härtelstr. 16-18, O-7010 Leipzig, FRG

231

RATIONAL USE OF AMPICILLIN: PHARMACOKINETIC CONSIDERATIONS V. Vlahov*, V. Kirkov*, Z. Gerova*, Markova*, R. Koytchev

The aim of this study was to investigate the ampicillin plasma concentrations after oral administration of a single dose of 750 mg. The comparison of the plasma concentrations with the MIC 90 for the most common pathogenic microorganisms could be used as a prognostic criterion for the effectiveness of antimicrobial therapy.

11 healthy oral volunteers participated in the study. Two liquid oral ampicillin German standard formulations were administered. Blood samples were taken before and at 15, 30, 45, 60, 90, 120, 150, 180, 240, and 300 min after the medication. The plasma concentrations were determined using an HPLC technique. There were no differences in the C_{max}, T_{max} and AUC of both preparations. The ampicillin concentrations after one of the preparations are shown in the following table:

Time period: (min)	15	30	45	60	90	120	150	180	240
Mean (µg/ml)	1.3	2.3	3.2	3.4	3.1	2.8	2.6	2.5	1.7
S.D.	0.2	0.9	1.1	1.4	1.6	1.3	0.9	0.5	0.4

The C_{max} is lower than the MIC 90 for E. coli, Proteus vulgaris, Klebsiella spec. and Enterobacter spec. The results illustrate that a daily dose of 3 g ampicillin could not be sufficient for effective antimicrobial therapy.

*Present address: Chair of Clinical Pharmacology, Medical Academy, Belo More str.8, 1040 Sofia, Bulgaria.
Cooperative Clinical Drug Research and Development, Edisonstrasse 63, O-1160 Berlin, FRG.

232

ASSESSMENT OF ANTINOCICEPTIVE EFFECTS IN MAN: COMPARISON OF IMIPRAMINE, TRAMADOL, AND ANPIRTOLINE
T. Hummel, C. Hummel, I. Friedel, and G. Kobal

The aim of the study was to compare the pain relieving properties of the three drugs, imipramine, tramadol, and anpirtoline. The investigational drug anpirtoline exhibits analgesia which is possibly mediated via serotonergic pathways in the CNS, whereas tramadol exerts its effects at opioid receptors. In the case of the antidepressant imipramine it is unclear, whether there is a genuine antinociceptive effect at all, despite its widespread use in pain therapy. The four fold-cross over, double blind, randomized, and controlled study was approved by the local ethics committee. 15 healthy, trained volunteers participated in four experiments. Drugs and placebo were administered orally (anpirtoline: 60 mg; tramadol: 150 mg; imipramine: 100 mg). Pain-related chemosomatosensory evoked potentials (CSSEP) were recorded after painful stimulation of the nasal mucosa with carbon dioxide. Subjects rated the perceived intensity of the stimuli by means of a visual analogue scale. In addition, acoustically evoked responses were recorded, the spontaneous EEG was analyzed in the frequency domain, and the subjects' performance was tested in a simple tracking task on a computer monitor. Moreover, side effects of the drugs were assessed. Anpirtoline and tramadol produced a significant decrease of both, CSSEP amplitudes and subjects' estimates. However, the analgesic effect of anpirtoline was more pronounced compared to tramadol. In contrast, after administration of imipramine no change of CSSEP amplitudes could be detected, whereas intensity estimates decreased significantly. This was accompanied by a significant decrease of arousal indicating that, in the case of imipramine, pain relief was majorily based on sedation. In conclusion, CSSEP may be a useful tool to differentiate between antinociceptive and sedative effects.

Department of Pharmacology and Toxicology, University of Erlangen-Nürnberg, Universitätsstr. 22, W-8520 Erlangen, FRG

233

B-HT 920 AND EMD 49980 - NOVEL DOPAMINE AUTORECEPTOR AGONISTS IN THE TREATMENT OF PATIENTS WITH SCHIZOPHRENIA

K.Wiedemann, A.Loycke, M.Kellner, J.-C. Krieg, and F.Holsboer

In an open clinical trial the azepine derivative B-HT 920 (6-allyl-2-amino-5,6,7,8-tetrahydro-4H-thiazolo-(4,5-d)-azepine) was administered to patients suffering from schizophrenia, paranoid type (according to ICD-9 and DSM-III R criteria), to examine whether dopamine autoreceptor stimulation exerts antipsychotic effects, as can be assumed by clinical studies with low dosed apomorphine. Twelve patients participated in the study and received the test drug orally for up to 28 days in a dose range from 0.3 to 1.2 mg/day. The following results emerged: in four patients a significant amelioration (reduction of the initial BPRS score by 50 % or more) of psychotic symptomatology was observed; eight patients remained without improvement of psychopathology. Psychomotor activation was observed in seven patients, and prompted termination of the trial in two cases. No other marked adverse effects including extrapyramidal symptoms were noted. Plasma prolactin concentrations were significantly reduced two hours after oral application of a single dose of the drug. - Since B-HT 920 has marked activating effects, which could be due at least in part to postsynaptic dopamine receptor stimulation, we applied in a further study the compound EMD 49980 (5-hydroxy-3-(4-phenyl-1,2,3,6-tetrahydropyridil-(1)-butyl)-indol), a dopamine autoreceptor agonist with very low postsynaptic potency. - EMD 49980 was administered in an open clinical trial to patients suffering from schizophrenia (according to ICD-9 and DSM-III R criteria), who showed predominantly negative symptoms. Ten patients participated in the study and received the test drug orally for up to 28 days in a dose range from 0.5 to 9.0 mg/day. In four patients a significant amelioration (reduction of the initial SANS score by 40 % or more) of negative symptoms was observed; one patient improved slightly, four patients remained without improvement of psychopathology. Worsening of psychotic symptomatology was observed in one patient. Treatment with EMD 49980 did not lead to any extrapyramidal symptoms which are characteristic for traditional neuroleptics. As already seen from B-HT 920, plasma prolactin concentrations dropped four hours after oral application of a single dose of the EMD 49980.Both compounds seem to have activating properties. It remains to be clarified whether the observed effects are related to dopamine autoreceptor stimulation, postsynaptic dopamine receptor effects or interaction with other neurotransmitter systems.

Max-Planck-Institute of Psychiatry, Kraepelinstraße 10, 8000 München, FRG

234

ß-CARBOLINES AS BIOLOGICAL MARKERS OF DRUG- AND ALCOHOL-DEPENDENCE

H. ROMMELSPACHER, S. LUTTER

The search for biological markers has been intensified since a genetic component of alcoholic risk had been established. Offspring of alcoholics are approx. five times more likely to develop alcohol-related problems than offspring of nonalcoholics (Pickens et al. Arch Gen Psychiat 48, 19, 1991). Biological trait-markers as well as so-called residual-markers in alcoholics and drug-dependent subjects might be useful for the understanding of the pathogenesis of dependence and the processes underlying the "point of no return" (Coper et al. Drug Alc Dep. 25, 129, 1990). We have found that norharman, an endogenous ß-carboline, is elevated in the blood plasma of alcoholics (n = 42) admitted to a psychiatric clinic. In a subgroup of alcoholics with delirium or hallucinosis, a slight increase of norharman during detoxication could be detected (p = 0.07; Rommelspacher et al., Alcohol Clin Exp Res 15, 1991). In a following study with heroin addicts (n = 11) an increased plasma concentration of norharman was detected as well. Also in 3 patients with an abuse history of cannabis increased levels of norharman were found   the day of admission to a psychiatric hospital. The concentration normalized in 1 patient but not in the others. The changes seem to correlate with the duration of abuse. As longer the drug has been abused as longer the levels of norharman remain elevated. The findings suggest that after the point of no return the levels don't return to normal concentrations. In this case norharman could be regarded as a residual-marker. We have some evidence that norharman modulates mesolimbic dopaminergic mechanisms which are part of the reward system. Since chronic intake of ethanol, opioids, and cannabis leads to an increased concentration of norharman, those changes might play a role for the initiation and maintenance of alcoholism and drug dependence.

Supported by DFG, AZ: HE 916/7-1.

Dept. Neuropsychopharmacology, Free University, Ulmenallee 30, 1000 Berlin 19

235

IN VITRO EFFECTS OF ETHANOL ON THE CHARACTERISTICS OF MONOAMINE OXIDASE (MAO, EC 1.4.3.4) IN PLATELETS OF ALCOHOLICS

T. May, S. Strauß, H. Damm, H. Rommelspacher

Recently Tabakoff et al. investigated the effect of 400 mM ethanol on the MAO activity of platelets (The New England Journal of Medicine 318, 134-139, 1988) from alcoholics and controls. They found a stronger inhibition in alcoholics with one substrate concentration ([^{14}C]phenylethylamine, 12 uM). The aim of the present study is to analyse the observed changes of the sensitivity of the MAO towards ethanol (K_m, V_{max}, type of inhibition, protein-dependence, 6 substrate concentrations instead of 2 etc.). Furthermore, a long-term study was designated to reveal whether the changes occur during the intoxication and withdrawal period only (state-marker) or remain detectable 3 and 6 months later (trait- and/or residual-marker).

The fluorometric assay for MAO activity demonstrated by utilizing kynuramine as substrate and potent and selective inhibitors of subtype A (clorgyline, brofaromine) and subtype B (L-deprenyl, pargyline) that human platelets contain MAO-B only. Ethanol acts as a competitive antagonist and has an apparent Ki of 270 mM. A significant increase of the Michaelis-constant (K_m) is detectable with 25 mM ethanol and higher concentrations.

In the clinical study we performed Lineweaver-Burk analyses in the presence and absence of 200 mM ethanol. This concentration induced a significant increase of the K_m of MAO in each group (p < 0.001): Controls (n = 10) about 68 %, patients before withdrawal (n = 15) 56 % and patients at the end of the withdrawal period 85 %. There were no significant differences concerning the K_m-values of the three groups, either with or without ethanol. The V_{max}-values showed no changes in all three groups in the presence of ethanol. However in the alcoholics before withdrawal the V_{max} were about 32 % lower than after one week withdrawal (p < 0.01) and about 30 % lower than in the control group (p < 0.05), regardless if ethanol was present or not. Whether the observed changes can serve as state-marker or trait-marker for alcoholism remains to be proved at the end of the study.

Supported by DFG, AZ: He 916/7-1.

Dept. of Neuropsychopharmacology, Free University, Ulmenallee 30, 1000 Berlin 19

236

DOUBLE-BLIND COMPARISON OF A COMBINATION ANALGESIC CONTAINING PARACETAMOL PLUS ACETYLSALICYLIC ACID PLUS CAFFEINE VS. PLAIN PARACETAMOL IN DENTAL SURGERY

D. Hellenbrecht and W.J. Müller

About 50% of dental prescriptions of analgesic drugs in Germany comprise combinations of 250 mg paracetmol plus 250 mg acetylsalicylic acid plus 50 mg caffeine. We compared this combination in a randomized double-blind closed sequential paired analysis with 500 mg of plain paracetamol in dental outpatients. They were medicated immediately before surgery, i.e. after onset of local anesthesia. Pain intensity was recorded hourly over four hours on two separate scales: (a) on a 100 mm visual analog scale and (b) on a five step verbal rating scale (VRS). The sums of pain intensity of each scale were used as parameters of analgesic efficacy among the paired patients. The null hypothesis of no difference between the two treatments with given 2α- (p=0.05) and 2β- (p=0.05) level was confirmed by the data of VAS after 20 treatment pairs. The data of the VRS (30 pairs) even tended to be in favor of plain paracetamol. The study was stopped then because of too many "ties" within this scale. There were several complaints of drowsiness reported from patients receiving the combination analgesic, but none after plain paracetamol.

Our results show that the analgesic efficacy of the combination used was at best additive:

1 + 1 < 2.

We conclude that in dental postsurgical pain plain paracetamol should be preferred over such combinations as those tested in our study.

Centre Pharmacol, Univ Clinics, Theodor-Stern-Kai 7, W-6000 Frankfurt/Main, GFR

237

CHRONOPHARMACOKINETICS OF RANITIDINE - A CROSSOVER STUDY
I.Mai, S.Unger, H.-G.Trautsch-Förster, H.Hüller

The circadian variations in gastric acid output are known. Different therapeutic schemes for ranitidine treatment take this variability into account. The aim of the study was to investigate the pharmacokinetic behaviour of a single dose of 150mg ranitidine after morning (7.00 a.m.) or evening (7.00 p.m.) administration to 12 healthy male subjects.
For the extent of absorption we estimated the area under the curve ($AUC_{0-\infty}$) and for the rate of absorption the maximum concentration and the plateau time of ranitidine in plasma. For each of the characteristic parameters we evaluated the ratio (percent) of morning and evening value with its confidence intervals (parametric and nonparametric). From the morning administration ranitidine seems to be absorbed faster and reaches higher peaks, the plateau time is somewhat shorter compared with evening administration. This interesting tendency requires further attention with increased sample size and correlation with pharmacodynamic parameters.

Institute of Clinical Pharmacology, Department of Medicine (Charité), Humboldt-University, Schumannstr. 20-22, O-1040 Berlin, Germany

238

LACK OF DIURNAL AND SEASONAL RHYTHMS OF N-ACETYLATION CAPACITY IN MAN
T. Riedel, W. Siegmund, G. Franke, S. Riedel

N-acetylation of isoniazid and procainamide in rats was found to be dependent on circadian rhythms (Bruguerolle, J Pharm Pharmacol 37: 654, 1985, Belanger, Drug Metab Dispos 17: 91, 1989). The following pharmacokinetic study in 8 male healthy slow acetylators (SA, 23-24 years, 63-78 kg) and 8 male rapid acetylators (RA, 20-29 years, 64-85 kg) was performed to describe variations of the metabolic fate of antipyrine (AP, 15 mg/kg bw, po) and sulfamethazine (SM, 500 mg, po) between day (07.00 a.m.) and night (07.00 p.m./SA and RA) as well as spring (March) and autumn (October/only RA). AP in serum and SM and its metabolite N-acetylsulfamethazine (AcSM) in serum and urine were measured photometrically according to Brodie et al. and Bratton/ Marshall, resp.
No marked seasonal and circadian variations of SM (Table) and AP were found in RA (* P<0.05)

SM-kinetics (RA)		day/spring	night	autumn
t_{max}	[h]	1.27±0.45	1.41±0.48	1.74±0.73*
c_{max}	[/ug/ml]	18.6±4.7	17.8±6.5	16.3±5.3
$t_{1/2}$	[h]	2.48±0.47	2.53±0.66	2.36±0.39
V_d	[l/kg]	0.22±0.02	0.22±0.06	0.21±0.03
Cl_{met}	[ml/kg/min]	1.00±0.24	0.84±0.17	0.98±0.32
AUC	[/ug*h/ml]	113±24	115±17	111±12

There were also no differences of SM- and AP-kinetics in SA between day and night. Further, no associations between acetylator status and elimination rates of AP could be found.

Dept. Clin. Pharmacol., University of Greifswald, Fleischmannstr., D O-2200 Greifswald

239

ENANTIOSELECTIVE METABOLISM OF AMITRIPTYLINE AND NORTRIPTYLINE IN RELATION TO CYTOCHROME P450 IID6 ACTIVITY IN MAN
U. Breyer-Pfaff, B. Pfandl, K. Nill, E. Nusser, C. Monney*, M. Jonzier-Perey*, D. Baettig* and P. Baumann*

Prior to amitriptyline (AT) therapy, 26 patients with major depression were phenotyped as extensive or poor metabolizers (EM or PM) via cytochrome P450 IID6 by measuring dextromethorphan and its oxidative metabolite dextrorphan in urine after a single oral dose. On day 8 of treatment with AT (150 mg/day), patients collected 24-h urine that was analysed for AT metabolites including the enantiomers of E- and Z-10-hydroxyamitriptyline and -nortriptyline (E- and Z-10-OH-AT and -NT). Though one patient only was classified as PM, there were highly significant negative correlations between the log metabolic ratio (log MR, dextromethorphan/dextrorphan) and the percent E-isomer in 10-OH-AT and -NT. This is in accordance with data on E- and Z-10-hydroxylation of NT in EM and PM volunteers (Mellström et al., Clin. Pharmacol. Ther. 30, 189, 1981). In addition, the log MR was highly correlated with the percent (-)-enantiomer in unconjugated and conjugated E-10-OH-NT and in conjugated E-10-OH-AT (r between - 0.8 and - 0.9). The enantiomer composition of Z-10-OH-NT was not correlated with the log MR. This indicates that the hydroxylation reaction in (-)-E-10-position of AT and NT which is the preferred reaction in EM subjects is dependent on cytochrome P450 IID6 to a larger extent than hydroxylations in the three other positions.
The same conclusion was arrived at when 4 volunteers with EM status took 25 mg NT without and with concomitant quinidine administration and urine collected within 72 h was analysed. Quinidine, a specific blocker of cytochrome P450 IID6, selectively reduced the production of (-)-E-10-OH-NT, while the excreted quantities of the (+)-enantiomer and of (-)- and (+)-Z-10-OH-NT were unchanged or increased. The excretion of the phenol 2-OH-NT was reduced by quinidine.

Institut für Toxikologie der Universität, D-W-7400 Tübingen, *Clinique Psychiatrique Universitaire, CH-1008 Prilly-Lausanne

240

TISSUE DISTRIBUTION AND INDUCTION OF HEPATIC ETHOXYRESORUFIN O-DEETHYLASE ACTIVITY IN RATS AFTER INTRAVENOUS ADMINISTRATION OF 2,3,7,8-TETRACHLORODIBENZO-P-DIOXIN.
Keisuke Yamashita, Georg Golor, Klaus Abraham, Ralf Krowke, and Diether Neubert.

Several polyhalogenated dibenzo-p-dioxins and dibenzofurans (especially those with > 6 Cl-atoms) are poorly absorbed orally. 2,3,7,8-Tetrachlorodibenzo-p-dioxin (TCDD) has been shown to be well absorbed after s.c.-injection (Abraham et al. Arch Toxicol 62:359, 1988), but maximal concentrations and effects were not observed earlier than 3 days after the application. We have therefore attempted to inject ^{14}C-TCDD i.v. (100 μl/rat in corn oil/0.9% NaCl-emulsion, 1+9 v/v) and compared TCDD concentrations and activity of ethoxyresorufin O-deethylase (EROD) with those seen after s.c.-injection. Highest TCDD concentrations were found in liver (Table).

300 ng TCDD/kg body wt	i.v.	s.c.
	Mean ± S.D.	
TCDD concentrations:		
peak (liver) after	3 hrs	3 days
peak in liver (ng/g)	4.5 ± 1.1	4.7 ± 0.9
peak (adipose tissue) after	1 week	1 week
peak in adipose tissue (ng/g)	0.9 ± 0.1	0.8 ± 0.1
peak in thymus (ng/g)	0.6 ± 0.1	----
hepatic EROD activity:		
peak after	1 day	7 days

Our data indicate that biological effects of TCDD can be assessed after i.v.-injection if rapid absorption is required for the study. Furthermore, EROD activities correlated well with target tissue (hepatic) concentrations regardless of the route of administration. However, TCDD concentrations in the brain were found to be very low (< 0.1 ng TCDD/g wet weight), also after i.v.-injection.

Supported by the grant # 07VDX019 from the Federal Ministry for Research and Technology (BMFT). Institut für Toxikologie und Embryopharmakologie, Freie Universität Berlin, Garystr. 5, 1000 Berlin 33, Germany

241

ON THE GLUCURONIDATION OF HIGHER ALIPHATIC ALCOHOLS
S.Iwersen, A.Schmoldt, C.Augustin,

Only little is known about the metabolism of higher aliphatic alcohols which are usually present in many alcoholic drinks in much lower concentrations than ethanol. Besides oxidation reactions which lead to aldehydes, ketones, and carboacids conjugation reactions like glucuronidation and sulfation have to be considered as important metabolic pathways.
The aim of the present study was to investigate the glucuronidation of some higher aliphatic alcohols by rat liver UDP-glucuronosyltransferases (UDP-GT).
Kinetic constants like K_M- and V_{max}-values were determined by means of Lineweaver Burk plots. Obviously, the affinity of the alcohols to microsomal UDP-GTs depends on their chain-length, hexanol and heptanol exhibiting lower K_M-values than butanols and pentanols.
The glucuronidation of the alcohols could not be increased by inducing the animals with phenobarbital or 5,6-benzoflavone.
When different UDP-GT enzyme forms were separated by chromatofocusing chromatography activities toward testosterone and toward 3-methyl-butanol or hexanol-1 coeluted, thus leading to the conclusion that the 17β-OH-steroid-GT mainly is responsible for the glucuronidation of higher aliphatic alcohols.

Institut für Rechtsmedizin der Universität Hamburg, Butenfeld 34, D-2000 Hamburg 54, FRG.

242

DEVELOPMENT OF A CAPSULE FOR BUCCAL APPLICATION OF NICOTINE
C. Conze, G. Scherer and F. Adlkofer

A gelatine capsule has been developed which releases 4 mg nicotine in 0.8 ml of an alkaline (pH 10) buffer solution into the mouth after breaking the capsule's wall (Conze et al (1991), In: 'Effects of Nicotine on Biological Systems'; Birkhäuser Verlag, pp 63-68)]. Administration of this capsule to smokers and non-smokers produced peak nicotine plasma levels of 4 to 10 ng/ml within 10 min. Heart rate and blood pressure slightly increased and fingertip temperature slightly decreased after capsule application. Detection of the excretion of major nicotine metabolites in urine suggests that about 1 mg of nicotine was buccally absorbed form one capsule. The capsule was well tolerated. No differences were observed between smokers and non-smokers with respect to pharmacokinetics, physiological and subjective responses. Although a relatively fast buccal absorption of the alkaloid was obtained, the attained plasma levels and cardiovascular responses after the use of one capsule were much lower than those after smoking a cigarette. To obtain a higher nicotine plasma concentration, the capsule buffer concentration was increased yielding pH 9-10 saliva for 4 min following administration. The use of this capsule increased the nicotine plasma level to 10-15 ng/ml. When a second capsule was administered 15 min later, the nicotine plasma level was further increased to 20-30 ng/ml producing similar levels to those found in smokers. Nicotine uptake, which is similar to that achieved on smoking may be useful for the investigation of the alkaloid's role in smoking behaviour as well as for therapeutic studies.

Analytisch-biologisches Forschungslabor Prof. Dr. F. Adlkofer, Goethestr. 20, 8000 München 2, Germany

243

INCREASED COTININE ELIMINATION AND METABOLISM BY PHENOBARBITAL INDUCTION IN RAT
H. Foth, J. Aubrecht, M. Höhne, H. Neurath, and G.F. Kahl

Estimation of nicotine exposure during active or passive smoking by monitoring the nicotine plasma concentrations is hindered by the fast metabolic elimination of nicotine. Usually, the main metabolite of nicotine, cotinine, is used as a parameter of nicotine consumption or abstinence. We studied the kinetics and metabolic fate of cotinine in phenobarbital (PB)-induced and non-induced isolated perfused rat lung and liver as well as in isolated hepatocytes of rats.
The clearance of ^{14}C-cotinine was low in isolated rat lung (0.16 $\pm$ 0.04 ml/min) compared to the values of liver (0.57 $\pm$ 0.05 ml/min). Although the rat lung is known to metabolize nicotine very effectively the pulmonary activity to convert the metabolite cotinine is relatively low. The pulmonary kinetics of cotinine were not affected by pretreatment with PB while the hepatic parameters were increased 8fold. The latter effect was paralleled by an increased formation of cotinine-N-oxide. Only trace amounts of trans-3'-hydroxy-cotinine were found in the perfusate of non-induced as well as PB-induced livers. In isolated hepatocytes obtained from PB-treated rats the rate of cotinine conversion to cotinine-N-oxide was increased 3 - 4fold. After addition of 100 μM metyrapone the formation of cotinine-N-oxide returned to control levels. The results indicate that the N-oxidation of cotinine is markedly induced by PB which is of importance for the use of cotinine as a parameter of nicotine consumption.

Department of Pharmacology and Toxicology, University of Göttingen, D 3400 Göttingen, FRG.

244

INFLUENCE OF SMOKING AND ORAL CONTRACEPTIVES ON THE PHARMACOKINETICS AND ANALGESIC EFFICACY OF S(+)-IBUPROFEN IN FEMALE VOLUNTEERS.
J. Warnecke, R. Pentz, and C.-P. Siegers

S(+)-ibuprofen is the pharmacologically-active enantiomere of racemic ibuprofen. In 24 female volunteers (age range: 18-40 y) with primary dysmenorrhea the influence of smoking (> 10 cig/die) and oral contraceptives on the pharmacokinetics and analgesic properties of 200 mg S(+)-ibuprofen-lysinate was investigated. Smoking did not alter the bioavailability of S(+)-ibuprofen as compared to non-smokers. Intensity of pain (IP value) was initially higher in smokers as compared to non-smokers; in both groups (n=12 each) a marked decrease of the IP values (<10% of initial value) was observed between 1 an 6 hrs after drug intake. In patients taking oral contraceptives (n=12) significant differences in the pharmacokinetic parameters were found: Maximum plasma concentration (t_{max}) was reached already at 25 min as compared to 45 min in patients without contraceptive treatment, half-life of the terminal elimination phase was shorter (1.71 h vs 2.06 h) and oral bioavailability was reduced (AUC-values: 45.7 vs 65.1 mg/l x 12 h). Patients taking contraceptives again showed a higher initial IP value as compared to those without contraceptives; in both groups S(+)-ibuprofen caused a prompt and long-lasting (up to 6 hrs) reduction of pain (<10% of initial IP value). These investigations indicate a significant influence of oral contraceptives on the bioavailability of S(+)-ibuprofen, probably as a consequence of an induction of microsomal-drug-metabolizing enzymes; however, these effects on the pharmacokinetics of S(+)-ibuprofen did not alter the analgesic efficacy.

Institut für Toxikologie der Medizinischen Universität zu Lübeck, Ratzeburger Allee 160, 2400 Lübeck

245

DOES HYDROCHLOROTHIAZIDE INFLUENCE THE PHARMACOKINETICS OF ENALAPRIL IN ELDERLY PATIENTS ?   K. Weisser, J. Schloos, S. Jakob, W. Mühlberg, D. Platt, and E. Mutschler

In a randomised cross-over study including 19 elderly hypertensive patients (aged 62-84 years, BP_{syst} > 160 mm Hg, BP_{diast} > 100 mm Hg, CL_{cr}: from 93.2 to 11.0 ml·min^{-1}) the pharmacokinetics of the ACE inhibitor enalapril was compared after a single oral dose of either 10 mg enalapril alone (I) or 10 mg enalapril + 25 mg hydrochlorothiazide (HCTZ) (II).
Similar to the observations with elderly healthy subjects (1), after treatment I AUCo->24h (mean ± SD: 1062 ± 822 ng·h·ml^{-1}), C_{max} (86.8 ± 46.5 ng·ml^{-1}), and t_{max} (6.0 ±2.6 h) of enalaprilat were higher and CL_{ren} (62.0 ± 43.7 ml·min^{-1}) was smaller than it is described for young healthy subjects (1). Correspondingly, after both treatments AUCo->24h was closely related to the individual renal function (CL_{cr}).
After II compared to I, AUCo->24h (1330 ± 1018 ng·h·ml^{-1}, p<0.05) and C_{max} (102.9 ± 65.2 ng·ml^{-1}) of enalaprilat were increased, CL_{ren} (42.6 ± 37.8 ml·min^{-1}, p<0.05) was decreased whereas t_{max} (6.1 ± 2.2 h) was unaffected. These changes occurred independent of the individual degree of renal impairment. The increased serum levels of enalaprilat after II were completely reflected by the corresponding values of serum ACE inhibition.
For enalapril, C_{max} (II vs. I: 124.7 ± 60.2 vs. 119.4 ± 53.0 ng·ml^{-1}), t_{max} (1.4 ± 0.6 vs. 1.1 ± 0.7 h), AUCo->∞ (270 ± 235 vs. 289 ± 221 ng·h·ml^{-1}), and k_{el} (1.14 ± 0.52 vs. 1.06 ± 0.62 h^{-1}) were similar in both treatments.
In conclusion, the coadministration of 25 mg HCTZ to 10 mg enalapril in elderly hypertensives lead to a decrease in renal clearance of enalaprilat resulting in higher serum levels. This might be either due to an initial reduction in GFR by HCTZ or to an interference in tubular secretion of both drugs. Whether this observation is persistent after chronic treatment requires further examination.
(1) Hockings et al. 1986, Br. J. clin. Pharmac. 21, 341-348

Zentrum der Pharmakologie, Klinikum der J.W.-Goethe-Universität, Theodor-Stern-Kai 7, D-6000 Frankfurt/M.

246

INVESTIGATIONS ON THE KINETICS OF 5-FLUOROURACIL AND FOLINIC ACID IN THE PRESENCE OF INTERFERON ∝-2 B ON TUMOR PATIENTS

F.Baumann, M.Matthias, E,.D.Kreuser, and R.Preiss*

A HPLC method for the simultaneous elimination of 5-fluorouracil (5-FU) and folinic acid in the plasma of tumor patients was developed. RP 18 columns (4.6 mm x 25 cm) were used for a gradient operation with bromodeoxyuridine as internal standard for 5-FU estimation. The components were detected at 280 nm. Patients with colon carcinoma received a 3-4 hour intravenous infusion of 5-FU in the presence and absence of interferon ∝-2 B preceded by a bolus injection of leucovorin one hour before the start of the 5-FU infusion. The first results without coadministration of interferon ∝-2 B showed a steady state plasma concentration for 5-FU from 3 to 6 µM and an elimination half-life in the range from 4 to 10 minutes. The elimination half-life of folinic acid ranged from 4 to 6 hours.

*Present address: Department of Clinical Pharmacology, University of Leipzig, Härtelstr. 16-18, O-7010 Leipzig, FRG

247

PHARMACOKINETICS OF COUMARIN AND ITS METABOLITES AFTER INTRAVENOUS AND PERORAL ADMINISTRATION OF HIGH DOSE COUMARIN IN NORMAL HUMAN VOLUNTEERS.
S. Sharifi, E. Lotterer, H.C. Michaelis, J. Bircher

Coumarin (1,2-benzopyrone) in high oral doses either as a single agent or in combination with cimetidine has demonstrated antitumor activity in vivo against human malignant melanoma and renal cell carcinoma (Marshall et al., J Clin Oncol 5(6):862, 1987; Zänker et al., Drugs Exp Clin Res X(11):767, 1984).
In order to clarify the pharmacokinetics of coumarin and its metabolites 7-hydroxycoumarin (7-HC), 7-hydroxycoumarin glucuronide (7-HCG) and 3-hydroxycoumarin (3-HC) after high dose administration, we evaluated the bioavailability and disposition of coumarin and its metabolites in human volunteers.
Ten healthy, male subjects were given 1 g and 2 g coumarin p.o. or 250 mg coumarin i.v. on three randomized testdays after an overnight fast. No food or drink was permitted for 2 h after dosing. Venous blood samples (10 ml) were obtained through an indwelling cannula immediately before and during 6 h after the dose. All subjects collected urine for 48 h after coumarin administration. Plasma concentrations of coumarin, 7-HC and 7-HCG and urine concentrations of 7-HC, 7-HCG and 3-HC were determined by high-performance liquid chromatography.
The plasma coumarin concentration-time profiles after i.v. administration of 250 mg showed two phases of elimination. The median terminal half-life was 97 min (range:56-200 min). Coumarin was rapidly metabolized to 7-HC and 7-HCG. The maximal plasma concentrations of these metabolites were reached after about 18 min respectively. However the plasma concentrations of 7-HCG were 10fold higher than those of 7-HC (median peak concentration of 7-HC: 760 ng/ml, range: 550-2050 ng/ml). No coumarin was detected after oral administration of 1 g. After an oral dose of 2 g, plasma concentrations (above 36 ng/ml) with values up to 2300 ng/ml were detectable in 6 patients. The median systemic availability of the 2 g dose was 1.3% (range:0-10.8%). The urine analyses showed that 36% (range:20-39%) of the total coumarin administered was recovered within 48 h as 7-HCG independent of dose and of route of administration. The urinary excretion of 3-HC after oral administration of coumarin was less than 1%. After i.v. administration of coumarin no 3-HC could be found in urine.
In conclusion coumarin had an extremely poor oral bioavailability probably due to extensive first- pass metabolism. The primary metabolite of coumarin, 7-HC, reaches significant plasma concentrations and may be responsible for the observed clinical effects of coumarin. Coumarin is likely to be a prodrug, 7-hydroxycoumarin presumably being its active component and pharmacodynamic studies with 7-HC are needed.

Dr. med. Sheida Sharifi, Department of Clinical Pharmacology, University of Göttingen, Robert-Koch-Str. 40, D-3400 Göttingen, FRG

248

ELIMINATION OF COUMARIN (VENALOT®) IN PATIENTS WITH DIFFERENT DEGREES OF LIVER DISEASE
H. Kraul, J. Truckenbrodt, A. Otto, R. Brix, and A. Hoffmann

There exist only few information concerning the in-vivo-elimination of coumarin in patients with liver diseases via P450Coh.
17 healthy men (Control) and 27 patients with liver diseases, divided into 7 with fatty liver (FL), 7 with chronic active hepatitis (CAH), and 13 with liver cirrhosis (Cirr), received 5 mg coumarin orally (Venalot®). Urine was collected 1, 2, 4, and 24 hrs after administration. 7-OH-coumarin (7HC), the main metabolite in humans, was determined in the urine fluorometrically after β-glucuronidase hydrolysis and chloroform extraction.

	Control	FL	CAH	Cirr
7HC excreted within 4 hrs (mg)	2.86 (0.51)	3.26 (0.59)	3.43 (0.56)	2,33[a,b] (0.67)
7HC excreted within 24 hrs (mg)	3.13 (0.51)	3.58 (0.68)	3.81 (0.64)	3.08[b] (0.72)
"coumarin test" (%)	82.3 (9.0)	80.4 (7.7)	65.3 (28.7)	64.6* (18.9)
range (%)	71-98	72-93	3.3-84	31-93

U-test; a:FL-Cirr, b:CAH-Cirr, *:Control-Cirr; p<0.05; $\bar{x}$(SD).
The preliminary results (Table) show the predominant excretion of 7HC during the first 4 hours. The amount of 7HC excreted was reduced in Cirr compared to FL and CAH. The percentage of excreted 7HC during the first two hours related to the total amount excreted within four hours ("coumarin test") was only diminished in Cirr compared to Control.
We conclude that at least patients with Cirr have a reduced ability to hydroxylate coumarin.

Institute of Clinical Pharmacology, Friedrich Schiller University, Bachstraße 18, O-6900 Jena, F.R.G.

249

INVESTIGATIONS ON THE ORAL BIOAVAILABILITY OF AMBAZONE IN TUMOR PATIENTS. J.Teichert[+], R. Schmidt, F. Baumann, H. Fischer, K. Hambsch and R. Preiss

In a phase-I study to estimate the bioavailability after a single oral dose of 50mg (4 patients) and 100mg (4 patients) ambazone administered to patients suffering from non-Hodgkin lymphoma, the renal elimination of ambazone and its main metabolite dihydroambazone was followed over a period of 48 hours.
Urine samples were applied to reversed-phase column without prior extraction. Ambazone was detected by measuring UV absorbance, whereas dihydroambazone was determined by reversed-phase ion-pair chromatography using sodium hexanesulfonate as counter ion and by electrochemical detection. Detection limits were 0.5 µg/ml for ambazone and 5ng/ml for dihydroambazone. The urinary elimination amounted to 49.4 ± 23.4% (50mg dose) and 45.3 ± 19.1% (100mg dose) of the orally administered dose. The ratio of ambazone to dihydroambazone in urine was 1:4.5. The mean t_{max}-values in urine were found to 3.06 ± 1.7 h for ambazone and 3.25 ± 1.49 h for dihydroambazone.
Everything points to the fact that resorption is independent of dose. Over an observation time of 3 days no side effects were observed with the exception of one case of urticarial reaction after 100mg dose.

[+]Present address: Department of Clinical Pharmacology. University of Leipzig. Härtelstr. 16-18, O-7010 Leipzig, FRG

250

BIODISTRIBUTION OF TRANS-1,2-DIAMINOCYCLOHEXANE-TRIMELLITATO-PLATINUM (II) ATTACHED TO MACROMOLECULAR CARRIERS
B. Šrámek, J. Drobník, and J. Květina

Two types of macromolecular drug forms of the second generation platinum antitumor drug 4-carboxyphthalato-(trans-1,2-diaminocyclohexane) platinum (II) (TMC) were prepared with non-biodegradable carrier derived from racemic poly (N[+]-substituted) aspartamide (A-type) and with biodegradable carrier derived from (N[+]-substituted) glutamine (G-type): following AN and/or GN type was prepared from N-(2-hydroxyethyl) and AR and/or GR type from N-(2-hydroxypropyl) derivative by acylation with trimellitato residues, thus yielding primary and secondary esters respectively.
Macromolecular carrier based on glutamine is splitted especially by pronase. Biodegradability by other types of enzymes can be increased by co-polymerisation with different amino acids.
Plasma levels, urinary excretion and organ deposition of platinum were followed after administration in rats. When compared with free TMA all types of macromolecular forms showed a retardation effect in platinum pharmacokinetics with the most pronounced differences using AR-type. Urine excretion of total platinum after the administration of polymeric drug forms was more gradual, while the total amounts excreted were not significantly different (in the range of 64 - 105 % of the dose administered) with the exception of GR-type (35 %). Considering all possible biodegradable bonds in the polymeric drug forms the nature of the drug-polymer link seemed to play an important role in the kinetics of drug release as revealed by the differences between compounds tested.

Present address: Institute of Experimental Biopharmaceutics, Czechoslovak Academy of Sciences, Heyrovského str., CS 500 05 Hradec Králové, Czechoslovakia.

251

PHARMACOKINETICS IN THE RAT OF A GADOLINIUM CHELATE USED AS A BILIARY CONTRAST AGENT FOR MAGNETIC RESONANCE IMAGING
G. Schuhmann-Giampieri, T. Louton, H. Schmitt-Willich

Because of its high level of hepatic uptake the Gd-EOB-DTPA complex consisting of the lanthanide ion gadolinium (Gd) with a derivative of the chelating agent DTPA, ethoxybenzyl-DTPA (EOB-DTPA), has been developed for intravenous administration in liver tumor detection by magnetic resonance imaging .
The pharmacokinetics of Gd-EOB-DTPA was studied in female rats (Han-Wistar) weighing 100-250 g. Low (0.05 mmol/kg) and high (0.5 mmol/kg) doses were applied intravenously to investigate the plasma concentration-time profile and the pattern of elimination. In addition biliary excretion and bile flow were examined after application of both low and high doses. To investigate the possibility of an enterohepatic circulation, Gd-EOB-DTPA was administered intraduodenally (0.25 mmol/kg) and biliary excretion was measured. Biodistribution studies were performed after intravenous administration of 0.25 mmol/kg. Binding of Gd-EOB-DTPA to rat, monkey and human plasma was determined in vitro by ultrafiltration at 1 mmol/L. Quantitative measurements were performed either radiometrically (153-Gd) or by inductively coupled plasma atomic emission spectrometry at 342.247 nm.
The values obtained for binding of Gd-EOB-DTPA to rat, monkey and human plasma were 10.3 ± 1.4%, 17.5 ± 1.0% and 10.0 ± 1.9%, respectively. Dose-dependent pharmacokinetics were observed with Gd-EOB-DTPA in the rat. After the low dose, renal and fecal elimination were 23.9 ± 2.98 and 73.4 ± 5.95 % of the dose, respectively, and the area under the plasma concentration versus time curve was 17.7 ± 2.09 µmol*h/L; after the high dose renal and fecal elimination values were 45.6±5.73 and 48.6±5.18, respectively, and the area under the curve was 315±41. The dose-dependent behavior must be due to a capacity-limited step in biliary excretion since whilst dose-dependency was also found in biliary clearance it was not observed in renal clearance of Gd-EOB-DTPA. Bile flow increased significantly (p < 0.01) after intravenous application of Gd-EOB-DTPA when compared with the control group and the bile/liver Gd-EOB-DTPA concentration ratios were over 500. Enterohepatic circulation can be almost completely excluded since, after intraduodenal application, biliary excretion was very little (< 0.2% of the dose). Biodistribution studies 7 d after intravenous application revealed minimal retention of Gd in the body of the rat (< 1%) indicating that the necessary elimination of the compound from the body is achieved.

Address: Forschung Diagnostika, Kontrastmittel für Kernspintomographie, Schering AG, Müllerstrasse 170-178, D-1000 Berlin 65, Germany

252

FIRST DATA ON THE FECAL EXCRETION OF POLYCHLORINATED DIBENZO-P-DIOXINS AND DIBENZOFURANS IN A 3-MONTH-OLD BREAST-FED INFANT.
Birgit Jödicke, Manfred Ende*, and Hans Helge.

It is well-established that breast-fed infants are exposed to considerable amounts of polychlorinated dibenzo-*p*-dioxins and dibenzofurans (PCDDs/PCDFs) via their mother's milk. Up till now, nothing is known about the rate of enteral absorption of the various PCDDs/PCDFs from the human milk. We have measured the concentrations of PCDDs/PCDFs in the stool of a 3-month-old breast-fed infant. From a pooled stool sample of 3.8 g after lyophilization 0.34 g of fat were recovered. The data of a GC-MS analysis from this first sample are presented in the table for some of the congeners. Because of the small amount of stool available, some of the congeners were below the detection limits.

		pg/g fat (ppt)
2378	-T4CDD	< 2
23478	-P5CDF	11
123478	-H6CDF	
+123678	-H6CDF	13
123678	-H6CDD	37
1234678	-H7CDF	31
1234678	-H7CDD	152
	OCDD	1367
I-TE		**14**

In the, possibly small, amount of alimentary fat escaping absorption and remaining in the feces, remarkable concentrations of some of the PCDD/PCDF-congeners, especially the higher chlorinated ones, were found. Expressed as International Toxicity Equivalents (I-TE) the amount in stool fat was found to be about ½ of the concentration to be expected in the fat of the breast milk.
Although we have proven that PCDDs/PCDFs are excreted in the stool of breast-fed infants, further quantitative evaluations on the correlation between ingestion and the fecal elimination are essential, and are under way, in order to assess the exact absorption rate of PCDDs/PCDFs from breast milk.

Supported by grant # 0765002 from the Federal Ministry for Research and Technology (BMFT).

*Kinderklinik (Kaiserin Auguste Victoria Haus), Freie Universität Berlin, Heubnerweg 6, 1000 Berlin 19, and *Staatliches Chemisches Untersuchungsamt Oldenburg, Germany*

253

EFFECT OF PHORBOL ESTERS AND INHIBITORS OF PROTEIN KINASE C ON HISTAMINE RELEASE FROM MAST CELLS

B.H. Löffler and K. Gietzen

Histamine release from mast cells is caused by certain stimulants. Compound 48/80 and calcium ionophore A23187 lead to a release by enhancing the intracellular calcium concentration, concanavalin A imitates the physiological receptor coupling and phorbol esters cause an activation of the protein kinase C.

Our experiments show that phorbol esters (TPA, PDD, PDB) produce a histamine release from rat peritoneal mast cells up to 60% of the total histamine content in a concentration (4-400ng/ml) and time dependent (up to 70 min) manner. At higher concentrations there results a decrease of histamine liberation. Only TPA causes at concentrations above $1\mu g/ml$ a cytotoxic release. The non-toxic release is inhibited by K-252a and staurosporin (inhibitors of protein kinase C). If phorbol esters are combined with compound 48/80 or calcium ionophore A23187 (fixed concentrations) there is a synergistic effect, but the decrease at higher phorbol ester concentrations remains. Combining phorbol esters and concanavalin A results in a synergism, but higher concentrations lead to an inhibition of the histamine release. This inhibition does not refer to activation of protein kinase C and is not influenced by K-252a or staurosporin.

Department of Pharmacology and Toxicology, University of Ulm, Albert-Einstein-Allee 11, W-7900 Ulm, Germany

254

THE INFLUENCE OF SYMPATHOMIMETIC AGENTS ON THE HITAMINE RELEASE FROM HUMAN MAST CELLS

Bent S, Voss T, Braam U, Schmutzler W

Sympathomimetic agents are known to inhibit mediator release from mast cells in allergic and pseudo-allergic conditions. Because of the known species and organ differences of mast cells we tested the influence of sympathomimetic agents on mast cells from human adenoidal tissue and skin. Human adenoidal mast cells were isolated mechanically, cutaneous enzymically using hyaluronidase and collagenase. The aliquots contained about 10000 adenoidal or 15000 cutaneous mast cells which were incubated with the test substance for 5 min. Histamine release was stimulated with Concanavalin A (ConA; $50\mu g/ml$), Compound 48/80 (Comp 48/80; 10 $\mu g/ml$) or Substance P $(10^{-5}M)$ for 10 min. Histamine was determined by the double isotope method.
Procaterol and reproterol inhibited dose-dependently the ConA stimulated histamine release from adenoidal mast cells from $\geq 10^{-8}$ M concentration on. The spontaneous histamine release was not affected by those substances.
In contrast, in the human cutaneous mast cells reproterol in the concentration of $10^{-5}M$ was necessary to achieve a slight inhibition of Comp 48/80 induced histamine release or a significant inhibition of ConA induced histamine release.
The relative resistance of cutaneous mast cells corresponds to the rather poor effects of sympathomimetic amines in cutaneous allergies.

Institut für Pharmakologie und Toxikologie der RWTH Aachen, Wendlingweg 2, 5100 Aachen, FRG

255

INFLUENCE OF PAF-ANTAGONISTS ON THE DEGRANULATION OF ACTIVATED RAT MAST CELLS (pRMC) IN VITRO

R. Grupe, T. Ziska, E. Göres

The platelet activating factor (PAF) is capable of stimulating many different types of cells. Since both the PAF induced activating processes of the most varied types of cells, and the degranulation processes of mast cells, initiated in the most varied ways via Ca^{2+}-mobilization are linked to the activating of the phospholipase (PL) A2 and/or PLC, the fact that the PAF antagonists can interfere with stimulus induced mast cell (MC) degranulation via these mechanismus cannot be ruled out.
Therefore we investigated to see if PAF antagonists were capable of influencing the non-cytotoxic, protamine (mobilization of internal Ca^{2+}-pools of MC) or A 23187 induced (activation by Ca^{2+}-influx in the MC) and/or the cytotoxic triton X-100 triggered release of histamine from unpurified pRMC. The PAF antagonists BN 52021, ketotifen (an antihistamine with PAF-antagonistic qualities), WEB 2086 and triazolam inhibit in this order with decreasing activity the release of histamine from pRMC activated with protamine and in the order WEB 2086 $\approx$ triazolam > ketotifen the A 23187 induced degranulation of pRMC. BN 52021 is ineffective in the last reaction. Both orders do not agree with the order of their inhibitory activity on PAF induced aggregation of human platelets. That implies, that the inhibition of the MC degranulation caused by PAF antagonists does not occur via PAF receptors. None of the compounds suppress the triton X-100 triggered release of histamine.
We conclude, that WEB 2086, triazolam and ketotifen are able to inhibit both the mobilization of internal Ca^{2+}-pools and the Ca^{2+}-influx in the pRMC, but BN 52021 only the first mechanism.

Biopharm Co. Ltd., A.-Kowalke-Str. 4, O-1136 Berlin

256

INFLUENCE OF ENZYMATIC SPLEEN- AND THYMUS-HYDROLYSATES ON PHAGOCYTIC ACTIVITY OF HUMAN POLYMORPHONUCLEAR LEUKOCYTES

H. Krasowski, P. Stehle[*], P. Fürst[*] and W. Kraus

Recently, clinical investigations suggest that enzymatic hydrolysates of spleen as well as thymus proteins may be therapeutically used as effective immunomodulating drugs. However, there are only few informations concerning possible mode of action on cellular level.
The effect of commercially available preparations of enzymatic calf spleen (Splen-Uvocal[R]) and thymus (Thym-Uvocal[R]) protein hydrolysates on the phagocytic activities of human polymorphonuclear leukocytes (PMNL) were investigated in vitro. As a comparison the biological active peptides Tuftsin and Thymopentin as well as one untreated thymus preparation, Thymostimulin, were tested.
At a chosen concentration of 200 µg/ml, all products studied exhibited a significant increase of PMNL activity, when Lucigenin-amplified chemiluminescence was measured. This effect was markedly enhanced with Tuftsin, Thymopentin and Splen-Uvocal[R] peptides compared to the thymus preparations.
In parallel experiments, phagocytosis of opsonized Zymosan was investigated by light microscopy. Only spleen derived peptides showed significant stimulation at a low concentration of 200 µg/ml, whereas all samples enhanced phagocytosis at 1000 µg/ml.
These observations point out that spleen and thymus protein hydrolysates influence PMNL activity by substrate-specific mechanism. Furthermore, the results indicate that short chain peptides are the effective compounds in these preparations.

Department of Chemistry, [*]Department of Biological Chemistry, University of Hohenheim, Garbenstr. 30, D-7000 Stuttgart 70, FRG

257

EFFECTS OF LIGANDS FOR PERIPHERAL TYPE BENZODIAZEPINE BINDING SITES ON CELL GROWTH OF HUMAN LYMPHOCYTES AND A HUMAN LYPHOMA CELL LINE
B. E. E. Alexander, E. Roller* and U. Klotz

Peripheral type benzodiazepine binding sites (PBR) are involved in the regulation of different physiological effects but the mechanisms of receptor function are not yet known. After characterization of the PBR on human lymphocytes and several human lymphoma cell lines using radioligand-binding-studies, we found the human lymphoblastoid cell line CCRF-CEM suitable as a cell model for further studies on PBR.

To evaluate the pharmacological specificity of binding to human lymphocytes and CCRF-CEM cells we tested different ligands in a concentration range from 10^{-10} to 10^{-4} M in displacement studies with the radioligand [^{3}H]1-(2-chlorophenyl)-N-methyl-N-(1-methylpropyl)-3-isoquinolinecarboxamide ([^{3}H]Pk 11195). Their ability to inhibit binding of [^{3}H]Pk 11195 to human lymphocytes corresponded to that for CCRF-CEM cells. Pk 11195 was found to be the most potent inhibitor followed by 4'-chlorodiazepam (Ro5-4864) and diazepam (inhibition constants from 7 to 365 nM), whereas ligands specific for the central type receptor like clonazepam and flumazenil had no inhibitory potency in the tested concentration range.

To study the influence of receptor ligands on cell growth and survival in vitro, we used a quantitative colorimetric assay (MTT). CCRF-CEM cells were exposed to different ligand concentrations (10^{-10} to 10^{-4} M) for two days, phytohaemagglutinine (PHA)-stimulated lymphocytes for four days respectively. Ligands which bind selectively to PBR inhibited cell growth in vitro, however half effective concentrations were in the micromolar range (EC_{50} values between 13 μM (Pk 11195) and 30 μM (Ro5-4864)) and above therapeutic in vivo concentrations. There was no distinct relationship between displacement potency and doses to inhibit cell proliferation of the ligands tested, although clonazepam and flumazenil showed no significant influence on cell growth nor had both any displacement capacity. The discrepancy between binding parameters and effective doses to inhibit cell proliferation might be due to the binding of benzodiazepines to serum proteins. Therefore we are testing serumfree media in growth experiments.

Supported by the Robert-Bosch-Foundation Stuttgart

Dr. Margarete Fischer-Bosch-Institut für Klinische Pharmakologie, Auerbachstraße 112, W-7000 Stuttgart 50, FRG; *Abteilung für Hämatologie, Onkologie und Immunologie, Robert-Bosch-Krankenhaus, Stuttgart, FRG

258

LYMPHOPENIA OCCURRING IN WOMEN DURING PARTURITION.
Reinhard Neubert, Sarah Pegg, Isabella Delgado, Joachim W. Dudenhausen* and Diether Neubert

We have studied whether a physiological "stress" situation in humans will alter the subpopulation pattern of peripheral lymphocytes, thus creating an altered basis for the action of medicinal products. Blood samples were taken within 30 minutes post partum or after C-sections. The first results of our ongoing studies reveal a pronounced decrease in the relative and absolute number of lymphocytes during births under labour, but not during primary sections. This is correlated with a change in the absolute number of certain lymphocyte subpopulations:

	Spont. deliveries	Primary C-sections	Controls
n =	9	4	4
Cells / μl	*Mean values ± SD*		
leucocytes	20644 ± 5893*	7775 ± 988	7325 ± 1590
% of lymphocytes	6.3 ± 1.4*	18.8 ± 2.1*	34.1 ± 7.8
lymphocytes	1248 ± 220*	1448 ± 127*	2450 ± 480
CD4+ cells	487 ± 96*	738 ± 239	1188 ± 176
CD4+CDw29+high density	160 ± 81*	206 ± 117*	529 ± 174
CD4+CDw29+low density	277 ± 97*	478 ± 295	516 ± 215
CD20+ cells	171 ± 99	87 ± 20	202 ± 141
CD4+/CD8+ ratio	1.5 ± 0.6	2.6 ± 1.3	1.8 0.6

* p < 0.05 (vs controls)   Mann-Whitney test

At present it cannot be decided whether the effects seen are caused by mediators such as glucocorticoids, endorphins or other substances, the levels of which are known to be altered during parturition. However, the results show that very pronounced changes in the composition of peripheral lymphocyte subpopulations occur under physiological extreme situations. It is feasible that these changes may modify the ability of such women to recover from infections and alter the potency and action of drugs given during this period.

Institut für Toxikologie, und *Frauenklinik, Univ.-Klinikum Rudolf Virchow, Freie Universität Berlin, Garystr. 5, 1000 Berlin 33, Germany

259

T-CELL SUBPOPULATIONS IN HUMAN CORD BLOOD.
Reinhard Neubert, Sarah Pegg, Isabella Delgado, Joachim W. Dudenhausen*, Diether Neubert.

It has been reported that blood from the umbilical cord lacks CD4+CDw29+ ("memory") lymphocytes and contains a high percentage of CD4+CD45RA+ ("naive") cells (Pirruccello et al. Clin Immunol Immunopath 52: 341-345, 1989). In the course of studies aimed at analysing drug effects on cord blood cells in vitro we have reinvestigated this problem, and arrived at quite different results (Table):

Lymphocyte subtypes		Fraction of total lymphocytes
n = 13		
		Median and Range
Total lymphocytes		4901 (3097-9000)
% CD4+ cells		55.2 (33.1-66.0)
% CD4+CDw29+	low density**	44.5 (28.8-64.0)
% CD4+CDw29+	high density	3.0 (0.3-7.9)
% CD4+CD45RA+	low density**	2.0 (1.1-4.4)
% CD4+CD45RA+	high density	0.0 (0.0-0.0)
CD4+/CD8+	ratio	2.1 (1.1-3.6)

** about 5×10^3 to 5×10^4 epitopes/cell

Further investigations using three colour analysis show that of the CD4+ subpopulation about 75% express CDw29 and less than 5% express CD45RA exclusively; 10% bear both epitopes leaving 10% showing neither.

The CD4+CDw29+ cells with low CDw29 epitope density can be converted in vitro by incubation with lectins (poke weed mitogen, concanavalin A, phytohemagglutinin) to high epitope density (5×10^4 to 7×10^5 epitopes/cell).

Human cord blood represents a convenient substrate to study maturation processes of T-lymphocytes in vitro.

Institut für Toxikologie, and *Frauenklinik, Univ.-Klinikum Rudolf Virchow, Freie Universität Berlin, Garystr. 5, 1000 Berlin 33, Germany

260

CELL PROLIFERATION IN POPLITEAL LYMPH NODES IN MICE AFTER FOOT PAD INJECTION OF DIFFERENT STIMULANTS AND INHIBITION OF THIS REACTION BY IMMUNOSUPPRESSIVES.
Andrej Schmidt, Hans-Jürgen Stroh, Maria Korte, Ralf Stahlmann and Diether Neubert

Cells in popliteal lymph nodes in mice proliferate after injection of suitable agents into the foot pad. The reaction can be suppressed by drugs or chemicals which affect the immune system. We studied the effects of cyclophosphamide (CP; 4 x 100 mg/kg body wt), cyclosporine A (CA; 4 x 75 mg/kg body wt) and 2,3,7,8-tetrachlorodibenzo-p-dioxin (TCDD; 1 x 3 μg/kg body wt) on the cell proliferation induced by injection of streptozotocin into the right foot pad (R). The left side remained untreated (L). After mechanical desintegration of the lymph nodes in phosphate buffered saline (PBS) the number of cells were determined with a cell counter. Cell numbers and the quotient of the results ("index") are given in the following table [mean ± SD]:

Stimulant[1] (No. of rats)	Test comp.[2]	Cell No. (L) ($\times 10^3$/μl PBS)	Cell No. (R) ($\times 10^3$/μl PBS)	Cell index (R/L)
[untreated] (19)	--	3.0 ± 1.4	3.4 ± 1.6	1.3 ± 0.7
concanavalin A (14)	--	2.0 ± 1.5	10.6 ± 4.4	7.2 ± 5.3
pokeweed (10)	--	3.6 ± 3.4	18.5 ± 6.6	7.1 ± 3.1
streptozotocin (14)	--	2.3 ± 1.4	18.4 ± 12.3	10.4 ± 7.8
streptozotocin (26)	TCDD	3.8 ± 2.3	19.4 ± 12.7	6.0 ± 3.9
streptozotocin (16)	CP	1.3 ± 1.1	4.6 ± 2.6	5.4 ± 4.7
streptozotocin (15)	CA	2.7 ± 1.4	3.0 ± 1.4	1.6 ± 1.6

1 = injected into the right foot pad; 2 = test compound was injected s.c. once one week before the test (TCDD) or several times (cf. text) during the week the test was performed (CP + CA)

Streptozotocin (0.5 mg/20 μl) induced the best proliferation of all stimulants tested. The reaction was clearly suppressed by treatment with cyclophosphamide or cyclosporine A, but not after pretreatment with TCDD. Since the variability of the index values is higher than that of the cell number in the stimulated lymph node we suggest evaluating the immunosuppressive action of chemicals on the basis of this variable.

Studies were supported by grant no. 0765002 from the Federal Ministry for Research and Technology (BMFT).

Institut für Toxikologie und Embryopharmakologie der Freien Universität Berlin, Garystr. 5, D 1000 Berlin 33, Germany

261

EFFECTS OF IMMUNOSUPPRESSIVE AGENTS ON THE STREPTOZOTOCIN-INDUCED CELL PROLIFERATION IN THE POPLITEAL LYMPH NODE IN RATS.

Hans-Jürgen Stroh, Andrej Schmidt, Maria Korte, Ralf Stahlmann and Diether Neubert

The "popliteal lymph node assay (PLNA)" performed in mice has been proposed as a simple method to screen for immunotoxic compounds. We studied the suitability of this method in rats, which is the more often used species for toxicological studies. Streptozotocin (strep) proved to be a suitable agent to induce cell proliferation in a popliteal lymph node after injection into a foot pad (5 mg in 40 μl). One week after this challenge lymph nodes from both legs were prepared, weighed and the cell numbers were determined after mechanical desintegration in phosphate buffered saline (PBS) with a cell counter (Digitana). The quotient of the results obtained from both lymph nodes ("index") was calculated. The results were compared with those from animals which were treated with the test compound or with their vehicle (saline, toluene/DMSO) before or during the week the test was performed. The following results were obtained (mean ± SD):

Number of rats	Substance (dose)	Treatment*	Weight index	Cell index
9	cyclosporin A	3 x 75 mg/kg	1.2 ± 0.4	1.1 ± 0.6
14	cyclosporin A	1 x 75 mg/kg	1.2 ± 0.4	2.0 ± 1.4
15	cyclophosphamide	2 x 100 mg/kg	1.3 ± 0.5	1.7 ± 1.4
30	TCDD**	1 x 3000 ng/kg	9.4 ± 2.3	29.9 ± 14
10	NaCl 0.9 %	3 x 6.0 ml/kg	7.1 ± 3.4	28.9 ± 20
20	toluene/DMSO	1 x 0.1 ml/kg	9.9 ± 5.5	26.6 ± 20
20	no treatment	- - -	7.1 ± 1.9	29.0 ± 15

* rats were treated s.c. one to three times before or after the foot pad injection of strep.
** 2,3,7,8-Tetrachlorodibenzo-p-dioxin

Our results indicate that by injection of streptozotocin (5 mg in 40 μl) into a foot pad an approximately 30fold cell proliferation can be induced in the popliteal lymph node of rats which is reducible by treatment of immunosuppressive agents.

Studies were supported by grant no. 0765002 from the Federal Ministry for Research and Technology (BMFT).

Institut für Toxikologie und Embryopharmakologie der Freien Universität Berlin, Garystr. 5, D 1000 Berlin 33, Germany

262

DOSE-DEPENDENT STIMULATIVE OR INHIBITORY ACTIONS OF TCDD ON T-LYMPHOCYTES IN PERIPHERAL BLOOD OF MARMOSETS.

Reinhard Neubert*, Georg Golor, Ralf Stahlmann, Hans Helge*, and Diether Neubert

2,3,7,8-Tetrachlorodibenzo-p-dioxin (TCDD) was found in previous studies to reduce the number of a defined CD4+ cell subpopulation in *Callithrix jacchus* after a single dose of as little as 10 ng TCDD/kg body wt (Neubert et al. Arch Toxicol 64: 345-359, 1990). We have now studied the effects of even smaller doses of TCDD given over a period of several months. Weekly doses of 1.5 ng TCDD/kg body wt, accumulating to effective doses of 5-10 ng TCDD/kg, produced the same reduction in the percentage and absolute number of CD4+CDw29+ cells as described before after the single applications. However, during the dosing with weekly 0.3 ng TCDD/kg body wt (accumulating to an actual effective dose of about 2.5 ng TCDD/kg body wt) an opposite effect was observed, namely an *increase* in the CD4+CDw29+ subpopulation ("helper-inducer" cells) and a *decrease* in the percentage of CD4+CD45R+ cells. For an easy overview the ratios of these subpopulations are given in the table:

Cumulative, effective dose of TCDD (ng TCDD/kg body wt)	n =	Ratio: CD4+CDw29+/CD4+CD45R+	
		M ± SD	Mann-Whitney test
Controls	5	1.6 ± 0.5	
about 2.5*	7	5.4 ± 3.9	p = 0.02
5 - 10**	7	0.7 ± 0.1	p = 0.006

* 0.3 ng TCDD/kg bw weekly (19 weeks), ** 1.5 ng TCDD/kg bw weekly (6 weeks)

Since in the still growing marmosets used by us there is a steady increase in the percentage and number of CD4+CDw29+ ("memory") cells in the venous blood during the several months of the study, this physiological change seems to be intensified by very small doses of TCDD.

*Institut für Toxikologie und Embryopharmakologie, Garystr. 5, 1000 Berlin 33 and *Kinderklinik, Univ.-Klinikum Rudolf Virchow, Freie Universität Berlin, Germany*

263

PYROGEN INDUCED FEVER: INFLUENCE ON INULIN-, SORBITOL-, PENICILLIN- AND SATERINONE CLEARANCE IN RABBITS

H. Iven and H. Meink

During a phase-I-study on the bioavailability of oral saterinone - a PDE-III-inhibitor with positive inotropic and vasodilatory activity - one of the volunteers presented with chills and fever two hours after dosing (common cold). Despite an increase in body temperature up to 39 °C no antipyretic was given and blood sampling was continued. Since his saterinone plasma concentrations were unexpectedly high, studies on the influence of pyrogen induced fever on the clearance of saterinone and penicillin were started in six male rabbits. Inulin was included as a marker for glomerular filtration rate and sorbitol as an indicator for hepatic blood flow. Steady state conditions were achieved by bolus injection (except saterinone) and continuous infusion for all compounds. After 2 h 1 μg/kg pyrogen was injected i.v. resulting in an increase (2.2 °C) in body temperature within 3 h. The rabbits served as their own controls (with and without pyrogen in randomised order). Urine was sampled by an indwelling catheter in 30-min-fractions and 1ml blood was taken every 15 min. Saterinone and penicillin were quantified by HPLC, inulin with the anthrone reagent and sorbitol with an enzymatic assay.

During the first 2 h steady state concentrations were reached for all the compounds and there was no significant change during the next 3 h under control conditions. Total (Cl-tot; 140 ml/min) and renal sorbitol clearance (Cl-ren; 12 ml/min) were not influenced by fever. In the penicillin experiments Cl-tot inulin (12 ml/min) was reduced by 25 % in fever. During control experiments Cl-ren increased over the 5 h observation period and was close to Cl-tot at the end of the experiment. Fever resulted in a decrease of Cl-tot, while Cl-ren remained at the level reached before giving the pyrogen. In saterinone experiments Cl-tot inulin was significantly higher (20 ml/min, pharmacodynamic effect of saterinone) than in penicillin experiments but also decreased by 30 % in fever. Fever increased Cl-tot penicillin (40 - 50 ml/min) by 20 %, predominantly due to an increase in extrarenal clearance. In contrast fever decreased Cl-tot saterinone (100 ml/min) by 40 % mainly due to a decrease in extrarenal clearance.

Institut für Pharmakologie der Medizinischen Universität zu Lübeck, Ratzeburger Allee 160, 2400 Lübeck, FRG.

264

CIRCULATING AUTOANTIBODIES FROM PATIENTS WITH ALLERGIC ASTHMA INTERFERING WITH β_2-ADRENOCEPTOR STIMULATION IN CULTURED NEONATAL RAT HEART MYOCYTES

G. WALLUKAT and A. WOLLENBERGER

The serum γ-globulin fraction from patients with allergic bronchial asthma (8/8), in contrast to that from healthy control subjects (10/10), was found to inhibit the positive chronotropic action of the β_2-selective adrenergic agonist clenbuterol on cultured neonatal rat heart myocytes pretreated with 1 mM pyruvate or 3 mM L(+)-lactate. No inhibition was exerted on the positive chronotropic response to prenalterol, which acted via β_1 adrenoceptors. The inhibitory effect of the asthmatic γ-globulins was concentration-dependent. It could nearly be abolished by immunoprecipitation with anti-human γ-globulin and anti-human IgG, but not with anti-human IgM. This means that the inhibitory immunoglobulins of the asthmatic patients were chiefly autoantibodies of the IgG isotype, capable of cross-reacting with chronotropic β_2 adrenoceptors on the cultured rat cardiomyocytes. In 4 patients investigated the immunogenic determinant could in every case be localized to the third extracellular loop of the β_2 adrenoceptor. These findings offer for the first time acceptable evidence for an autoimmune mechanism as a factor in the diminished β-adrenergic responsiveness in human allergic bronchial asthma.

Institut für Herz-Kreislauf-Forschung, O-1115 Berlin-Buch, FRG

265

THE RAT FEMALE PROTEIN, A NEW PENTRAXIN OF IMMUNOPHARMACOLOGICAL INTEREST

R. Schade, W. Bürger, A.-M. Ladhoff, C. Pfister

The C-reactive protein (CRP) is the major acute
phase protein (APP) in humans which binds lectin-
like to different membraneous structures and
exerts an important function in non-specific defense.
Because of a pentameric molecular symmetry CRP as
well as serum amyloid P component (SAP) and hamster
female protein (FP) was merged into a special
protein family named pentraxins. In rats a protein
was found close related to hamster FP concerning
the hormonal regulation and APP-nature, referred
to as rat FP. Based on this conformity the molecular structure of rat FP was analyzed and a
pentameric structure could be found, too.
Furthermore, the response of rat CRP and FP on
adrenal hormones was investigated. The results
indicate a neuroendocrine control because both
proteins were significant influenced by dexamethasone and epinephrine but each in a different
way. Using FITC-labelled lectin the exposition
of galactose-containing membraneous structures
could be demonstrated in carbon tetrachloride
injured liver tissue in contrast to controls.
These binding sites are in accordance with
increased FP-binding shown by immunofluorescence
histochemistry. Thus, lectin-like properties
may be ascribed to rat FP comparable to CRP
and SAP activity.

Institut of Pharmacology and Toxicology,
Institut of Microbiology and
Institut of Anatomy of the Department of Medicine
(Charité) of the Humboldt University of Berlin.

266

FETALES ALKOHOLSYNDROM UND IMMUNSYSTEM : NEUROIM-MUNOLOGISCHE EFFEKTE B. GÜNTHER, P. CLAUSING

Beim Fetalen Alkoholsyndrom (FAS) handelt es sich
um eine besondere Form des psychoorganischen Syn-
droms, einer klinisch bedeutsamen kindlichen Ver-
haltensstörung mit gestörter adrenerger bzw. nor-
adrenerger Transmission. Pädiatrische Befunde und
erste Tierexperimente weisen darauf hin, daß das
FAS mit einer gestörten Immunantwort verbunden ist.
Wir untersuchten den zellulären Immunresponse (Delayed Type Hypersensitivity (DTH)-Reaktion) von
C57BL/6-Mäusen, die pränatal Ethanol (ETH)-expo-
niert waren (2x täglich 1 ml/kg Körpermasse 20%-
iges Ethanol vom 14.-18. Tag p.c.). Die Kontakt-
sensibilität (DTH-Reaktion) wurde anhand der Ohr-
schwellung der Mäuse nach Sensibilisierung und
Challenge mit Pikrylchlorid beurteilt. Ähnlich wie
die unmittelbare Verabreichung von adrenergen-Ago-
nisten (Clonidin, Noradrenalin) an erwachsene Mäuse
führte pränatale ETH-Gabe zu einer verstärkten DTH
-Reaktion. Die Verabreichung von Isoprenalin (β-
adrenerger Agonist) an adulte Tiere führte zu einer DTH-Suppression. Bei pränatal ETH-exponierten
Tieren kompensierte die Applikation von Isoprenalin und Yohimbin (α-adrenerger Antagonist) die erhöhte DTH-Reaktion. Der vermutlich erhöhte Noradre-
nalinspiegel bei den Nachkommen Alkohol-behandel-
ter Mütter scheint die Freisetzung und/oder Akti-
vierung von T-Zellen in lymphatischen Organen zu
beeinflussen.

Institut für Mikrobiologie und experimentelle
Therapie, Beutenbergstr. 11, 6900 Jena/BRD

267

INHIBITORY EFFECTS OF SALAZOSULFAPYRIDINE ON A CONTACT HYPERSENSITIVITY REACTION IN MICE AND ON THE EXPERIMENTAL ALLERGIC ENCEPHALOMYELITIS IN RATS

Karin Schmidt, R. Hirschelmann, M. Kurowski, and Anke Brandt

Salazosulfapyridine (SASP) is widely used for the treatment of
inflammatory diseases such as ulcerative colitis and Crohn's
disease. Not until recently SASP has gained a position as a
second line antirheumatic drug, mainly through the work of
Mc Conkey et al. (e.g. Br. Med. J. 280, 1980, 442-4). But the
mode of action of this drug in rheumatoid arthritis is not fully
understood.
In our study we examined the effect of SASP on the contact
hypersensitivity reaction to picryl chloride in mice and on the
experimental allergic encephalomyelitis (EAE) in rats. When
administered daily from sensitization up to challenge in a dose of
500 mg/kg p.o. SASP inhibited the ear edema to picryl chloride.
In EAE, SASP (250 mg/kg p.o.) showed a suppressive effect when
given daily from the day of immunization. For comparison,
ciclosporine A caused a stronger inhibition at 10 mg/kg p.o.
Furhermore we investigated the effects of the main metabolites
of SASP, i.g. 5-aminosalicylic acid and sulfapyridine.

Our results indicate that SASP may act as an immunosuppressive
agent by inhibiting the function of cell populations involved in
the pathogenesis of cellular immunological reactions.

In summary we may state, immunosuppression could be a part of
the mode of action of SASP and perhaps of further disease
modifying antirheumatic drugs, too.

Dept. Pharmacology, Fac. Pharmacy, Martin-Luther-University,
Weinbergweg 15, O-4050 Halle/Saale, FRG

268

INHIBITION OF ACETYLATING FORMATION OF PAF (PLATELET-ACTIVA-TING FACTOR) BY SOME POLYETHYLENE GLYCOLS AND BITUMINOSUL-FONATES

Dragica Cerinski-Hennig and Franz v. Bruchhausen

Since there is evidence for participation of platelet-acti-
vating factor (PAF) in some dermatic diseases and early fertilization stage, we studied the influence of some ethylene
oxide compounds and bituminosulfonates used in local skin
creams or in topical anticontraceptive creams on PAF biosynthesis. Using microsomal enzyme preparations of AcCoA: lyso
PAF-acetyltransferase [EC 2.3.1.67] of ovine intestinal
lymph nodes, we found formerly effective inhibition by gos-
sypol, a male contraceptive substance (v. Bruchhausen et
al., Arch. Pharmacol. 342, R6, 1990). With the same preparation we now found the inhibitory actions of the following
compounds [in parenthesis given the repeating ethylene oxide
number as EO; IC_{50} value in mg/ml or n.i. (no inhibition by
< 0.6 mg/ml) respectively]:
Alkyl ethylene glycols: Lauryl [EO 9; 0.06 mg/ml ~ polidoca-
nol]; oleoyl [EO 5; n.i.]; oleoyl [EO 10; n.i.].
Alkyl phenyl ethylene glycols: Nonoxynol [EO 4; n.i.]; nonoxynol [EO 5; n.i.]; nonoxynol [EO 6; 0.075 mg/ml]; nonoxynol [EO 10; 0.21 mg/ml]; nonoxynol [EO 15; 0. 11 mg/ml];
tert. octyl phenoxy ethylene glycol [EO 10; 0.05 mg/ml].
Ammonium bituminosulfonate (Ichthyol[R]) [IC 50: 0.02 mg/ml].
This compound and polidocanol revealed reversible inhibition
type (by a washing out approach) and a noncompetitive inhibition type for both substrates (AcCoA; lyso PAF) in a Lineweaver Burk diagram. So some of these compounds tested had
in vitro inhibitory actions for the main step in the biosyn-
thetic pathway of PAF formation in concentration which are
reached in topical applications.

Institut für Pharmakologie, Freie Universität Berlin, Thielallee 67-73, D-1000 Berlin 33

269

NEURONAL CELL CULTURES AS A TEST SYSTEM FOR THE NEUROTOXICITY OF IMMUNSUPPRESSIVE DRUGS
F. Boegner*, G. Stoltenburg+, U. Kunzendorf#, H.-J. Brockmöller°, P. Marx*

Cell cultures have become increasingly important in replacing animal studies in pharmacological investigation. Because of the growing use of immunsuppressive drugs in transplantation medicine and in particular the neurotoxicity we attempted to test the effectiveness of cell cultures for the analysis of such phenomena.
Pure neuronal, pure glial and mixed cultures were prepared from dorsal root ganglia (DRG) of 8 day old chick embryos (E8) and cultivated in serum containing F12-medium with nerve growth factor (NGF) and the neurotrophic matrix factor B 82 (NTF B 82). After two days in culture the immunsuppressive drugs were applied. We analysed the selective vulnerability of different parts of the nervous system by comparing the type of damage observed in DRG cells with that in sympathetic ganglia, myelon and brain. Evaluation was carried out with the help of phase contrast microscopy, light microscopy and scanning electron microscopy.
The gliatoxicity of iv. cyclosporine which we could demonstrate corresponds to the documented changes of white matter shown by computed tomography (CT) and magnetic resonance tomography (MRT).

*Department of Neurology, Klinikum Steglitz, Free University Berlin, F.R.G.
+Institute of Neuropathology, Klinikum Steglitz, Free University Berlin, F.R.G.
#Department of Internal Medicine, Klinikum Steglitz, Free University Berlin, F.R.G.
°Institute of Clinical Pharmacology, Klinikum Steglitz, Free University Berlin, F.R.G.

270

THE IMMUNOSUPPRESSIVE ACTION OF GLUCOCORTICOIDS ON MOUSE SPLEEN CELLS IN VITRO IN DEPENDENCE ON THE IMMUNOLOGICAL STATE
B. Tiefenbach and S. Wichner*

Dependent on time of the application, organophosphate (OP) pesticides may either suppress or stimulate the formation of antibodies in mice. The immunomodulatory effects of the OP tested were mainly induced by the release of glucocorticoids, therefore their direct action on mice spleen cells in vitro was studied dependent on the antigen-stimulation state of cells.
For that reason hydrocortisone (H), dexamethasone (D) and prednisolone (P) were added to antigen-stimulated (SBRC) spleen cell cultures. Varying concentrations of steroids and time of administration were used: simultaneously with the antigen, 1 or 2 days after antigen stimulation. Viability (trypan-blue-exclusion test) and antibody expression (plaque forming cells, PFC) of spleen cells were tested.
H, D and P inhibit both viability and antibody expression in concentrations between 10^{-12} and 10^{-5} mol/l. Viability was reduced stronger than formation of the PFC. D was the the most potent inhibitor. The glucocorticoids tested exert their action only in case of the simultaneous addition with the antigen. The extent of the immunodepression was reduced or even cancelled when steroids were added 1-2 days later.
So it can be concluded that the immunosuppressive capacity of glucocorticoids depends on the antigen-induced stimulation state of mouse spleen cells.

Institute of Pharmacology and Toxicology and *Institute of Biochemistry, University of Rostock, Leninallee 70, O-2500 Rostock, FRG

271

ISOLATION OF IMMUNOSUPPRESSIVE RAPAMYCIN METABOLITES AFTER IN VITRO METABOLISM M. Sattler, U. Christians, H.M. Schiebel, H. Radeke, K.-Fr. Sewing.
The macrolide rapamycin (Rp) is currently under investigation as an immunosuppressant after transplantation. As for today nothing is known about its metabolism, it was the aim of this study to metabolize Rp by human liver and rat small intestinal microsomes, to isolate the metabolites, characterize their structures and evaluate their immunosuppressive activity. Rp was incubated with human liver or rat small intestinal microsomes and an NADPH regenerating system, the metabolites were purified by solid-liquid extraction and isolated by semi-preparative HPLC. Rp and its metabolites (RpM) were eluted in 25 fractions from the 500 x 10 mm RP8 column by a concave acetonitrile/water gradient. Column temperature was 75°C, the flow 5 ml/min and the detection wavelength 276 nm. The detection limit was 5 ng. The immunosuppressive activity was tested in a PHA-stimulated human lymphocyte assay (3 different donors, n=4).
Rp is metabolized by the liver cytochrome P450 system, and after an incubation period of 20 min with 0.75 mg/ml human liver microsomal protein the initial Rp concentration was reduced by 89 ± 4%. Metabolism of Rp was inducible by dexamethasone. At least 6 fractions proved to contain RpM. Their structures were characterized by FAB-MS and DCI-MS. One of the metabolites was identified as 41-O-desmethyl-Rp by analysis of its fragmentation pattern. The other RpM were demethylated and/or hydroxylated in unknown positions. Metabolism of Rp by rat small intestinal microsomes yielded at least five RpM, which were identical with those isolated from human liver microsomes. Two metabolites retained an immunsuppressive activity with an IC_{50} of 1 nmol/l (41-O-desmethyl-Rp) and of 1.5 nmol/l ((hydroxy-Rp) which is 10 % and 7 % of that of Rp (IC_{50}: 0.1 nmol/l).
It is concluded that Rp is metabolized by the liver and small intestine cytochrome P450 system to at least two immunosuppressive metabolites.

Supported by DFG grant Pi 48/11-4, project D5.
Institut für Allgemeine Pharmakologie, Medizinische Hochschule Hannover, Konstanty-Gutschow-Str. 8, 3000 Hannover 61, FRG, Institut für Molekularpharmakologie, Medizinische Hochschule Hannover, and Institut für Organische Chemie, TU Braunschweig, FRG.

272

INDIVIDUALISATION OF IMMUNOSUPPRESSIVE THERAPY AFTER RENAL TRANSPLANTATION
H.G. Trautsch-Förster, P. Glander, K. Schröder*, G. Stamminger**, and I. Mai

The mechanisms of action of the usual immunosuppressive drugs are very complex. The consequence is a wide interindividual variation of the obtained immunosuppressive effect. In order to get an information about the individual cluster of immunosuppression we were interested in some pharmacokinetic and -dynamic parameters.
We investigated 34 renal transplant patients (from 0.5 to 7 years after transplantation). All patients were on triple therapy with cyclosporine A (2.1 - 5.2 mg/kg/day), azathioprine (0.3 - 2.5 mg/kg/day) and prednisolone (0.05 - 0.21 mg/kg/day). Blood was taken of at 7.00 a.m. immediately before intake of Cyclosporine A and prednisolone and 4 hours later. Following parameters were investigated: concentrations of thioguaninenucleotides, prednisolone, Cyclosporine A and of endogenous cortisol, as well as the counts of neutrophilic granulocytes and lymphocytes.
The highest values observed exceed the lowest one from 6 to 25 times. The results should be further systematized to reach a good fit between the obtained immunosuppressive effect and the individual need.

Institute of Clinical Pharmacology, Clinic of Urology* and Institute of Pathological Biochemistry**, Department of Medicine (Charité), Humboldt-University, Schumannstr. 20-22, O-1040 Berlin, FRG

273

FOLLOW-UP STUDY OF ANTIOXIDATIVE DEFENSE MECHANISM
IN LYMPHOCYTES OF RATS WITH COLLAGEN-II-INDUCED
ARTHRITIS
S. Böckmann and I. Paegelow

It is generally accepted that reactive oxygen species (ROS) produced by several sources are involved
in cell-mediated immune responses.
To evaluate the importance of this enzymatic antioxidative defense system in immunocompetent cells,
a collagen type II (C II) arthritis in Lewis rats
was induced in comparison to an arthritis induced
with complete Freund's adjuvans (CFA) as a control.
In lymphocytes and thymocytes of these rats the
activities of the superoxide dismutase (SOD), glutathione peroxidase (GPx), glutathione reductase
(GR) and the content of the glutathione (GSH) were
determined during the course of the inflammation.
No significant different enzyme activities were
found in these cells derived from rats with C II
arthritis in comparison to the controls (CFA).
However, the level of the GSH content correlated
with the course of the enzyme activities (GPx,GR):
The lowest GR activity and GSH content and the
highest GPx values were found between day 10 and 15
after the immunization. These findings demonstrate
that lymphocytes and thymocytes have an enzymatic
antioxidative defense system comparable with that
existing in granulocytes.
To evaluate further the pathophysiological role of
the ROS in lymphocytes, the influence of the H_2O_2-
generating system (glucose/glucose oxidase) will be
investigated in cell cultures.

Institute of Pharmacology and Toxicology
University of Rostock
Leninallee 70, D-2500 Rostock, FRG

274

THE HIV-1 SURFACE PROTEIN GP120 AND TRANSMEMBRANAL T-CELL
SIGNALLING. IS THERE ANY EFFECT OR NOT?
R. Kaufmann (1), D. Laroche (2), K. Buchner (3), F. Hucho
(3), C. Rudd (4), C. Lindschau (5), P. Ludwig (6), A. Höer
(7), E. Oberdisse (7), I.-J. Körner (8), J. Kopp (8), V.
Kalyanaraman (9), and H. Repke (2)

The hypothesis that a direct immunmodulatory effect of HIV
proteins substantially contribute to the development of the
immune deficiency syndrome is attractive but controversial.
Previously published data provided evidence for a stimulatory effect of the viral envelope protein gp120 on a variety
of effector systems in lymphocytes. The validity, however,
of some of these data has recently been questioned.
This study was performed to contribute to a resolution of
this issue by using well characterized gp120 preparations:
we predominantly used gp120 isolated from HIV-1 infected
cells and different preparations of recombinant gp120. The
results obtained indicated no effects of gp120 on phosphoinositide and arachidonic acid metabolism, intracellular
calcium concentration, protein kinase C activity, tyrosine
phosphorylation and cAMP generation in different T-cell
lines, T-cells and peripheral blood mononuclear cells. In
conclusion, we did not find any evidence for a lymphokine-
like action of gp120 regardless of the cell type and the
gp120 preparation used. Taken together with previously published reports, it appears unlikely that gp120-induced
transmembranal signalling plays a significant role in AIDS
pathogenesis.

(1) Institute of Pharmacology and Toxicology, (6) Institute
of Physiological and Biological Chemistry, Humboldt University Berlin, (3) Institute of Biochemistry, (5) Medical Clinic, Klinikum Steglitz, (7) Institute of Pharmacology , Free
University Berlin, (8) Institute of Molecular Biology, Berlin, (2) Division of Human Retrovirology, (4) Division of
Tumor Immunology, Dana Farber Cancer Institute, Boston, MA,
USA, (9) Advanced Bioscience Labs., Kensington, MD, USA

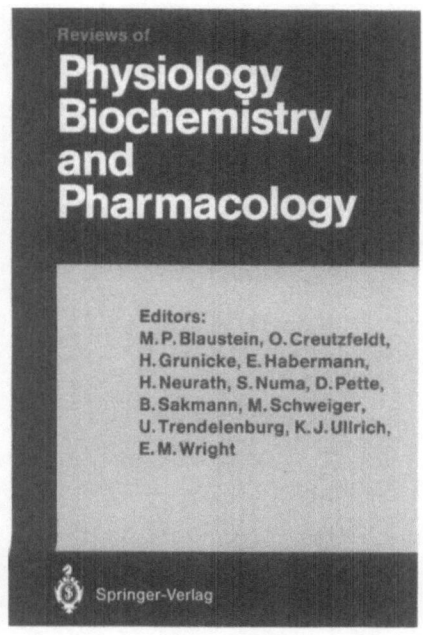

Reviews of

Physiology Biochemistry and Pharmacology

Editors:
M. P. Blaustein, O. Creutzfeldt,
H. Grunicke, E. Habermann,
H. Neurath, S. Numa, D. Pette,
B. Sakmann, M. Schweiger,
U. Trendelenburg, K. J. Ullrich,
E. M. Wright

Springer-Verlag

Volume 117

1991. VI, 274 pp. 18 tabs.
Hardcover DM 148,–
ISBN 3-540-53663-9

Contents: *R. Seifert, G. Schultz:* The
Superoxide-Forming NADPH Oxidase
of Phagocytes: An Enzyme System
Regulated by Multiple Mechanisms.

Volume 115

1990. V, 140 pp. 24 figs. 4 tabs.
Hardcover DM 118,–
ISBN 3-540-51712-X

Contents: *B. Neumcke:* Diversity of
Sodium Channels in Adult and Cultured Cells, in Oocytes and in Lipid Bi-
layers. - *H.-A. Kolb:* Potassium Channels
in Excitable and Non-Excitable Cells. -
F. Dreyer: Peptide Toxins and Potassium
Channels.

Volume 114

1990. VI, 268 pp. 21 figs. 9 tabs.
Hardcover DM 148,–
ISBN 3-540-51693-X

Contents: *H. Glossmann, J. Striessnig:*
Molecular Properties of Calcium Chan-
nels. - *D. Pelzer, S. Pelzer, T. F. McDonald:*
Properties and Regulation of Calcium
Channels in Muscle Cells. - *H. Porzig:*
Pharmacological Modulation of Voltage-
Dependent Calcium Channels in Intact
Cells.

Prices are subject to change without
notice.

Volume 113

1989. VI, 146 pp. 12 figs. 5 tabs.
Hardcover DM 104,– ISBN 3-540-50948-8

Contents: *A. Kurtz:* Cellular Control of
Renin Secretion. - *U. Walter:* Physiological Role of cGMP and cGMP-Dependent Protein Kinase in the Cardiovascular System. - *E. Ozawa:* Transferrin as a
Muscle Trophic Factor.

Volume 112

1989. V, 265 pp. 26 figs. 11 tabs.
Hardcover DM 164,–
ISBN 3-540-50947-X

Contents: *L. Stjärne:* Basic Mechanisms
and Local Modulation of Nerve Im-
pulse-Induced Secretion of Neurotrans-
mitters from Individual Sympathetic
Nerve Varicosities. — *P. Illes:* Modula-
tion of Transmitter and Hormone
Release by Multiple Neuronal Opioid
Receptors. — *A. Rothstein:* The Na+/H+
Exchange System in Cell pH and
Volume Control.

Volume 111

1988. V, 231 pp. 32 figs. 10 tabs. Hardcover DM 128,– ISBN 3-540-19156-9

Contents: *A. Philippou:* Regulation of
Blood Pressure by Central Neurotrans-
mitters and Neuropeptides. - *J. H. Exton:*
The Roles of Calcium and Phospho-
inositides in the Mechanisms of
α_1-Adrenergic and Other Agonists.

Volume 109

1987. V, 183 pp. 14 figs. Hardcover
DM 112,– ISBN 3-540-18108-3

Contents: *J. R. Keast:* Mucosal Innerva-
tion and Control of Water and Ion
Transport in the Intestine. -
D. A. S. G. Mary: Exercise Training and
Its Effect on the Heart. - *H. Thoenen,
C. Bandtlow, R. Heumann:* The Physio-
logical Function of Nerve Growth
Factor in the Central Nervous System:
Comparison with the Periphery.

Volume 108

1987. V, 211 pp. 19 figs. 16 tabs. Hardcover DM 98,– ISBN 3-540-17778-7

Contents: *N. Katunuma, E. Kominami:*
Abnormal Expression of Lysosomal
Cysteine Proteinases in Muscle-Wasting
Diseases. - *T. Saheki, K. Kobayashi,
I. Inoue:* Hereditary Disorders of the
Urea Cycle in Man: Biochemical and
Molecular Approaches. - *R. v. d. Heydt:*
Approaches to Visual Cortical Function.
- *B. Damerau:* Biological Activities of
Complement-Derived Peptides.

Volume 107

1987. V, 230 pp. 23 figs. 6 tabs. Hardcover DM 128,– ISBN 3-540-17609-8

Contents: *L. A. Walker, J. C. Frölich:*
Renal Prostaglandins and Leukotrienes.
- *K. Starke:* Presynaptic α-Autorecep-
tors. - *S. Bhakdi, J. Tranum-Jensen:*
Damage to Mammalian Cells by
Proteins that Form Transmembrane
Pores.

Volume 106

1987. V, 182 pp. 57 figs. Hardcover
DM 98,– ISBN 3-540-17608-X

Contents: *B. Fischer:* The Preparation of
Visually Guided Saccades. - *W. Waespe,
V. Henn:* Gaze Stabilization in the
Primate. The Interaction of the Vesti-
bulo-Ocular Reflex, Optokinetic Nystag-
mus, and Smooth Pursuit. - *H. Caspers,
E.-J. Speckmann, A. Lehmenkühler:*
Direct Current Potentials of the Cere-
bral Cortex. Seizure Activity and
Changes in Gas Pressures.

Volume 105

1986. V, 264 pp. 74 figs., some in color.
Hardcover DM 128,–
ISBN 3-540-16874-5

Contents: *J. T. Shepherd, G. Mancia:*
Reflex Control of the Human Cardiovascular System. - *R. Hainsworth:*
Vascular Capacitance: Its Control and
Importance. - *U. Zimmermann:* Electrical Breakdown, Electropermeabilization
and Electrofusion.

Volume 104

1986. V, 270 pp. 16 figs. Hardcover
DM 124,– ISBN 3-540-15940-1

Contents: *T. Simmet, B. A. Peskar:* Eico-
sanoids and the Coronary Circulation. -
H. Koepsell: Methodological Aspects of
Purification and Reconstitution of
Transport Proteins from Mammalian
Plasma Membranes. - *W. Jelkmann:*
Renal Erythropoietin: Properties and
Production.

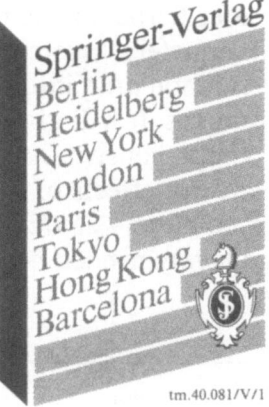

Springer-Verlag
Berlin
Heidelberg
New York
London
Paris
Tokyo
Hong Kong
Barcelona

□ Heidelberger Platz 3, W-1000 Berlin 33, F. R. Germany □ 175 Fifth Ave., New York, NY 10010, USA □ 8 Alexandra Rd., London SW19 7JZ, England
□ 26, rue des Carmes, F-75005 Paris, France □ 37-3, Hongo 3-chome, Bunkyo-ku, Tokyo 113, Japan
□ Room 701, Mirror Tower, 61 Mody Road, Tsimshatsui, Kowloon, Hong Kong □ Avinguda Diagonal, 468-4° C, E-08006 Barcelona, Spain

tm.40.081/V/1

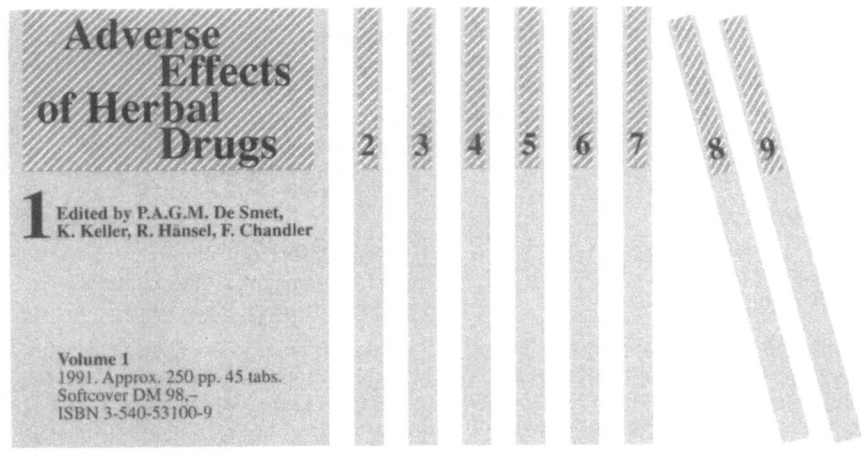

Adverse Effects of Herbal Drugs

1 Edited by P.A.G.M. De Smet, K. Keller, R. Hänsel, F. Chandler

Volume 1
1991. Approx. 250 pp. 45 tabs.
Softcover DM 98,–
ISBN 3-540-53100-9

A complete description of herbal remedies in a new multi-volume work!

Adverse Effects of Herbal Drugs

Editors:
P.A.G.M. De Smet, The Hague;
K. Keller, Berlin; **R. Hänsel,**
Munich; **F. Chandler,**
Dalhousie University, Halifax,
N.S.

The new series **Adverse Effects of Herbal Drugs** will be an indispensable supplement to other more general works, since herbal medicines are not adequately covered in the common drug information sources. It will give a comprehensive overview of the adverse effects of botanical medicines – an overview which is sorely needed because of the enormous rise in the use of herbal remedies.

The series will consist of nine volumes and provide approximately 150 monographs on herbal remedies and plant-derived drugs that are or have been used in the Western world. Each monograph gives introductory information about botany and chemistry, but the major focus is on pharmacology and clinical data. The sections describing uses are followed by adverse reaction profiles subdivided according to organ and function.

Volume 1
1991. Approx. 250 pp. 45 tabs.
Softcover DM 98,–
ISBN 3-540-53100-9

Contents: Toxicological outlook on the quality assurance of herbal remedies. – Allium Sativum. – Aristolochia species. – Asafetida. – Berberin. – Cinnamomum species. – Cymbopogon species. – Eucalyptus species. – Foeniculum vulgare. – Gaultheria procumbens. – Hedeoma pulegioides and Mentha pulegium. – Marsdenia condurango. – Medicago sativa. – Mentha piperita / M. spicata. – Panax ginseng. – Sesquiterpene lactones. – Arnica montana. – Chamomilla recutita. – Laurus nobilis. Tanacetum parthenium. – Pyrrolizidine alkaloids. – Cynoglossum officinale. – Petasites species. – Senecio species. – Symphytum species. – Tussilago farfara.

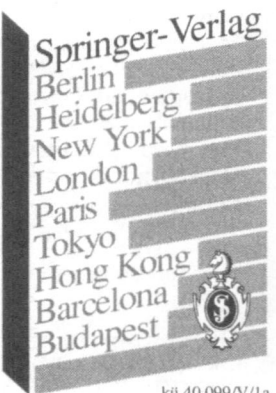

Springer-Verlag
Berlin
Heidelberg
New York
London
Paris
Tokyo
Hong Kong
Barcelona
Budapest

Heidelberger Platz 3, W-1000 Berlin 33, F. R. Germany

kü.40.099/V/1a